ANNALS OF
THE NEW YORK ACADEMY
OF SCIENCES

Volume 620

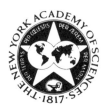

EDITORIAL STAFF

Executive Editor
BILL BOLAND

Managing Editor
JUSTINE CULLINAN

Associate Editor
MARION GARABEDIAN

The New York Academy of Sciences
2 East 63rd Street
New York, New York 10021

WINDOWS ON THE BRAIN

NEUROPSYCHOLOGY'S TECHNOLOGICAL FRONTIERS

ANNALS OF THE NEW YORK ACADEMY OF SCIENCES
Volume 620

WINDOWS ON THE BRAIN

NEUROPSYCHOLOGY'S TECHNOLOGICAL FRONTIERS

Edited by R. A. Zappulla, F. Frank LeFever, Judith Jaeger, and Robert Bilder

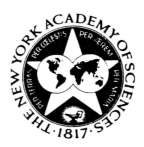

The New York Academy of Sciences
New York, New York
1991

Library of Congress Cataloging-in-Publication Data

Windows on the brain: neuropsychology's technological frontiers/
    edited by R.A. Zappulla . . . [et al.].
        p. cm. — (Annals of the New York Academy of Sciences, ISSN
0077-8923 : v. 620)
    Grew out of conference held jointly by the New York
Neuropsychology Group and the New York Academy of Sciences, in New
York, N.Y., Mar. 14, 1987.
    Includes bibliographical references and index.
    ISBN 0-89766-555-4 (cloth : alk. paper). — ISBN 0-89766-556-2
(pbk. alk. paper)
    1. Neuropsychology—Methodology—Congresses. 2. Neurophysiology—
Methodology—Congresses. I. Zappulla, R. A. II. New York
Neuropsychology Group. III. New York Academy of Sciences.
IV. Series.
    [DNLM: 1. Brian—physiology—congresses.
2. Electroencephalography—methods—congresses.
3. Magnetoencephalography—methods—congresses. 4. Neuropsychology—
methods—congresses. W1 AN616YL v. 620/WL 141 W765 1987]
Q11.N5 vol. 620
[QP360]
500 s—dc20
[612.8'2]
DLC
for Library of Congress   91-11165
                                                                          CIP

PCP
Printed in the United States of America
ISBN 0-89766-555-4 (cloth)
ISBN 0-89766-556-2 (paper)
ISSN 0077-8923

ANNALS OF THE NEW YORK ACADEMY OF SCIENCES

Volume 620
April 24, 1991

WINDOWS ON THE BRAIN[a]
NEUROPSYCHOLOGY'S TECHNOLOGICAL FRONTIERS

Editors and Conference Organizers
R. A. ZAPPULLA, F. FRANK LeFEVER, JUDITH JAEGER, AND ROBERT BILDER

CONTENTS

[a] This volume grew out of the New York Neuropsychology Group's Eighth Annual Conference entitled Windows on the Brain: Neuropsychology's Technological Frontiers, in a joint meeting with the Psychology Section of the New York Academy of Sciences, which was held on March 14, 1987 in New York, New York.

Introductory Remarks

R. A. ZAPPULLA[a] AND F. FRANK LeFEVER[b]

[a]Department of Neurosurgery
The Mount Sinai Medical Center
New York, New York 10029

[b]Neuropsychology Laboratory
Helen Hayes Hospital
West Haverstraw, New York 10993

The last two decades have seen the introduction and development of new technologies for the investigation of the human nervous system. The advances and promises these technologies hold for the future of the brain sciences have been formally recognized by the governmental designation of the 1990s as the "decade of the brain." In a large part the technical advances in the brain sciences have been driven by the technical revolution in other fields. The development of magnetic sensors, solid-state analog amplifiers, and methods of isotope production represent some of the methodologies that have been employed to investigate functional aspects of cerebral activity. Of equal importance are the recent advances in computer technology that have been employed for efficient acquisition, reduction, analysis, and display of the large amount of data generated by these technologies.

The advances in anatomical imaging, computerized axial tomography (CAT), and magnetic resonance imaging (MRI) have been complemented by quantified electrophysiology, positron emission tomography (PET), magnetoencephalography (MEG), and cerebral blood flow measures. It is the functional aspects of these technologies, illustrated by specific examples in Parts I and II, that offer the greatest opportunity for investigating the physiologic basis of cognitive activity.

Part III includes descriptions of a variety of techniques, some new and some old but with proposed new neuropsychological applications. They tend to be simpler than those described in Parts I and II, but as the introductory paper argues, they may offer advantages that can be exploited in many clinical settings, or that can complement the work done with techniques described in Parts I and II—for example, measures of cerebral blood flow that lack the spatial resolution or broad integration of techniques described in Parts II but have superior temporal resolution, which might help determine optimal times for obtaining the finer spatial map.

However, with new applications of old techniques or with the advent of any new technique, one must be aware of potential artifacts arising from the peculiarities of the technology. This requires an appreciation of the electronic, chemical or physical characteristics of the technology and, in the early stages of technical development, a close collaboration with professional personnel with special expertise in these disciplines.

Although initial technological results may indicate significant advances in the understanding of particular aspects of brain function, confirmation of these findings requires replication by multiple centers. This depends upon the proliferation of the technology and time for researchers to develop a working knowledge of the advantages and limitations of the technology. It is by experimental replication and corroboration with the results from established and proven techniques that a new technology can be accurately applied to the study of brain function.

The present volume reviews the recent advances in technologies that relate to the study of brain activity. The contents of this book are expanded from a previous conference on this subject held by the New York Neuropsychology Group and the Psychology Section of the New York Academy of Sciences. Although this collection of papers is not exhaustive on any of the new technologies being applied to the study of brain activity, it is the feeling of the editors that the reader will be able to gain an appreciation of the contributions of each of the technologies to the study of brain function.

Fundamentals and Applications of Quantified Electrophysiology

R. A. ZAPPULLA

Department of Neurosurgery
The Mount Sinai Medical Center
New York, New York 10029

INTRODUCTION

Quantified electrophysiology refers to the computer-based acquisition, display, storage, and analysis of EEG or stimulus-evoked responses (ER). The data can be evaluated in the time domain or converted to the frequency domain. The latter permits analysis of the EEG and ER based upon the frequency components of the signal. The spatial distribution of the dependent variables are frequently presented as two-dimensional topographic color maps.

Quantified electrophysiology has been advocated as an adjunct to traditional EEG and ER recordings. It offers a method by which to quantify aspects of the EEG that have been routinely evaluated qualitatively. The unique and promising advantage of quantified electrophysiology is the ability to quantify aspects of the EEG and evoked response that are not observable from visual inspection of the time-domain record and that may convey information concerning cerebral function, correlates of cognitive activity, neurophysiologic mechanisms, spatial localization of cortical generators, and diagnostic classification. The data lends itself to statistical analysis for evaluating objectively within-subject changes during experimental manipulation or individual comparisons to age-adjusted normative databases.

The emergence of quantified electrophysiology has been driven, in part, by the recent advances in microprocessor technology. The hardware and software requirements for signal acquisition, display, analysis, and storage that were once only available on expensive mainframe systems have been implemented on low-cost personal computers. This has resulted in an increase in the accessibility of this technology and an expansion of the clinical and experimental applications of quantified electrophysiology.

Along with the proliferation of this technology are controversies concerning various aspects of the methodology and its application.[1-6] These issues relate to data acquisition techniques, the physiological significance of the variables derived from spectral analysis, the spatial relationship between scalp potentials and cortical generators, the limitations of topographic mapping, and the appropriate statistical analysis of the multiple variables derived from quantitative electrophysiology.

The present paper will review the methodology and applications of quantified electrophysiology. The techniques of data acquisition will be presented from the perspective of their effects on frequency analysis measures: power, coherence, and phase. The advantages and limitations of topographic mapping as a technique for the spatial

1

localization of dipole sources will be discussed. Finally, statistical strategies for individual and group comparisons will be presented.

DATA ACQUISITION

The acquisition of EEG for quantitative analysis should adhere to the standards established for traditional EEG and should include the ability to view the EEG during collection on a polygraph or high resolution video display. This permits the identification of artifacts and insures the integrity of the input data. Most applications use the 10-20 international system of electrode placement for EEG acquisition. Larger number of electrodes have been advocated by some workers to increase spatial resolution and to meet the mathematical assumptions of data manipulation and analysis. Additional electrodes to monitor extracerebral contaminants of the EEG such as eye movement, EKG, and muscle activity are essential.

Amplification, filtering, and digitization determine the frequency characteristics of the EEG and ER and the source of potential artifacts. The acquisition parameters must be chosen with an understanding of their effects on signal acquisition and subsequent analysis. Amplification increases the amplitude of the EEG or ER signal from the microvolt level at the scalp to the amplitude range (volts) of the analog to digital (A/D) converter. The resolution of the A/D converter is determined by the smallest amplitude steps that can be sampled. This is calculated by dividing the voltage range of the A/D converter by 2 to the power of the number of bits of the A/D converter. For example, an A/D converter with a range of $\pm$ 5 V with 12-bit resolution can resolve samples as small as $\pm$ 2.4 mV. Appropriate matching of amplification and A/D converter sensitivity permits resolution of the smallest signal while preventing clipping of the largest signal amplitudes.

The bandwidth of the filters and the rate of digitization determine the frequency components of the EEG and evoked response. The filter bandwidth is adjusted to insure that frequency components of interest are passed, while other frequencies outside the band of interest that may represent potential artifacts, such as aliasing,[7] are rejected. A filter's characteristics are determined by the rate of amplitude decrease of frequencies at the bandwidth's upper and lower edges. Proper digital representation of the analog signal depends on the rate of data sampling, which is governed by the Nyquist theorem that states that data sampling should be at least twice the highest frequency of interest.

In addition to the information available from the spontaneous electrical activity of the EEG, the brain's electrical response to sensory stimulation can contribute data as to the status of cortical and subcortical regions activated by sensory input. Due to the relatively small amplitude of a stimulus-evoked potential as compared to the spontaneous EEG potentials, the technique of signal averaging is used to enhance the stimulus-evoked response. Stimulus averaging takes advantage of the fact that the brain's electrical response is time-locked to the onset of the stimulus and that the non-evoked background potentials are randomly distributed in time. Consequently, the average of multiple stimulus responses will result in the enhancement of the time-locked activity, while the averaged random background activity will approach zero. The result is an evoked response that consists of a number of discrete and replicable peaks that occur, depending upon the stimulus and recording parameters, at predicted latencies from the onset of stimulation. The spatial localization of maximum peak amplitudes has been associated with cortical generators in primary sensory cortex. The scalp topographic map in FIGURE 1 is constructed at the first cortical peak (N20) of the somatosensory evoked response. The maximum amplitude of the peak is localized to the scalp overlying the primary sensory cortex contralateral to median nerve stimulation.

The quality and number of responses needed to obtain a stimulus-evoked response depend upon the signal-to-noise ratio. This ratio can be enhanced by filtering techniques that reduce the size of the background activity, while maintaining the frequency response in the range of the evoked response as in the cases of brainstem auditory and somatosensory evoked responses. The intensity, duration, and rate of stimulation can affect signal strength and alter the signal-to-noise ratio. Increases in signal strength

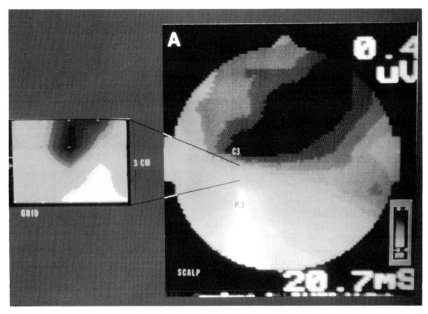

FIGURE 1. Cortical and scalp topographic maps constructed by linear interpolation at the N20 peak of a somatosensory evoked response elicited by stimulation of the right median nerve. Both responses are from the same individual. The scalp activity was recorded from electrodes in the 10-20 configuration, and the cortical activity from a rectangular grid array (4 × 5 electrodes) on the surface of the sensorimotor cortex. Color key: Red, maximum positivity; white, maximum negativity.

occur with increases in stimulus intensity, thereby reducing the number of responses needed to elicit an evoked response. In addition to peak amplitude, stimulus conditions can also affect the peak latency of the evoked response. FIGURE 2A depicts the decrease in peak amplitude and increase in peak latency of the brainstem auditory evoked response (BAER) with decreases in the intensity of auditory stimulation. As the stimulus intensity approaches auditory threshold, waveform components are difficult to ascertain on visual inspection of the evoked tracings. The change in the BAER with decreasing stimulus intensity is quantitatively represented by a decrease in spectral power for the frequency components of the BAER (FIG. 2C). These stimulus-dependent changes in the evoked response emphasize that ER comparisons based on peak amplitude or latency should be performed on ERs collected under the same stimulus conditions.

Extracerebral potentials, such as muscle activity, are a source of contamination that can reduce the efficiency of averaging. This has been addressed by the use of hardware or software strategies that automatically eliminate artifactually contaminated responses from the average based upon voltage threshold criteria. The presence of time-locked electrical interference from recording equipment can also be a source of contamination that can sometimes be identified by comparing the evoked potentials elicited under stimulus and no-stimulus conditions.

As the foregoing discussion demonstrates, proper signal acquisition techniques are essential for accurate interpretation of EEG and evoked response data and to prevent

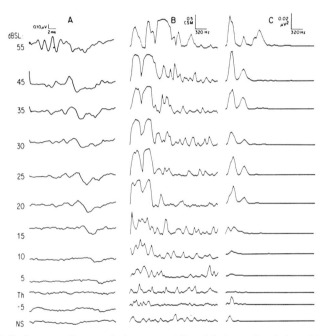

FIGURE 2. Brainstem auditory evoked responses (**A**) and their associated phase (**B**) and spectral plots (**C**) collected at varying auditory stimulus levels. Phase is plotted as 1 minus the phase variance. Th indicates auditory threshold; NS, no-stimulus condition. (From Greenblatt et al.[12] Reprinted by permission from *Audiology.*)

the confounding that can occur from artifactual signal or spectral components arising from improper data collection.

FREQUENCY ANALYSIS

Traditionally, EEG and evoked responses have been evaluated in the time domain, that is, with time on the x-axis and voltage on the y-axis, the standard polygraphic record. Alternatively, EEG and evoked responses can be converted into the frequency domain by the application of the fast Fourier transform (FFT) and can be quantitatively described by the frequency, amplitude, and phase of a number of sinusoidal waveforms. The resolution and range of frequencies are determined by the time period of the EEG analyzed and the sampling frequency. The quantitative measure derived from the FFT is the amplitude spectrum of the EEG, which is presented as microvolts for each frequency or for groups of frequencies such as the traditional frequency bands of delta, theta, alpha, and beta. In some instances the alpha and beta bands are divided into high and low frequencies to increase specificity. An alternative measure, which is consistent with engineering applications, is the square of the amplitude spectrum. This is referred to as the power spectrum whose units are squared microvolts (μV^2).

The duration of EEG that is required to represent accurately spectral activity is governed by the lowest frequency of interest and the amount of continuous artifact-free EEG available. The length of the EEG segment determines the low-frequency components that can be resolved. A 2-sec segment of EEG allows resolution of frequencies down to 0.5 Hz, a value approximating the high pass filters used in most commercial instruments. With longer periods of EEG, there is a greater probability that artifacts will be introduced into the record, thereby confounding the spectral pattern. A compromise solution is to segment the EEG into epochs of shorter duration (2-3 sec). In this way segments of EEG containing artifacts can be rejected from analysis. The power spectrum of a period of EEG is presented as an average value calculated by performing FFTs on the remaining artifact-free epochs. This strategy requires that the EEG collected be longer in duration than the period of EEG analyzed in order to allow for rejections of some epochs. The duration and number of segments that adequately describe the spectral signature of an EEG record depend upon the variability of the EEG during the recording. If, for example, the EEG is relatively stationary, then several seconds of EEG may be adequate to demonstrate the posterior distribution of alpha activity in the eyes-closed condition (FIG. 3). In contrast, if the EEG is non-stationary due to transient changes within a record arising from abnormal discharges, changes in arousal, or experimental manipulation, then the average spectral power may not reflect these transient changes. Since these transient changes may convey relevant clinical or experimental information, it is of value to display the spectral results for each epoch so that they can be correlated with the time-domain data. In addition, the variance around the mean offers a measure of variability within the EEG record.

There are conditions in the EEG and ER, for example, spike activity, peaks of the ER, where the spectral components are changing so rapidly that it is difficult to define an epoch length short enough for the signal to be more or less stationary. In addition, the use of very short time intervals to isolate these phasic events reduces the frequency range of the power spectrum. Consequently, there is a compromise between time and frequency resolution. Several approaches have been applied to define a time-varying spectrum that reflects the changes in the power spectrum over time. Initial attempts included computing spectra for closely overlapping epochs. An alternative measure is to develop a joint function of time and frequency based on the distribution of both variables that describes simultaneously for time and frequency the intensity of a signal.[8] In this regard, the Wigner distribution has been demonstrated to yield information regarding time and frequency locations of signal energy of the evoked response.[9]

In addition to absolute power derived directly from the power spectrum, other measures calculated from absolute power have been demonstrated to be of value in quantifying various aspects of the EEG. Relative power expresses the percent contribution of each frequency band to the total power and is calculated by dividing the power within a band by the total power across all bands. Relative power has the benefit of reducing the inter-subject variance associated with absolute power that arises from inter-subject differences in skull and scalp conductance. The disadvantage of relative

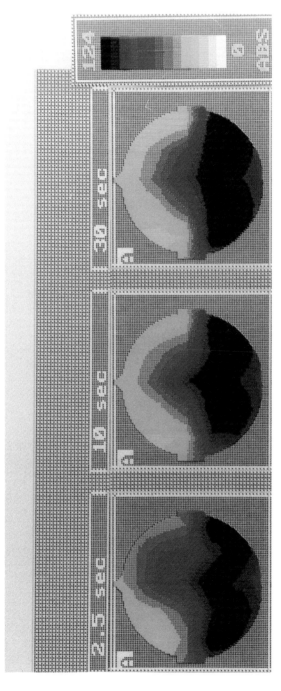

FIGURE 3. Topographic maps constructed for absolute alpha activity for 2.5, 15, and 30 sec of continuous EEG activity.

power is that an increase in one frequency band will be reflected in the calculation by a decrease in other bands.

Other workers have reported directional shifts between high and low frequencies associated with changes in cerebral blood flow and metabolism.[10] Power ratios between low (delta and theta) and high (alpha and beta) frequency bands have been demonstrated to be an accurate estimator of changes in cerebral activity during these metabolic changes.

Another measure evaluates the difference in power between leads and is referred to as amplitude asymmetry. This measure is derived by calculating the difference in power between two leads, expressed either as a ratio or as the difference in power between two leads. When the amplitude asymmetry is calculated for homologous left- and right-sided electrodes, it gives a measure of lateralized differences.

In addition to frequency and amplitude, phase is another measure derivable from the FFT. Phase represents the relationship between the component frequencies of a complex waveform and the beginning of the analysis epoch. For a single channel of data, the phase along with the frequency spectrum is essential for reliable reconstruction of the waveform from the FFT components as in the case of digital filtering.

Phase conveys limited descriptive information for EEG where the beginning of the analysis epoch may be arbitrary. In contrast, for sensory evoked potentials where the onset of each evoked response is time-locked to the stimulus onset, phase describes the temporal relationship of frequency components of each response to the onset of the stimulus. Where the frequency components reflect the peaks of the evoked potential, phase is an objective quantitative measure of peak latency. The phase variance between individual evoked responses or groups of responses, calculated for a group of frequency components that describe an evoked response, has been demonstrated to yield quantitative information regarding the replicability of an evoked response, where replicability in the time domain is based upon the congruence of peak latencies across responses.[11] FIGURE 4 is a plot of groups of brainstem auditory evoked responses (BAERs) to auditory stimulation at 10 and 60 dB above auditory threshold. Visual inspection of both groupings demonstrates the poorer replication, that is, variability of peak latencies across replications, at the low intensity stimulation. This lack of replicability is reflected by a larger phase variance for the low-intensity stimulus. Phase variance has been used as an objective measure for determining auditory thresholds where peak identification becomes difficult at low-stimulus intensities.[12] FIGURE 2B is a plot of one minus the phase variance for subgroups of BAERs collected at decreasing stimulus intensities. This plot demonstrates the increase in phase variance with decreasing stimulus intensity. The increase in phase variance with decreasing stimulus intensity quantitatively reflects the decrement in the configuration of the BAER (FIG. 2). Similar increases in phase variance of the BAER have been described for structural lesions disrupting brainstem auditory pathways.[13,14]

Although the power spectrum quantifies activity at each electrode, other variables derivable from the FFT offer a measure of the relationship between activity recorded at distinct electrode sites. Coherence, calculated from the cross-spectrum analysis of two signals, is similar to cross-correlation in the time domain and expresses the degree of synchrony between broad-band or individual frequency components of two signals. Coherence values range from 1 to 0, indicating maximum or no synchrony, respectively, and are independent of power. The temporal relationship between two signals is expressed by phase, which is a measure of the lag between two signals for common frequency components or bands. Phase is expressed in units of degrees, 0° indicating no time lag between signals or 180° if the signals are of opposite polarity. Phase can also be transformed into the time domain, giving a measure of the time difference between two frequencies.

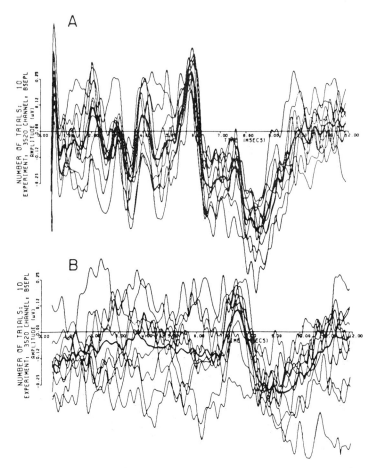

FIGURE 4. Overlapping plots of 10 brainstem auditory evoked response averages (200 sweeps per average) collected at (*panel A*) high and (*panel B*) low intensity stimulation. (From Greenblatt *et al.*[12] Reprinted by permission from *Audiology*.)

Coherence and phase represent measures that can be employed to investigate the cortical interactions of cerebral activity. Short (intracortical) and long (cortico-cortical) pathways have been proposed as the anatomic substrate underlying the spatial frequency and patterns of coherence.[15] Therefore, discrete cortical regions linked by such fiber systems should demonstrate a relatively high degree of synchrony, whereas the time lag between signals, as represented by phase, quantifies the extent to which one signal leads another.

Broad-band coherence has been found to be highly correlated with interelectrode distance.[16] Thatcher[15] reported that while coherence decreases with interelectrode distance, there are anterior-posterior directional differences in coherence for the same interelectrode distances. According to Thatcher, this spatial inhomogeneity argues against a volume-conduction model of coherence in favor of coherence reflecting the extent of connectivity between spatially distinct cortical regions. He has proposed a two-compartmental model to explain the spatial distribution of coherence in terms of varying fiber lengths.

The difficulties inherent in scalp recordings, such as distortion of the current conducting pathways through the bone and scalp as well as spatial averaging at electrode sites, may obscure the differences in activity at discrete cortical sites and bias coherence measures. Cortical surface recordings offer a method whereby coherence can be evaluated in the absence of these confounding factors. The same decrease in coherence with increasing interelectrode distance has been reported using closely spaced cortical electrodes in animals.[17] The rate of decrease in coherence is frequency dependent with a greater rate of change in coherence at higher frequencies. We have demonstrated from cortical recordings in the rat that while coherence decreases as a function of interelectrode distance, the rate of decline for the same interelectrode distances differs between functionally discrete cortical regions (FIG. 5). This finding reflects a spatial inhomogeneity of coherence at the cortical level and supports the assumption that coherence reflects the extent of connectivity between discrete cortical regions.

The performance of coherence and phase as measures of cerebral connectivity has been investigated in a number of studies. Both measures have been found, in some instances, to predict the pattern and direction of spike propagation between discrete cortical and subcortical regions with established connections.[18-24] Alternatively, we have demonstrated in a group of patients with focal cerebral lesions disrupting cortex and adjacent subcortical white matter a decrease in coherence between the activity over the site and surrounding electrodes (FIG. 6).

Coherence has also been used to investigate the functional relationships between cerebral areas during various cognitive tasks and between subject groups with different

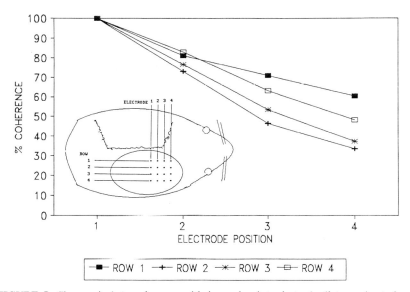

FIGURE 5. Changes in beta coherence with increasing interelectrode distance (posterior to anterior) for closely spaced (1 mm) cortical electrodes in the rat. Coherence was calculated between electrode 1 and all electrodes (1-2, 1-3, 1-4) in the same row. Each coherence value is the mean from eight animals. The change in coherence with distance differed among rows of electrodes.

behavioral and psychiatric profiles. The results of these studies suggest that coherence patterns may be specific for gender,[25] arousal,[26] laterality,[26,27] cognitive processing,[25] and psychological profiles.[28] French and Beaumont,[29] in a review of studies of hemisphere function using EEG coherence, raise the issue of lack of replicability across studies. These authors emphasize that methodological problems related to the use of a cephalic reference may account for the discrepancies in these studies. They, as well as other authors,[30] have discussed the difficulty in interpretation of coherence data because of an active reference electrode and emphasize the need for reference-free recording techniques.

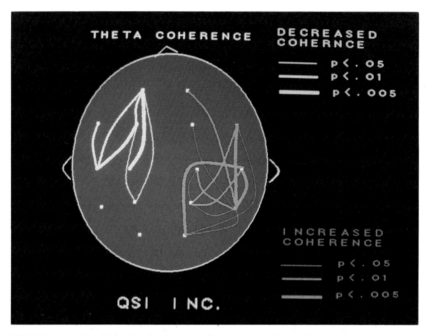

FIGURE 6. Intrahemispheric coherence plot for a patient with a left frontal tumor. The significance values are derived from comparisons with an age-adjusted normative database.

TOPOGRAPHIC MAPPING

Computerized axial tomography (CAT) and magnetic resonance imaging (MRI) have demonstrated the impact of spatial displays on data interpretation and analysis. Similarly, mapping techniques have been applied to electrophysiologic data to depict the spatial information available from multielectrode recordings. This effort has been assisted by the development and implementation of low-cost, high-resolution graphic displays on micro- and mini-computer systems. The data are frequently presented as two-dimensional topographic color maps. In the time domain, color values depict the changes in potential across the scalp at each time point. This is exemplified by mapping peaks of an evoked potential or the spatial distribution of an epileptic spike (FIG. 1). Temporal changes in the spatial distribution of voltage can be presented graphically as a series of maps constructed at adjacent time points or by cartooning the topographic maps over the time interval of interest. In the frequency domain, color coding can be used to map spatially power, coherence, phase, and Z-score values. These maps may be constructed for broad-band activity or for selective frequency components.

Unlike CAT and MRI displays where each picture element or pixel value represents real data, most of the pixels comprising an EEG and ER topographic map consist of interpolated values. This is because the activity from a finite number of electrodes represents a sampling of the spatial activity over the scalp. Consequently, the remaining values of the map located outside the electrode positions must be estimated from this sampled activity. One technique for deriving these values is linear interpolation. In the case of four-point interpolation, the map is divided into boxes whose corners are defined by real data. The interpolated points within the boxes are calculated by the weighted sum of the four real data points, based on their distance from the interpolated point. Although linear interpolation is the most popular technique, polynomial regression[31-33] and surface spline interpolation[34,35] have been employed as alternative procedures. These methods reduce the discontinuities inherent in linear interpolation and offer better estimates of extreme values. The differences between the interpolation methods can be visually appreciated by comparing the somatosensory topographic maps in FIGURE 1 (linear interpolation) and FIGURE 7 (surface spline). Polynomial regression has the additional advantage of permitting quantitative comparisons between maps by taking into account the topographic information represented in the map.[36]

Maps can be presented in any of several projections to assist in interpretation. The most common projection is the top view which presents the spatial distribution of variables from all leads simultaneously. Lateral, posterior, and anterior projections highlight local areas of interest (FIG. 7). Although mapping presents a method by which spatial information can be efficiently communicated, it is important to be alert to the artifacts that can arise from map construction and manipulation. Neuer and Jordan[37] have reported a series of topographic spatial artifacts that can lead to misinterpretation. These include ring enhancement around a spike using source-derivation references, spatial aliasing arising from linear interpolation which causes maximal activity to be mapped at electrode sites, the enhancement of activity away from the midline, and the attenuation of midline activity on amplitude asymmetry maps (centrifugal effect).

The quality of the spatial information derivable from EEG and ER recordings depends upon the number of recording electrodes, the choice of the reference electrode, and the conductive properties of intracranial and extracranial structures. The localization of cortical activity from scalp recordings assumes that the potentials recorded from the scalp reflect cortical activity generated in proximity to the recording electrode. Therefore, the greater the density of recording electrodes, the more accurate the estimate of the spatial distribution of scalp potentials and the localization of cortical generators. Nunez,[38] however, points out that the distance between the cortical source and recording electrode, as well as the low conductivity of the skull, results in a selective attenuation of small dipole fields. He proposes, on theoretical grounds, that most available EEG information can be obtained with an average scalp-electrode spacing of 2 cm.

The relationship between cortical and scalp potentials is demonstrated in FIGURE 1. The somatosensory ER to left median nerve stimulation is depicted topographically for scalp and cortical electrodes in the same patient. A comparison of both maps demonstrates that although the posterior/anterior dipole is diffuse over the scalp, it is confined to approximately 3 cm on the cortical surface in the region of the sensorimotor cortex (FIG. 1).

Topographic maps are constructed from monopolar electrodes referenced to a common cephalic (linked ears or mandible, chin and nose) or noncephalic (linked clavicles or a balanced sternum-vertebra) electrode. Although the reference electrode

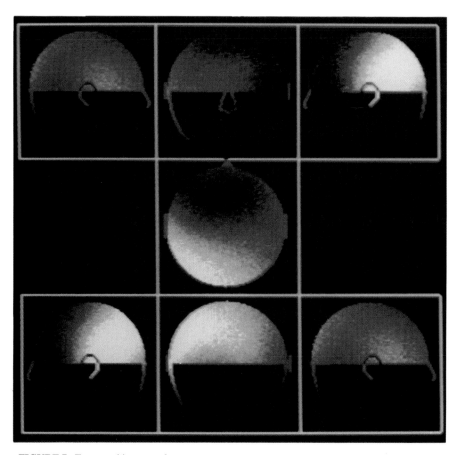

FIGURE 7. Topographic maps of somatosensory evoked response to right median nerve stimulation constructed at the N20 peak using the surface spline technique. The dipole at the central sulcus is seen on the left hemisphere and top projections. Color key: White, maximum negativity; red, maximum positivity.

should be free of any EEG activity, in practice most cephalic electrodes contain some EEG activity, while noncephalic electrodes are a potential source of EKG or muscle activity. Differential amplification of an EEG-contaminated reference electrode can decrease or cancel similar activity in neighboring electrodes, while at electrodes distant from the reference, the injected activity will be present as a potential of opposite polarity. Similarly, noncerebral potentials can be injected into scalp electrodes and misinterpreted as cerebral activity. Therefore, a non-neutral reference electrode can result in misleading map configurations. Several techniques have been applied to circumvent this problem. The construction of multiple maps using several different reference electrodes can sometimes assist in differentiating active and reference electrode activity.[39] This can be accomplished by acquiring serial EEG records using different references. Alternatively, various references can be acquired simultaneously during acquisition, and various montages can be digitally reconstructed, post hoc.

A more computationally intensive method for localizing a source at an electrode is that described by Hjorth.[40,41] The source derivation technique calculates the local source activity at any one electrode based on the average activity of its neighbors, weighted by their distance from the source. The technique has the advantage of suppressing potentials that originate outside the measurement area. Hjorth has presented the weighting factors for implementing source deviation techniques for each of the electrodes in the 10-20 system.

Another reference technique popularized by Lehmann,[42,43] the average head reference, uses the average activity of all active electrodes as the common reference. He emphasizes that the activity at any one electrode will vary depending upon the activity at the site of the reference electrode, which can be anywhere on the recording montage. Therefore, for N number of recording electrodes, each being a potential reference, there are N-1 possible voltage measurements at each instant of time for each electrode. Maps constructed using the average head reference represent a unique solution to the problem of active reference electrodes in that the average reference produces an amplitude-weighted, reference-free map of maximal and minimal field potentials. Lehmann points out that power maps constructed from the average reference best depict the spatial orientation of the generating field, and the areas with extreme values are closest to the generating processes. Other workers,[44,45] however, present evidence that the average head reference favors tangential rather than radial dipoles, an effect that can result in underestimating local generators.

Topographic maps represent an efficient format for displaying the extensive amount of data generated by quantitative analysis. However, for reasons discussed above, the researcher and clinician must be cautious in deriving spatial and functional conclusions from mapped data. Although the replicability of map configurations across subjects or experimental conditions may represent a useful basis for experimental and diagnostic classification, judgments concerning the localization of cortical generators or functional localization of cerebral activity are less certain and more controversial. Research continues on defining models and validating assumptions that relate scalp potentials to cortical generators in an attempt to arrive at accurate mathematical solutions that can be applied to mapping functions.

STATISTICAL ANALYSES

An extension of quantitative electroencephalography (QEEG) is the opportunity for statistical interpretation of within-subject EEG changes associated with experimental or pharmacologic manipulations and dynamic pathological cerebral processes. These within-subject statistics have the advantage of control over or knowledge of the experimental or clinical event of interest and the lack of inter-individual variability associated with EEG measures. Alternatively, inter-subject analysis, such as the statistical comparison of individual EEG measures to a normative database, presents different problems. The assumptions underlying the use of normative databases are that electrophysiologic measures represent specific neurophysiologic processes and that certain of these measures are consistent between individuals, thereby permitting the establishment of normative parameters by which individual variations can be statistically assessed and diagnostically categorized. Of course, standardization in the collection of the data is imperative. Concurrent with the positive reports of normative databases are a number of controversies concerning the definition of a normal population, statistical techniques for handling the large number of parameters generated by quantitative electrophysiology, and the relationship between quantitative electrophysiology and functional and anatomic localization. A familiarity with these statistical methods and controversies is important in understanding the QEEG literature and formulating strategies for experimental or clinical application of QEEG.

Valid statistical comparisons of electrophysiologic data depend not only on choosing the proper statistic and meeting statistical assumptions but also on the quality of the input data. This requires maintaining consistency in the recording parameters, state of the subject (e.g., eyes closed or eyes open), electrode positions, rejection of artifacts, and, in the case of ERs, consistency in stimulation parameters and reduction of ambient sensory noise that can alter stimulus threshold.

The effect of recording parameters on EEG activity has been discussed above. Inter- or intra-individual spectral comparisons of EEG collected with different recording parameters (e.g., filter bandwidth) reflect response differences of the recording equipment rather than a change in EEG spectral power.

Alteration of the EEG due to the mental state of the subject has been long recognized. Indeed, state-dependent EEG changes have been used as statistical measures of mental state and performance.[46,47] Consequently, control over the patient's state must be enforced to eliminate spectral shifts caused by such changes from being interpreted as significant clinical or experimental effects.

Because of the inhomogeneous spatial distribution of spectral activity, statistical comparisons are sensitive to electrode position. The individual difference in the amount and distribution of spectral power between scalp electrodes can be greater than between individuals for homologous electrodes. Therefore, the development of normative statistics for multiple-lead montages requires that electrode placement be consistent across subjects. Although standard electrode placements based on skull measurements, as in the 10-20 international system, reduce electrode position variability, the presence of skull asymmetries account, in part, for asymmetric placement. A recent study reported substantial variability in 10 of 107 left-sided and 12 of 102 right-sided electrode positions (10-20 system) and underlying cerebral structures as demonstrated by CAT scanning in subjects with minimal skull asymmetry.[48] However, despite the variability, even in patients with skull symmetries, 80% of the leads were grouped within homologous anatomic/functional structures.

A frequently discussed problem is the elimination of artifactual data that can confound analysis. Artifacts can occur during acquisition from eye movements, muscle activity, EKG, or electrode popping. Automated techniques for eliminating artifacts by voltage or frequency thresholds have been reported. However, these techniques can result in the distortion of meaningful EEG data, such as spike activity, that may have the same morphology as artifacts. Eye movements can give rise to slow activity distributed in the frontal leads. The use of periorbital electrodes and digital modeling as well as subtraction techniques have been used to eliminate eye-movement potentials from the EEG record.

The most frequently used strategy for identifying artifacts is the visual review and editing of the raw EEG.[49] Segments of EEG that contain artifacts are edited out from the record before analysis. Since artifacts can occur for variable durations, this technique can lead to arbitrary discontinuity in the edited record, resulting in unpredictable spectral results. This problem has been addressed by segmenting the EEG into fixed-length epochs and excluding the entire epoch that contains the artifact. The criteria of what constitutes an EEG artifact have implications on the incidence of false-positive and false-negative classifications when comparing individual EEG records that may not have been subjected to the same artifactual criteria that were used to construct the database.

In addition to the artifacts arising during acquisition, other artifacts have been introduced by the quantitative analysis performed. One such artifact is the artificial increase in frequencies that occurs as a result of performing a frequency analysis on an EEG epoch whose beginning and end points are above baseline. This can be partially corrected by multiplying the EEG epoch by a cosine function (Hanning window filter), thereby reducing the beginning and end data points to zero.[50]

Statistical comparisons that involve normative databases frequently employ parametric statistics. However, misleading conclusions can occur if the assumption of normality is violated. The lack of normality of QEEG variables has been corrected by applying transformations to the data. The most successful transforms for constructing a normal or Gaussian distribution for most of the broad-band parameters have come from the application of various logarithmic transformations to the data.[51–53] The transforms log x and log [x/(1-x)] for absolute and relative power, respectively, have resulted in a significant decrease in skewness and kurtosis in the population distribution of these variables and have been used in the construction of normative databases. FIGURES 9 and 10 are plots of the frequency distributions of absolute alpha activity at the PZ electrode before and after a log transformation, respectively, for a population of 122 normal adults. The skewed distribution of the untransformed data (FIG. 8) was normalized after a log transformation of the data (FIG. 9).

Of major importance in the statistical analysis of the EEG is the assumption that any one EEG recording adequately reflects the state of cerebral activity.[54] This is reflected in the consistency of EEG activity between testing sessions. Test-retest reliability has been reported to be .83 with a one week retesting interval. There were less significant test-retest differences for relative (2%) than absolute power (12%).[51] Test-retest has been shown to be frequency-specific with alpha activity having a higher retest reliability than delta activity in children during a resting condition.[55] The steady decrease in replicability in children over longer retest (.68 at 2.5 yr) intervals has been attributed to age-related changes in the EEG.[51]

The changes in EEG with age have been used as a technique for quantifying the normal development of the central nervous system. Gasser et al.[56] reported non-linear changes in absolute and relative power in 158 normal children aged 6-17 yr. Absolute power decreased with age in all bands except alpha$_2$ (9.5-12.5 Hz), while for relative power there was a decrease in slow activity and an increase in fast activity. A decrease in relative theta activity was supplanted after a lag by an increase in alpha$_2$ activity. The same group[16] reported an age-related change in the topographic distribution of spectral band power. Maturation (increase) of theta, alpha$_1$, and alpha$_2$ occurred earliest in the posterior region before proceeding in an anterior direction. John et al.[51] proposed the concept of maturational lag/lead, based on the age-related EEG changes. This is calculated as the difference between the physiologic age based on a multivariate EEG statistic and the chronologic age of the subject. A maturational lag exists when the physiologic age is less than the chronologic age of the subject, whereas the converse indicates a maturational lead.

Although the evidence is clear for age-related EEG changes in the younger population, the results for the adult population are less certain. Pollock et al.[52] failed to show

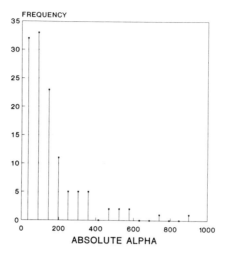

FIGURE 8. Frequency plot of absolute alpha power at the PZ electrode (untransformed data). N = 122 subjects.

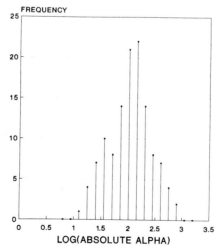

FIGURE 9. Frequency plot of log transformed data of FIGURE 8.

a correlation between age and log-transformed, broad-band amplitude in an adult population. In contrast, Duffy *et al.*[47] reported a significant decrease in delta and theta activity and an increase in beta activity with age. Both of these studies present evidence against the popular notion that aging is associated with an increase in slow activity. The differences between the studies can be explained by several factors[52] including the age range of the population studied, the criteria used to select normal subjects, and the downward shifts in frequency with age which may be minimal and concealed by broad-band analysis.

Age-related changes in the EEG represent not only a technique for measuring normal development and aging of the central nervous system, but also a source of potential error when individual comparisons to a normative database fail to adjust for age effects. Therefore, age-adjusted comparisons are important in preventing misclassification based on normal age changes of the EEG. This adjustment has been performed by the use of polynomial age-regression equations or by comparisons to a database consisting of normative values from multiple, narrow-range age groups.

Duffy *et al.*[57] popularized the use of significance probability mapping (SPM) as a means of statistically evaluating the variables derived from EEG spectral analysis and ER time points. The technique converts each of the variables to a Z-score, which represents the number of standard deviations a variable deviates from normative values. The number of univariate statistics generated from each EEG or ER record is formidable. An analysis of an EEG record with 19 electrodes (10-20 system) for which relative and absolute power, coherence, phase, and amplitude asymmetry are calculated within each of six spectral bands will produce over 600 variables. Evoked potential analysis can translate into thousands of variables when each time point from multiple leads is compared to a normative database. Several authors have raised the issue that chance alone will result in significant differences when large numbers of variables are compared post hoc, particularly if the p value is not reduced to compensate for the large number of comparisons.[1,3] In response to this criticism, Duffy[58] points out that QEEG is an exploratory technique rather than diagnostic or confirmatory and should be used in conjunction with conventional EEG and ER analysis. Principal component analysis[16] and composite variables in a multivariate statistic[51] have been advanced as alternative techniques for managing the large number of variables. The use of discriminant functions based upon univariates or a multivariate subset of quantitative measures has been demonstrated to perform adequately in classifying various pathological groups.[59-62]

CONCLUSION

Quantified electrophysiology offers a method by which EEG and evoked responses can be quantitatively evaluated. The advantages and limitations of this methodology depend in large part upon proper data acquisition techniques. Frequency-domain measures complement and enhance traditional time-domain analysis of electrophysiologic data. The frequency spectrum, phase, and coherence have been used to evaluate various aspects of the electrophysiologic signal that are not available through visual inspection of the EEG or ER record.

Topographic mapping can efficiently display the spatial information available from scalp electrical activity and spectral measures using multichannel recordings. Caution must be exercised, however, with respect to cortical localization of scalp activity from mapped data. Spatial distortion due to bone and scalp conductive properties, an active reference electrode, limited spatial sampling from a finite number of recording electrodes, and restrictions of interpolation algorithms can result in misinterpretation of mapped activity.

Statistical comparisons of quantitative electrophysiologic measures afford the researcher and clinician the opportunity to evaluate objectively and quantitate within- and inter-subject differences. Transformation of quantitative EEG and ER measures is necessary to meet the assumption of normality required for the application of parametric statistical procedures. Individual comparisons to normative and diagnostic databases have been demonstrated to assist in subject classification.

REFERENCES

1. FISCH, B. J. & T. A. PEDLEY. 1989. The role of quantitative topographic mapping or "neurometrics" in the diagnosis of psychiatric and neurological disorders. Electroencephalogr. Clin. Neurophysiol. 73: 5-9.

2. JOHN, E. R. 1989. The role of quantitative EEG topographic mapping or "neurometrics" in the diagnosis of psychiatric and neurological disorders: the pros. Electroencephalogr. Clin. Neurophysiol. 73: 2-4.

3. OKEN, B. S. & K. H. CHIAPPA. 1986. Statistical issues concerning computerized analysis of brain waves topography. Ann. Neurol. 19: 493-494.

4. HARNER, R. N. 1988. Brain mapping or spatial analysis? Brain Topogr. 1(2): 73-75.

5. DUFFY, F. H. 1989. Comments on quantified neurophysiology: Problems and advantages. Brain Topogr. 1(3): 153-155.

6. NUWER, M. R. 1988. Quantitative EEG: I. Techniques and problems of frequency analysis and topographic mapping. J. Clin. Neurophysiol. 5(1): 1-43.

7. OKEN, B. S. 1986. Filtering and aliasing of muscle activity in EEG frequency analysis. EEG Clin. Neurophysiol. 64: 77-80.

8. COHEN, L. 1989. Time-frequency distributions: A review. Proc. Inst. Electr. Electron. Eng. 77: 941-981.

9. GEVINS, A. S. & S. L. BRESSLER. 1988. Functional topography of the human brain. In Functional Brain Mapping. G. Pfurtscheller & F. H. Lopes da Silva, Eds.: 99-116. Hans Huber Publishers. Lewiston, NY.

10. NAGATA, K. 1988. Topographic EEG in brain ischemia—Correlation with blood flow and metabolism. Brain Topogr. 1(2): 97-106.

11. FRIDMANN, J., R. A. ZAPPULLA, M. BERGELSON, E. GREENBLATT, L. I. MALIS, F. MORRELL & T. HOEPPNER. 1983. Application of phase spectral analysis for brain stem auditory evoked potential detection in normal subjects and patients with posterior fossa tumors. Audiology 22: 99-113.

12. GREENBLATT, E., R. A. ZAPPULLA, S. KAYE & J. FRIDMANN. 1985. Response threshold determination of the brain stem auditory evoked response: A comparison of the phase versus magnitude derived from the fast Fourier transform. Audiology 24: 288-296.

13. ZAPPULLA, R. A., E. GREENBLATT, S. KAYE & L. I. MALIS. 1984. A quantitative assessment of the brain stem auditory evoked response during intraoperative monitoring. Neurosurgery 15: 186-190.

14. GREENBLATT, E., R. A. ZAPPULLA & S. KAYE. 1988. Quantification of brainstem auditory evoked responses for patient monitoring. Int. J. Clin. Monit. Comput. 5: 147-153.

15. THATCHER, R. W., P. J. KRAUSE & M. HRYBYK. 1986. Cortico-cortical associations and EEG coherence: A two compartmental model. Electroencephalogr. Clin. Neurophysiol. 64: 123-143.

16. GASSER, T., C. JENNEN-STEINMETZ, L. SROKA, R. VERLEGER & J. MOCKS. 1988. Development of the EEG of school age children and adolescents. II. Topography. Electroencephalogr. Clin. Neurophysiol. 69: 100-109.

17. BULLOCK, T. H. & M. C. McCLUNE. 1989. Lateral coherence of the electrocorticogram: A new measure of brain synchrony. Electroencephalogr. Clin. Neurophysiol. 73: 479-498.
18. BRAZIER, M. A. B. 1972. Spread of seizure discharge in epilepsy: Anatomical and electrophysiological considerations. Exp. Neurol. 36: 263-272.
19. BRAZIER, M. A. B. 1973. Electrical seizure discharges within the human brain: The problem of spread. In Epilepsy, Its Phenomenon in Man. M. A. B. Brazier, Ed.: 153-170. Academic Press. New York, NY.
20. GOTMAN, J. 1983. Measurement of small time differences between EEG channels: Method and application to epileptic seizure propagation. Electroencephalogr. Clin. Neurophysiol. 56: 501-514.
21. GOTMAN, J. 1987. Interhemispheric interactions in seizures of focal onset: Data from human intracranial recordings. Electroencephalogr. Clin. Neurophysiol. 67: 120-133.
22. MARS, N. J. I. & F. H. LOPES DA SILVA. 1983. Propagation of seizure activity in kindled dogs. Electroencephalogr. Clin. Neurophysiol. 56: 194-209.
23. MARS, N. J. I., P. M. THOMPSON & R. J. WILKENS. 1985. Spread of epileptic seizure activity in humans. Epilepsia. 26: 85-94.
24. LIEB, J. P., K. HOGUE, C. E. SKOMER & X. SONG. 1987. Inter-hemispheric propagation of human mesial temporal lobe seizures: A coherence/phase analysis. Electroencephalogr. Clin. Neurophysiol. 67: 101-119.
25. RAPPELSBERGER, P. & H. PETSCHE. 1988. Probability mapping: Power and coherence analyses of cognitive processes. Brain Topogr. 1: 46-54.
26. SWENSON, R. A. & D. M. TUCKER. 1983. Multivariate analysis of EEG coherence: Stability of the metric, individual differences in patterning and response to arousal. Biol. Psychol. 17: 59-75.
27. SHAW, J. C., K. P. O'CONNOR & C. ONGLEY. 1977. The EEG as a measure of cerebral functional organization. Br. J. Psychiatry 130: 260-264.
28. COLTER, N. & J. C. SHAW. 1982. EEG coherence analysis and field dependence. Biol. Psychol. 15: 215-228.
29. FRENCH, C. C. & J. G. BEAUMONT. 1984. A critical review of EEG coherence studies of hemispheric function. Int. J. Psychophysiol. 1: 241-254.
30. FEIN, G., J. RAZ, F. F. BROWN & E. L. MERRIN. 1988. Common reference coherence data are confounded by power and phase effects. Electroencephalogr. Clin Neurophysiol. 69: 581-584.
31. ASHIDA, H., J. TATSUNO, J. OKAMOTO & E. MARU. 1984. Field mapping by unbiased polynomial interpolation. Comput. Biomed. Res. 17: 267-276.
32. TATSUNO, J. 1988. Pattern differences in two-dimensional EEG maps during mental calculation. In Functional Brain Imaging. G. Pfurtscheller & F. H. Lopes da Silva, Eds.: 3-10. Hans Huber Publishers. Lewiston, N.Y.
33. BUCHSBAUM, M. S., E. HAZLETT, N. SICOTTE, R. BALL & S. JOHNSON. 1986. Geometric and scaling issues in topographic electroencephalography. In Topographic Mapping of Brain Electrical Activity. F. H. Duffy, Ed. Butterworths: Boston, MA.
34. BERTRAND, O., F. PERRIN, J. F. ECHALLIER & J. PERNIER. 1988. Topographic and model analysis of auditory evoked potentials: Tonotopic aspects. In Functional Brain Imaging. G. Pfurtscheller & F. H. Lopes da Silva, Eds.: 75-82. Hans Huber Publishers. Lewiston, NY.
35. PERRIN, F., J. PERNIER, O. BERTRAND, M. H. GIARD & J. F. ECHALLIER. 1987. Mapping of scalp potentials by surface spline interpolation. Electroencephalogr. Clin. Neurophysiol. 66: 75-81.
36. TATSUNO, J., H. ASHIDA & A. TAKAO. 1988. Objective evaluation of differences in patterns of EEG topographical maps by Mahalanobis distance. Electroencephalogr. Clin. Neurophysiol. 69: 287-290.
37. NEUER, M. R. & S. E. JORDAN. 1987. The centrifugal effect and other spatial artifacts of topographic EEG mapping. J. Clin. Neurophysiol. 4: 321-326.
38. NUNEZ, P. L. 1988. Methods to estimate spatial properties of dynamic cortical source activity. In Functional Brain Imaging. G. Pfurtscheller & F. H. Lopes da Silva, Eds.: 3-10. Hans Huber Publishers. Lewiston, NY.
39. SAMSON-DOLFUS, S. & H. BENDOUKHA. 1989. Choice of the reference for EEG mapping

in the newborn: An initial comparison of common nose reference, average and source derivation. Brain Topogr. **2:** 165-169.

40. HJORTH, B. 1975. An on-line transformation of EEG scalp potentials into orthogonal source derivations. EEG Clin. Neurophysiol. **39:** 526-530.

41. HJORTH, B. 1980. Source derivation simplifies topographical EEG interpretation. Am. J. EEG Technol. **20:** 121-132.

42. LEHMANN, D. & W. SKRANDIES. 1980. Reference-free identification of components of checkerboard-evoked multichannel potential fields. Electroencephalogr. Clin. Neurophysiol. **48:** 609-621.

43. LEHMANN, D. 1984. EEG assessment of brain activity: Spatial aspects, segmentation and imaging. Int. J. Psychophysiol. **1:** 267-276.

44. DESMEDT, J. E., V. CHALKIN & C. TOMBERG. 1990. Emulation of somatosensory evoked potential (SEP) components with the three shell head model and the problems of "ghost" potential fields when using an average reference in brain mapping. Electroencephalogr. Clin. Neurophysiol. **77:** 243-258.

45. TOMBERG, C., P. NOEL, I. OZAKI & J. E. DESMEDT. 1990. Inadequacy of the average reference for the topographic mapping of focal enhancements of brain potentials. Electroencephalogr. Clin. Neurophysiol. **77:** 259-265.

46. PETSCHE, H., H. POCKBERGER & P. RAPPELSBERGER. 1986. EEG topography and mental performance. *In* Topographic Mapping of Brain Electrical Activity. F. H. Duffy, Ed.: 63-98. Butterworths. Boston, MA.

47. DUFFY, F. H., M. S. ALBERT, G. MCANULTY & A. J. GARVEY. 1984. Age related differences in brain electrical activity of healthy subjects. Ann. Neurol. **16:** 430-438.

48. HOMAN, R. W., J. HERMAN & P. PURDY. 1987. Cerebral location of international 10-20 system electrode placement. Electroencephalogr. Clin. Neurophysiol. **66:** 376-382.

49. COBURN, K. L. & M. A. MORENO. 1988. Facts and artifacts in brain electrical activity mapping. Brain Topogr. **1:** 37-45.

50. DUMERMUTH, G. & L. MOLINARI. 1987. Spectral analysis of EEG background activity. *In* Methods of Analysis of Brain Electrical and Magnetic Signals. EEG Handbook. A. S. Gevins & A. Remond, Eds. **1:** 85-129. Elsevier. Amsterdam.

51. JOHN, E. R., L. S. PRICHEP & P. EASTON. 1987. Normative data banks and neurometrics. Basic concepts, methods and results of norm constructions. *In* Methods of Analysis of Brain Electrical and Magnetic Signals. EEG Handbook. A. S. Gevins & A. Remond, Eds. **1:** 449-540. Elsevier. Amsterdam.

52. POLLOCK, V. E., L. S. SCHNEIDER & S. A. LYNESS. 1990. EEG amplitudes in healthy, late-middle-aged and elderly adults: Normality of the distributions and correlations with age. Electroencephalogr. Clin. Neurophysiol. **75:** 276-288.

53. GASSER, T., P. BACHER & J. MOCKS. 1982. Transformations towards the normal distribution of broad band spectral parameters of the EEG. Electroencephalogr. Clin. Neurophysiol. **53:** 119-124.

54. OKEN, B. S. & K. H. CHIAPPA. 1988. Short-term variability in EEG frequency analysis. Electroencephalogr. Clin. Neurophysiol. **69:** 191-198.

55. GASSER, T., P. BACHER & H. STEINBERG. 1985. Test-retest reliability of spectral parameters. Electroencephalogr. Clin. Neurophysiol. **60:** 312-319.

56. GASSER, T., R. VERLEGER, P. BACHER & L. SROKA. 1988. Development of the EEG of school-age children and adolescents. I. Analysis of band power. Electroencephalogr. Clin. Neurophysiol. **69:** 91-99.

57. DUFFY, F. H., P. H. BARTELS & J. L. BURCHFIEL. 1981. Significance probability mapping: An aid in the topographic analysis of brain electrical activity. Electroencephalogr. Clin. Neurophysiol. **51:** 455-462.

58. DUFFY, F. H. 1986. A response to Oken and Chiappa. Ann. Neurol. **19:** 494-496.

59. JOHN, E. R., L. S. PRICHEP, J. FRIDMAN & P. EASTON. 1988. Neurometrics: Computer-assisted differential diagnosis of brain dysfunctions. Science **239:** 162-169.

60. ZAPPULLA, R. A., B. Z. KARMEL & E. GREENBLATT. 1981. Prediction of cerebellopontine angle tumors based on discriminant analysis of brain stem auditory evoked responses. Neurosurgery **9:** 542-547.

61. ZAPPULLA, R. A., L. I. MALIS, E. GREENBLATT & B. Z. KARMEL. 1984. Utility of brainstem auditory evoked potentials in the diagnosis and treatment of tumors of the cerebellopontine angle. *In* Evoked Potentials II. R. H. Nodar & C. Barber, Eds.: 194-202. Butterworths. London.

62. PRICHEP, L. S. & E. R. JOHN. 1987. Neurometrics: Clinical applications. *In* Methods of Analysis of Brain Electrical and Magnetic Signals. EEG Handbook. A. S. Gevins & A. Remond, Eds. **2:** 153-170. Elsevier. Amsterdam.

Neurocognitive Networks of the Human Brain[a]

ALAN S. GEVINS AND JUDY ILLES

EEG Systems Laboratory
51 Federal Street
San Francisco, California 94107

INTRODUCTION

Among the techniques for studying brain-behavior relationships in humans, scalp-recorded neural potentials have been used widely for over 50 years. With the technological advances of the 1970s and 1980s, new recording and analysis tools have been developed for obtaining increasingly specific information about the spatial and temporal features of neurocognitive processes. Such advances have made possible neuroelectric recordings with many channels, well beyond the original 19 channels of the international 10-20 system proposed by Jasper[1] in the 1950s. These tools have also provided improved signal processing and means of correlating neuroelectric measures with anatomical information from magnetic resonance images. We will focus on these tools in the first part of this chapter; in the second part, we will describe how we have been applying the tools to study the split-second components of higher cognitive functions.

TOOLS OF THE TRADE

Improved Spatial Sampling

Electrode Arrays with 125 Channels

One of the requirements for extracting detailed information about cognitive processes from the scalp-recorded EEG is to have adequate spatial sampling. The 19 channels customarily employed in clinical recordings provide an interelectrode distance of about 6 cm. While this is sufficient for detecting signs of gross pathology, it is obviously insufficient for resolving functional differences within small cortical regions. To improve spatial resolution, we have been making 59-channel recordings for the past

[a] Supported by grants from the National Institute of Neurological Diseases, the National Institute of Mental Health, the Air Force Office of Scientific Research, and the National Science Foundation.

several years. This provides an interelectrode distance of about 3.5 cm on a typical adult head, which is still not good enough. To improve sampling, we recently developed a 125-channel recording system that provides an interelectrode distance of about 2.25 cm. Subjects wear a stretchable EEG recording cap, with electrodes placed on the cap according to an expanded version of the standard international 10-20 system.[2] Prior to each EEG recording session, the 3-D position of each electrode on the individual subject's head is measured precisely with a commercial 3-D digitizer (FIG. 1). To date 12 full-scale 125-channel recordings have been made from subjects receiving visual, auditory, and somatic stimuli.

Registration of Scalp-Electrode Positions with Underlying Anatomical Structures

To visualize the brain areas underlying the scalp electrodes, a procedure is needed for aligning scalp-electrode positions and underlying anatomical structures. This first requires producing an accurate anatomical representation of a subject's brain.

Distortion Correction of Magnetic Resonance Images. While magnetic resonance (MR) images are invaluable because of the anatomical differentiation they provide, they contain inherent distortion that, if not corrected, may cause quantitative measurements of position, length, area, and volume to be erroneous. The distortion can exceed 10% and commonly arises from calibration errors and inhomogeneities of the magnetic field gradients. We have been working on correcting this problem using both phantom calibration data and data recorded from human subjects wearing constructed helmets with spherical fiducial markers that are easily visualized on MR images. It is necessary to correct both image intensity and image position.

To test our methods, scans from a Diasonics MTS MR system were made on three subjects. The maximum total distortion measured on this machine was 8%. Variation between images with TR = 600 msec and TE = 20 msec and images with TR = 2000 msec and TE = 35 and 70 msec were found to be less than 2%. We compared the location of the spherical fiducial markers in coronal, sagittal, and axial images, and various image transforms were then used to bring the measured points into alignment. We found that by computing a separate scale factor for each direction combined with a translation and rotation, two sets of images could be brought into reasonably close alignment. An example of a set of Diasonics MRIs before correction is shown in FIGURE 2A. It is clear that the anatomical positions corresponding to the scalp and cranium do not line up. The coronal sections shown in blue are shifted to the left of their correct position. The sagittal sections shown in reddish brown are "stretched" by approximately 17% in the anterior/posterior direction compared to the horizontal or transaxial sections which are shown in dark green. The same images after correcting for distortion are shown in FIGURE 2B.

Alignment of EEG Electrode Positions with MR Surface Reconstructions. A linear transformation is calculated to superimpose electrode positions and the scalp-surface contours obtained from MR images. This transformation is initially determined by visually adjusting a graphical display of the electrodes and scalp contours. An optimal transformation is then calculated by a program that adjusts each parameter in the transformation until the average distance between all electrode positions and the closest scalp point is minimized (FIG. 3). The aligned surface model can also be superimposed onto composite MR images showing various orientations (FIG. 4). Additionally, surfaces may be constructed by manually tracing other structures on each MR image and then calculating the polygonal surface which fits these contours (FIG. 5).

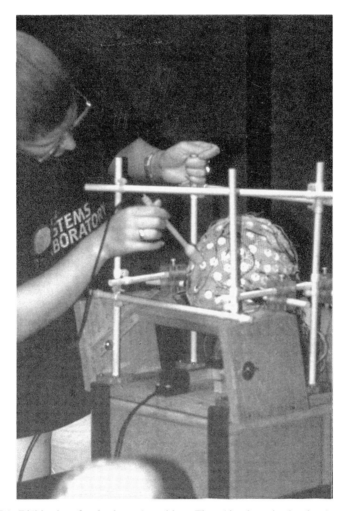

FIGURE 1. Digitization of scalp electrode positions. The subject is resting in a headrest designed to minimize head movement. The technician touches the stylus (which contains electromagnetic field sensors for x, y, and z axes) to each of the electrodes in turn. The 3-D coordinates of each electrode position are transmitted to the data collection and analysis computer.

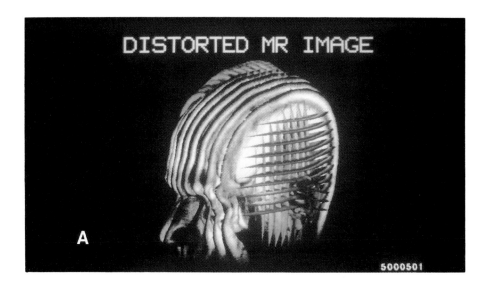

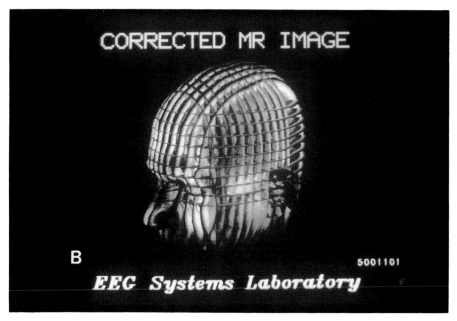

FIGURE 2. (A) Composite of distorted MR images in horizontal, sagittal, and coronal orientations as originally recorded. The location of the scalp is not consistent for different orientations. (B) Composite of the same images after transformation to correct for distortion. The scalp surface now appears at the same location in all orientations.

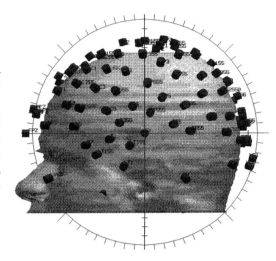

FIGURE 3. Rough sagittal view of 128-electrode montage constructed from horizontal MR images and positioned on the scalp surface. Also shown is the coordinate system with the origin located halfway between the T3 and T4 temporal electrodes. Some electrodes are not properly aligned with the scalp surface due to a mechanical problem that has been corrected.

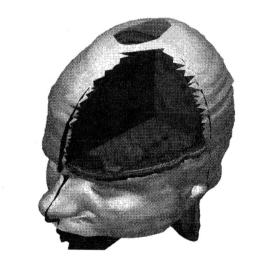

FIGURE 4. Rough surface reconstruction of the scalp from horizontal MR slices with a cutaway to show horizontal, sagittal, and coronal MR images of the left frontal lobe. In this early reconstruction, the sagittal and horizontal slices are not entirely aligned, causing the sagittal section to protrude from the surface.

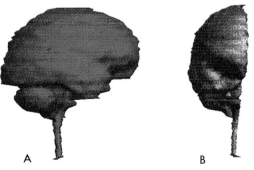

FIGURE 5. Reconstruction of the right hemisphere of the brain and spinal cord viewed from the (A) right and (B) anteriorly.

Reduction of Brain Potential Blur Distortion

Laplacian Derivation. Neuroelectric signals recorded at the scalp are principally distorted by transmission through the low-conductance skull. This distortion manifests as a spatial low-pass filtering which causes the potential distribution at the scalp to appear blurred or out of focus. There are a number of methods for reducing this distortion, among which the spatial Laplacian operator is perhaps the simplest and most effective. This method, which is often referred to as the Laplacian derivation, is derived by computing the second derivative in space of the potential field at each electrode. This converts the potential into a quantity proportional to the current entering and exiting the scalp at each electrode site, and eliminates the effect of the reference electrode used during recording. An approximation to the Laplacian derivation, introduced by Hjorth[3,4] assumes that electrodes are equidistant and at right angles to each other. Although this approximation is fairly good for some electrode positions such as midline central (Cz), it is less accurate for others such as midtemporal (T5). We have been using a more accurate estimate of the Laplacian derivation that is based on projecting the measured electrode positions onto a two-dimensional surface. Although this produces a dramatic improvement in topographic detail, some problems remain because of the assumptions that surrounding electrodes used to estimate the Laplacian of an electrode are near that electrode and that the current gradient is uniform over the region encompassed by the surrounding electrodes. Furthermore, it is not possible to estimate the Laplacian at peripheral electrodes because the surrounding electrodes are incomplete.

Spatial Deconvolution Using Spherical Head Model. By modeling the tissues between brain and scalp as surfaces with different thicknesses and resistances, we have performed a deblurring operation that, in principle, makes the potential appear as if it were recorded just above the level of the brain surface,[5] without assumptions about the actual (cortical or subcortical) source locations. The deblurring operation, however, requires detailed modeling of the tissues which, when the exact shape of the head is taken into account, is a great deal of work. The operation is even further complicated by the fact that a solution to calculating the local resistance of the skull precisely does not yet exist. With the conduction of potentials from a localized source spread over a considerable area of scalp, the summation of signals at any given scalp site may reflect many sources over much of the brain. In the context of a four-shell spherical head model, we have estimated the amount of spread—the "point spread"—for a radial equivalent dipole source in the cortex to be about 2.5 cm. If the conductance of the skull is known, a deblurring operation using a model-based deconvolution can, in principle, achieve a better signal enhancement than a Laplacian derivation when the distance between electrodes is less than approximately the point spread distance of 2.5 cm.

Finite Element Method. Another method of increasing spatial resolution for those cases for which the source generators can be modeled as current dipoles, and for which MR data is available, is the finite element method (FEM). The entire volume of the head, as found in MR images, is broken up into many small elements representing various tissues: the scalp, skull, and brain. By assigning each element a conductivity constant (obtained from textbook values) and one for a known source, it is possible to calculate the potential at each vertex of all the finite elements using Maxwell's equations. Because the number of vertices is approximately 10,000, an efficient algorithm is necessary to make this practical on a small computer. Using a SUN Sparc-1 workstation rated at about 12 MIPS, the initial matrix decomposition based on a set of finite elements takes about 90 min, while the potential computation for each source takes

6 min. If a practical method can be developed for estimating local skull conductance, the FEM deblurring method has the capability of producing highly enhanced representations of the current distribution on the exposed surface of the cortex.

Detecting Artifacts

The usual practice in evoked potential studies of cognition is to reject automatically artifacted trials in which the voltage of the eye-movement measurement channels exceeds a fixed threshold.[6] While this procedure catches large contaminants, it entirely misses small ones. This can lead to a spurious result if there are small, but consistent saccades or microblinks approximately time-locked to stimulus presentation. Although we also use an on-line artifact detection procedure to flag automatically portions of trials and individual electrodes that have unusually high or low amplitude, all data are examined visually on a graphics terminal to confirm and improve the computer's detections as needed. In our studies with clinically healthy, young adult subjects, there is about 10% data attrition due to artifacts.

Data Set Formation: Controlling for Spurious Sources of Variance

After the data have been cleared of instrumental and subject-related artifacts, data sets are usually formed in pairs to test specific hypotheses. In forming these data sets, it is imperative that the major difference between two sets be related to the hypothesis being tested. It is, of course, standard practice to try to eliminate spurious differences by careful experimental design, but there is always the chance that some remaining factors differ between sets. These uncontrolled factors can include small residual eye-movement contaminants, arousal level, and response movement parameters (e.g., force or reaction time), all of which are known to affect neuroelectric signals.

To ascertain that the major source of variance is actually related to the hypothesis, the two sets of artifact-free trials are submitted, usually on a subject-by-subject basis, to an interactive program that displays the means, *t* tests, and histogram distributions of up to 50 behavioral and physiological event variables. These include stimulus parameters, reaction time, movement magnitude and duration, error, EEG arousal index, eye-movement, muscle potential indices, and so on. The data sets are inspected for significant differences in variables which are not related to the hypothesis, and outliers are discarded. As an example, an unintentional difference between experimental conditions in response force may be present. In the data set with the larger response force, the associated movement-related potentials could overlap the P300 evoked potential peak causing a spurious between-condition difference in P300 amplitude. After careful balancing of the data sets for such movement parameters, valid assessments about P300 peak effects may be made. In balancing our data we are careful not to truncate the histogram distribution severely. The unrelated variables are reduced to a between-condition alpha significance of 0.2, or if this is not possible without seriously affecting the distribution, to just over 0.05. The net effect of these procedures is the certainty that when a neuroelectric difference between experimental conditions is found, the difference actually relates to the hypothesis under consideration.

Neurocognitive Pattern Analysis

We have been using the term "neurocognitive pattern analysis" (NCP analysis) to refer to our procedures for extracting task-related spatiotemporal patterns from the unrelated background activity of the brain. In the first of three generations of NCP analysis, we measured background EEG spectral intensities while people performed complex tasks, such as arithmetic problems lasting up to one minute. These patterns had sufficient specificity to identify the type of task,[7,8] but when the tasks were controlled for stimulus-, response-, and performance-related factors, they had identical, spatially diffuse EEG spectral scalp distributions.[7] This study suggested that complex tasks involving a variety of sensory, cognitive, and motoric processes activate large, wide-spread areas of cortex to a degree proportional to the subject's effort. It also strongly suggested that most studies of EEG correlates of cognitive activities, including those of hemispheric lateralization, may have confounded electrical activity related to limb and eye movements, stimulus properties, and task difficulty with those of mental activity per se.

In the second generation of NCP analysis, we measured cross-correlations between electrodes recorded during performance of simple visuomotor judgment tasks.[9] From this experiment, in which rapidly shifting focal patterns were extracted from two similar spatial tasks, it was clear that a split-second temporal resolution is imperative for isolating the rapidly shifting neurocognitive processes associated with successive information processing stages.

In the third generation, we extended our methods to include event-related covariances (ERCs). The ERC approach is based on the hypothesis that when regions of the brain are functionally related, their event-related potential (ERP, another name for evoked potential) components are related in shape and in time.[10] The idea is that the ERP waveform delineates the time course of event-related mass activity of a neural population, so that if two populations are functionally related, their ERPs should line up in time, perhaps with some delay. If so (and if the relationships are linear as they often appear to be), this could be measured by the lagged covariance between the ERPs, or portions of the ERPs, from different regions (FIG. 6). This is the event-related covariance method.

The procedures that are followed for ERC analysis are described here. Procedures 1–4 have been discussed in detail above.

1. A sufficient amount of data are recorded using as many electrodes as possible.
2. Data with artifact contamination are removed.
3. Pairs of conditions to be compared are selected, and trials with extreme values of behavioral variables are eliminated.
4. The Laplacian operator is applied to the potential distribution of each non-peripheral scalp-electrode location.
5. Analysis intervals and digital filter characteristics are determined. The analysis intervals are usually either centered on an ERP peak, or are positioned just before or after a stimulus or response.
6. Enhanced, filtered, and decimated averaged Laplacian ERPs for each condition are computed. (In an optional procedure, used when the signal-to-noise ratio is very low, a statistical procedure is used to identify trials with measurable event-related signals, and averages are formed only from those trials.[11])
7. Multilag cross-covariance functions are computed between all pairwise channel combinations of these averaged ERPs in each selected analysis window. The

magnitude of the maximum value of the cross-covariance function and its lag time are the features used to characterize the ERC. The covariance analysis interval is the width of one period of the band-center frequency of each filter. Down-sampling factors are determined by the 20 dB rejection point, and the covariance function is computed up to a lag time of one-half period of the high frequency for each band. For example, we often use a filter with 3 dB cutoffs at 4 and 7 Hz, and with 20 dB attenuation at 1.5 and 9.5 Hz. The filtered time series are decimated from 128 to 21 Hz for each covariance calculation. Covariance is estimated over a 187-msec window, which corresponds to one period of a 5.5-Hz sinusoid. Each window is lagged by up to 8 lags at the original undecimated sampling rate, i.e., one hundred-twenty-eighth of a second per lag.

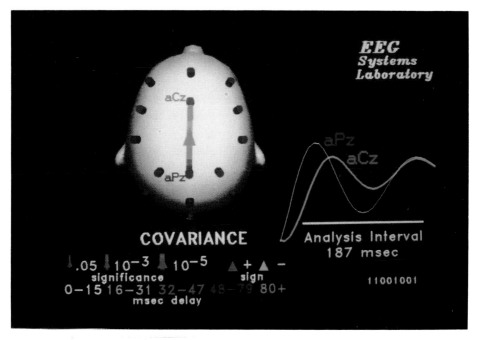

FIGURE 6. Schematic diagram showing the relationship of an event-related covariance (ERC) line on a top view of a model head (*left*) to the theta-band-filtered, averaged event-related Laplacian derivation waveforms (*right*). ERCs were computed over the indicated 187-msec analysis interval from the aPz and aCz electrode sites. The width of an ERC line indicates the significance of the covariance between two waveforms, with the scale appearing above the word "significance." The color of the line indicates the time delay in msec (lag time of maximum covariance) as shown in the scale above "msec delay." The color of the arrow indicates the sign of the covariance (same color as line = positive; skin color = negative). The arrow points from leading to lagging channel, unless there is no delay, in which case a bar is shown. The covariance between aPz and aCz is significant at $p < 10^{-5}$. The aPz waveform leads the aCz waveform by about 16-31 msec (*green line*), and the covariance is positive (*green arrow*) (From Gevins et al.[17])

8. The significance of ERCs is determined by reference to an estimate of the standard deviation of the "noise" ERC. The noise ERC is computed by averaging random intervals in each single trial of the ensemble of trials. ERC analysis is then performed on a filtered and decimated version of the resulting "noise" averages, yielding a distribution of "noise" ERCs. The threshold for significance is reduced according to the dimensionality of the data with Duncan's correction procedure. The number of channels is used as a conservative estimate of the number of independent dimensions. The most significant ERCs in each interval are graphed.

9. ANOVA and post-hoc t tests are used to compare ERC patterns between conditions. The similarity of appearance of two ERC graphs is measured with an estimate of the correlation between them. The estimate comes from a distribution-independent "bootstrap" Monte Carlo procedure,[12] which also yields a confidence interval for the estimates.

10. The between-subject variability of ERC patterns is tested by determining whether each pair of experimental conditions of a particular subject can be distinguished using discriminating equations generated on the other subjects.

11. The within-subject reliability is assessed by attempting to discriminate the experimental conditions for each session using equations generated on that subject's other sessions.

The tests of both between- and within-subject variability and reliability are performed on sets of single trials. This quantifies the extent to which the condition-specific patterns from the ERC analysis of the average ERPs can be observed in each trial. Although this procedure could be done with any type of discriminant analysis, we have developed the use of distribution-independent, layered, artificial "neural network" pattern classification algorithms for this purpose.[13,14] We have shown that this method has better sensitivity than stepwise or full-model linear or quadratic discriminant analysis.[15] The pattern recognition approach has the advantage of testing how well a subject's individual trials conform to those of the group in discriminating two behavioral conditions of interest. In the same way, the trials of each session of a subject are tested by conformity to trials from the other sessions of that subject. Requiring trial-by-trial discriminability is a strict condition for deciding between-subject variability and within-subject reliability.

Each subject's classification yields a score, which is the percent of trials that are correctly classified by the group discrimination equations. The score is assessed for significance by comparison to the binomial distribution.[15] A significant classification score for a subject indicates that the group equations are successful in discriminating the two conditions in his or her trials.

Within-subject (between-session) reliability is tested in a similar manner. The trial set (consisting of the two conditions) from each of a subject's sessions is tested with equations developed on the trial sets from his or her other sessions. The single-trial ERC values come from channel pairs that are significant in the ERC pattern formed from the average over all his or her sessions. Post-hoc comparisons are valuable in determining whether effects of learning and/or habituation are evident over sessions, by indicating which sessions are alike and where transitions occur between sessions.

FIGURE 7 is a block diagram of the data collection and analysis process discussed above. For studies not requiring pattern recognition analysis, the event-related covariances are computed on averaged event-related potentials after band-pass filtering.

In the next section, results of a study of bimanual visuomotor performance and a study of the effects of mental fatigue on human cognitive networks are presented. Preliminary results of a study of elementary language processes are also described.

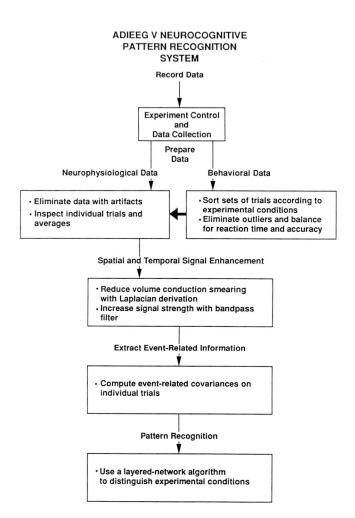

FIGURE 7. ADIEEG-V system for pattern recognition of event-related brain signals. Separate subsystems perform on-line experimental control and data collection, data selection and evaluation, signal processing and pattern recognition. Current capacity is 128 channels.

APPLYING THE TOOLS

Bimanual Visuomotor Task

One of the goals of the bimanual visuomotor experiment was to study prefrontal involvement while subjects prepared to perform a task accurately and used feedback about their accuracy to gauge their responses.[16–18]

Subjects and Task

Seven healthy, right-handed, male adults participated in this study. A visual cue, slanted to the right or to the left, prompted the subject to prepare to make a response pressure with the right or left index finger. One sec later, the cue was followed by a visual numeric stimulus (numbers 1-9) indicating that a pressure of 0.1 to 0.9 kg should be made with the index finger of the previously indicated hand. A two-digit number, presented 1 sec after the peak of the response pressure, provided feedback that indicated the subject's exact pressure. On a random 20% of the trials, the stimulus number was slanted in the opposite direction to the cue; subjects were to withhold their responses on these "catch trials." The next trial followed 1 sec after disappearance of the feedback. Each subject performed several hundred trials, with rest breaks as needed.

Recordings

Twenty-six channels of EEG data, as well as vertical and horizontal eye-movements and flexor digitori muscle activity from both arms, were recorded. All single-trial EEG data were screened for eye-movement, muscle potential, and other artifacts, and contaminated data were discarded.

Analysis and Results

Intervals used for ERC analysis were centered on major event-related potential peaks. ERCs were computed between each of the 120 pairwise combinations of the 16 nonperipheral channels. Intervals were set from 500 msec before the cue to 500 msec after the feedback. We first calculated the mean error (deviation from the required finger pressure) over all trials from the recording session. Individual trials were then classified as accurate (trial error less than mean error) or inaccurate (trial error greater than mean error).

ERC patterns during a 375-msec interval, centered 687 msec post-cue (spanning the late contingent negative variation—CNV), regardless of subsequent accuracy, involved left prefrontal sites, as well as appropriately lateralized central and parietal sites

(FIG. 8A and B). Inaccurate performance by the right hand was preceded by a very simple pattern, while inaccurate performance by the left hand was preceded by a complex, spatially diffuse pattern. The relative lack of ERCs preceding inaccurate right-hand performance may simply reflect inattention on those trials, while the strong and complex patterns preceding inaccurate performance with the left hand may reflect effortful, but inappropriate, preparation by the right-handed subjects.

ERC patterns related to feedback about accurate and inaccurate performances were similar immediately after the onset of feedback, but began to differ in an interval, centered at 375 msec, that spanned the P3 (FIG. 9A and B). The ERC patterns for feedback to accurate performance by the two hands were very similar (bootstrap correlation = 0.91 ± 0.01), involving midline anterocentral, central, anteroparietal, parietal, and anterooccipital sites; left anteroparietal and anterocentral sites; and right parietal, anteroparietal, anterocentral, and frontal sites. These accurate patterns involved many long-delay (32–79 msec) ERCs. The waveforms of the frontal and anterocentral sites lagged those of more posterior sites. For feedback to inaccurate performance, patterns for both hands were also very similar (bootstrap correlation = 0.90 ± 0.02) and involved most of the same sites as the accurate patterns, with the striking inclusion of the left and midline frontal sites. Again, frontal waveforms lagged those of the more posterior sites with which they covaried. There were even more long-delay ERCs than in the accurate patterns.

Summary

The pre-stimulus ERC patterns seem to characterize a distributed preparatory neural set that is related to the accuracy of subsequent task performance. This network involves distinctive cognitive (frontal), integrative-motor (midline precentral) and lateralized somesthetic-motor (central and parietal) components. The involvement of the left-frontal site is consistent with Teuber's[19] notions of corollary discharge and with other experimental and clinical findings suggesting the synthesis and integration of functional networks in prefrontal cortical areas.[20–23] A midline anterocentral integrative-motor component is consistent with known involvement of premotor and supplementary motor areas in initiating motor responses. The finding of an appropriately lateralized central and parietal component is consistent with evidence from primates and humans for neuronal firing in motor and somatosensory cortices prior to motor responses.

FIGURE 8. Preparatory event-related covariance (ERC) patterns (*colored lines*). Measurements are from an interval 500 to 875 msec after the cue for subsequently accurate (**A**) right-hand and (**B**) left-hand visuomotor task performance by seven right-handed men. The ERCs are superimposed for illustrative purposes over a horizontal MR scan. The thickness of a covariance line is proportional to its significance (from .05 to .005). A violet line indicates the covariance is positive, while a blue line is negative. ERCs involving left frontal and appropriately contralateral central and parietal electrode sites are prominent in patterns for subsequently accurate performance of both hands. The magnitude and number of preparatory ERCs are greater preceding subsequently inaccurate left-hand performance than those preceding inaccurate right-hand performance by the right-handed subjects. Inaccurate left-hand preparatory ERCs are more widely distributed compared with the left-hand accurate pattern. For the right-hand, fewer and weaker ERCs characterize subsequently inaccurate performance.

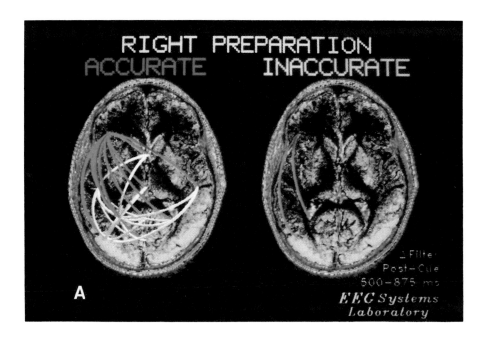

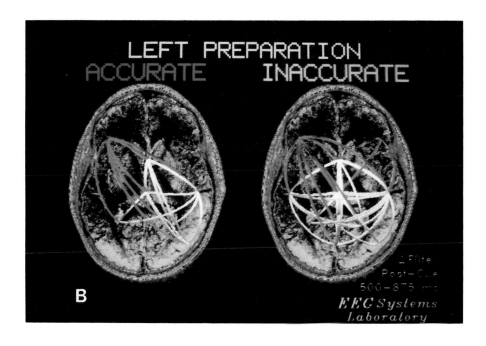

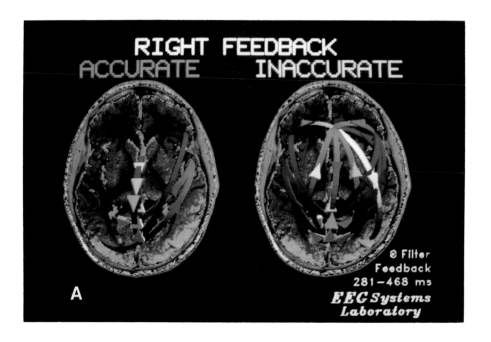

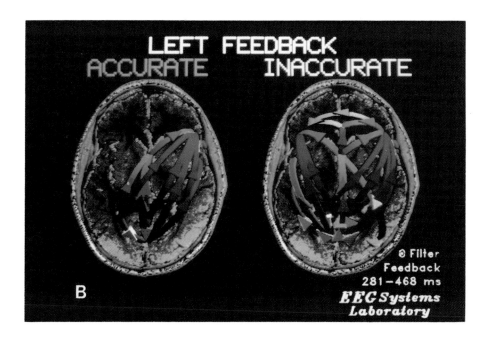

Since ERC feedback patterns of accurate or inaccurate performance (involving either hand) were more similar than those between accurate and inaccurate patterns for one hand, it may be inferred that the feedback patterns were related more to performance accuracy than to the hand used. The fact that ERC patterns following disconfirming feedback involved more frontal sites than did patterns following confirming feedback is consistent with the idea that greater resetting of performance-related neural systems is required following disconfirming feedback. Likewise, the front focus of these differences is consistent with the importance of the frontal lobes in the integration of sensory and motor activities.[20,23]

Effects of Mental Fatigue on Functional Brain Topography

In this study, the effects of mental fatigue on preparation and memory, stimulus recognition and stimulus processing were studied.[24]

Subjects and Task

Five healthy, right-handed, male subjects performed a task that required that they remember two continuously changing numbers, in the presence of numeric distractors, and produce precise finger pressures. Each trial consisted of a warning symbol, followed by a single-digit visual stimulus to be remembered, followed by the subject's finger-pressure response to the stimulus number presented two trials ago, followed by a two-digit feedback number indicating the accuracy of the response. For example, if the stimulus numbers in five successive trials were 8, 6, 1, 9, 4, the correct response would be a pressure of 0.8 kg when seeing the 1, 0.6 kg for the 9, and 0.1 kg for the 4. To increase the task difficulty, subjects were required to withhold their response on a random 20% of the trials. These "no-response catch trials" were trials in which the current stimulus number was identical to the stimulus two trials ago. Subjects were given ample practice to stabilize accuracy and reaction time.

Subjects performed the task over a 10-14 h period. Sets of trials with equally accurate performance and response movement parameters were selected from three periods: an early period during the first 7 h (Alert), a middle period just prior to any decline in overall performance accuracy (Incipient Performance Impairment), and a late period after performance had significantly degraded.

FIGURE 9. Most significant (top 2 SD) feedback ERC patterns elicted when subjects were given information about the accuracy of their finger pressure response by the right hand (**A**) and left hand (**B**). ERCs were derived from a 187-msec-wide interval, beginning 281 msec and ending 468 msec post-feedback, on theta-band-filtered, 7-subject-averaged evoked potential waveforms. The color of the covariance line indicates the lag time of maximum covariance between electrodes: yellow, 0-15 msec; green, 16-31 msec; blue, 32-47 msec; red, 48-79 msec; purple, 80+ msec. A major difference between accurate and inaccurate patterns is that the left and midline frontal sites are only involved in the inaccurate patterns. The involvement of these sites may reflect greater processing after inaccurate performance in order to improve subsequent performance.

Recordings

EEGs were recorded with either 33 or 51 channels set in a nylon mesh cap. Vertical and horizontal eye movements were also recorded, as were the responding flexor digitori muscle potentials, electrocardiogram, and respiration. Three-axis magnetic resonance image scans were made of three of the five subjects.

Analysis and Results

Neuroelectric effects were observed during two fraction-of-a-second intervals when subjects (1) prepared to receive a new stimulus number while holding the two previous stimulus numbers in working memory (CNV interval), and (2) when they withheld their response in the instance where the current stimulus number was the same as the two-back stimulus number (P300 interval). Significant differences were seen between the early Alert period and the middle Incipient Performance Impairment (IPI) period ($p < 0.0001$). While the magnitude of the patterns was reduced during both preparatory and response inhibition intervals, the topographic distribution of the pattern was only affected during preparation (FIG. 10). The preparatory pattern shifted from one strongly focused on midline central and precentral sites to one focused primarily on right-sided precentral and parietal sites. It appeared as though extended task-performance altered the "neural strategy" used to perform the same behavior. Thus, prolonged mental work differentially affected two successive split-second information processing intervals.

The extent to which each subject's patterns corresponded to the group's and the extent to which it was possible to distinguish individual trials from the Alert and IPI periods of the session were determined next using pattern recognition analysis. ERCs common to the group (FIG. 10, left and middle) were considered as possible variables. For the preparatory interval, they consisted of ERCs computed over the 500 msec pre-stimulus epoch of each trial. For separate groups of three and two subjects whose resting EEG characteristics differed, five equations were formed on four-fifths of the trials, and tested on the remaining one-fifth. The average test set accuracy of Alert versus IPI discrimination was then computed and tested for significance by reference to the binomial distribution. Discrimination accuracy was 62% ($p < 0.001$). Individual-ized equations were generated on the subject with the most usable data, still using the variables from the group pattern. Discrimination accuracy climbed to 81% ($p < 0.0001$).

Summary

Striking changes occurred in the ERC patterns after subjects performed the difficult memory and fine-motor control task for an average of 7-9 h, but before performance deteriorated. Pattern strength was reduced in a fraction-of-a-second-long response preparation interval over midline precentral areas and over the entire left hemisphere. By contrast, pattern strength in a succeeding response-inhibition interval was reduced over all areas. The pattern changed least in an intervening interval associated with visual-stimulus processing. This suggests that, in addition to the well-known global reduction in neuroelectric signal strength, functional neural networks are selectively affected by sustained mental work in specific fraction-of-a-second task intervals. For practical application, these results demonstrate the possibility of detecting leading indicator neuroelectric patterns which precede degradation of performance due to sustained mental work.

Neurocognitive Analysis of Elementary Language Processes

Preliminary results of a recent experiment demonstrate good spatial and temporal differentiation of basic linguistic functions using 59-channel EEG recordings.

Subjects and Task

Nine right-handed, healthy male subjects performed a language task in which they had to judge whether the second visually presented stimulus of a given condition (S2) formed a match with the first stimulus (S1). There were four, fully randomized conditions in the experiment. In the graphic non-letter condition, the stimuli were characters of Katakana, a Japanese script with which none of the subjects were familiar. Subjects were required to judge whether or not the stimuli were identical. In the phonemic condition, subjects were required to judge if the pronounceable but neologistic word stimuli sounded alike. In the semantic condition, subjects were required to decide if the high frequency, open-class monosyllabic words were opposite or not. Finally, in the grammatical condition, subjects judged if the verb of the S2 formed a meaningful and grammatically correct sentence with the S1 pronoun. Eighty-five percent of the trials were "match" trials and no response was required; subjects responded to the 15% mismatch trials with a button press using the left index finger.

Recordings

EEGs referenced to the midline anterior-parietal (aPz) electrode were recorded from 59 scalp electrodes. The montage was an extended 10-20 system,[2] and included the frontal sites aF1 and aF2, Fz, F3 to F8, and Fpz; the anterior central aCz, aC1 to aC6; central Cz, C3 and C4; anterior temporal aT5 and aT6; temporal T3 to T8; lower temporal lT1, lT2, lT5, lT6; ventral temporal vT5 and vT6; anterior parietal aP1 to aP6; parietal Pz, P3 to P6; anterior occipital aO1 and aO2; occipital Oz, O1 and O2; ventral occipital vO1 and vO2; and the inion (I) and both mastoids (M1 and M2). Vertical eye movements were recorded bipolarly from an electrode pair placed supra- and suborbitally; horizontal eye movements were recorded bipolarly between electrodes at the outer canthus of each eye. Other bipolar pairs were placed over flexor digitori muscles of left and right arms to record EMG and at the submentalis to record subvocal movements of the larynx and mouth. The EEG was amplified 8333 times, band-pass filtered from 0.5-50 Hz and recorded at 128 samples per sec.

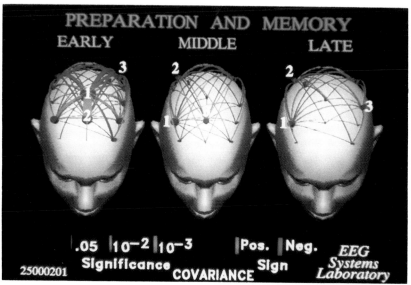

FIGURE 10. Pattern recognition analysis using an artificial, layered neural network that distinguished ERC neuroelectric patterns recorded during baseline (early), incipient performance impairment (middle), and impaired performance (late) periods from five Air Force test pilots performing a difficult visuomotor-memory task over a 14-h period. Baseline data were obtained during the first 7 hours; incipient performance impairment data during hours 7-10 preceding impaired performance; the impaired performance data were obtained during hours 10-14. The ERCs were measured during a 500-msec interval when the subjects were remembering two numbers and preparing for the next stimulus. ERCs greatly declined in magnitude from baseline (early) to incipient performance impairment (middle) to impaired performance (late) epochs. The patterns also changed, with the emphasis shifting from the (1) midline central, (2) midline precentral, and (3) left parietal sites to right hemisphere sites.

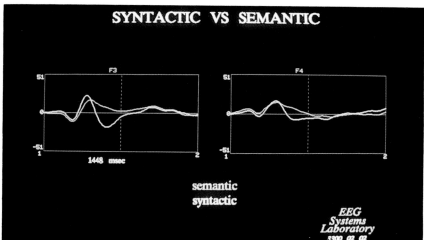

FIGURE 11. LD waveforms evoked by the first of two stimuli (syntactic and semantic) in an experiment designed to study elementary language processes. The waveforms are averaged across nine subjects. The major difference between the grammatic (syntactic) and semantic conditions is lateralized to the left hemisphere, where the grammatic condition has a substantial peak at 442 msec at left frontal and anterior central sites. The x-axis shows 1-sec beginning with the S1. The y-axis corresponds to ± 0.153 μV/sq cm.

Analysis and Results

Analysis of both ERP and ERC data is ongoing. Among the condition differences observed to date, for example, syntactic and nonsyntactic trials were clearly differentiated by ERP topography. After S1, the grammatic (syntactic) condition alone had a substantial peak at 442 msec at lateral frontal and anterior central sites. N442 was most robust at F3 (FIG. 11), F5, and aC1, where it was significantly larger than in the semantic condition (p < 0.05). After S2 (not shown), the grammatic condition was again distinguished from the semantic condition by a positive peak at 279 msec at left frontal and anterior central electrodes. At these sites, the grammatic P279 was larger in amplitude than in the semantic condition (p < 0.05). It was not significantly lateralized.

Summary

Stimuli in both the nonsyntactic and syntactic conditions in this experiment were words with similar physical characteristics. The main difference between them post-S1 was that the semantic (nonsyntactic) condition used open-class words (content words such as nouns and adjectives) and the grammatic (syntactic) condition used closed-class words (function words), in this case pronouns. It is possible that the N411 observed for the syntactic condition is related to processing the closed-class words, to the initiation of a "syntactic parser,"[25] or to both processes simultaneously. The location of the "syntactic" effect at left frontal sites (F3, F5, and aC3) after both S1 and S2 is consistent with neurophysiological observations of syntactic deficits and difficulties in handling closed-class words in aphasia patients whose lesions involve and extend deep to Broca's area.

CONCLUSIONS

Methodological

Advances in neuroelectric recording and analysis technology during the past two decades have significantly increased the sensitivity and specificity of measuring brain-behavior relationships. Sharper spatial resolution is provided by an increased number of electrodes and by use of the Laplacian derivation. Information about common activity and its temporal relationships is provided by the event-related covariance measure, while neural network pattern recognition analysis provides a powerful method of detecting neurocognitive signals in sets of single-trial data. The signs we have seen of rapidly shifting, functionally interdependent cortical networks are particularly intriguing in light of their consistency with both historical and contemporary, clinical and experimental findings about brain-behavior relationships. In our current research, we hope to further refine and elaborate these methodological and experimental paradigms.

Models of Neural Information Processing in Cognitive Electrophysiology

Because of the stimulus-response design inherent in most experimental designs, many models of cognitive functioning have a passive tone. The brain reacts to a given stimulus, and the stages leading to response are inferred from measures of reaction time, ERP peak latencies, and so on. However, we know from experience, observation, and inference that cognitive processes are highly interactive. Our environment is, in a sense, altered by our perception of it, because perception itself is a synthesis of sensation, current brain state, and past cognitive experience. This synthesis involves a continuously updated, dynamic internal representation of what we imagine our selves and

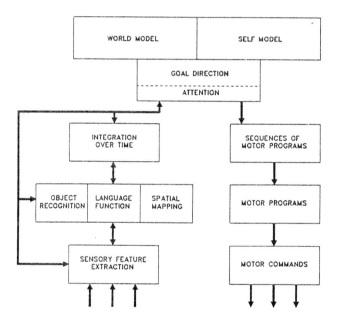

FIGURE 12. Sketch of parallel, sequential, hierarchically organized information processing in functional networks of the human neocortex. The previous moment's internal model influences the current moment's goal direction and attention, which in turn influences other stages of processing.

environment to be like at any given moment. Moreover, we use our effector and sensory systems to probe actively the environment for information relevant to maintaining and updating the self/world model (FIG. 12). Each perception, each action is incorporated into the internal model, and new perceptions and actions are in turn influenced through the model's role in directing attentional and conceptual processes. It is challenging, but not impossible, to design experimental situations which emphasize this dynamic and interactive nature of cognition. Two areas that have been of particular interest to us are preparatory processes, which precede the stimulus and are directed by the internal model, and feedback, which governs the updating of the model after behaviors. Although it is likely that the frontal cortex plays a pivotal role in both processes, it would be simplistic to consider the frontal lobes as a mere executor. Rather, it is likely that the entire brain is involved in a constellation of rapidly changing, functional networks that provide the delicate balance between stimulus-locked behavior and purely imaginary ideation. The pre-stimulus and the feedback-associated "processing networks" observed in our studies may be signs of such interrelated activity. With even further advances in brain imaging in neuropsychophysiology in the 1990s, we can hope to achieve increasingly detailed and direct measurements of the organization and interrelationships of sensory and higher cognitive behaviors in health and in disease.

ACKNOWLEDGMENTS

The authors gratefully acknowledge the efforts of their scientific collaborators Drs. S. Bressler, P. Brickett, B. Cutillo, R. Fowler-White, D. Greer, J. Le, N. Morgan, and B. Reutter for their contributions to the original research presented here.

REFERENCES

1. JASPER, H. H. 1958. The ten-twenty electrode system of the International Federation of Societies for Electroencephalography. EEG Clin. Neurophysiol. **10:** 371.
2. GEVINS, A. S. 1988. Recent advances in neurocognitive pattern analysis. *In* Dynamics of Sensory and Cognitive Processing of the Brain. E. Basar, Ed.: 88-102. Springer-Verlag. Heidelberg.
3. HJORTH, B. 1975. An on-line transformation of EEG scalp potentials into orthogonal source derivations. Electroenceph. Clin. Neurophysiol. **39:** 526-530.
4. HJORTH, B. 1980. Source derivation simplifies topographical EEG interpretation. Am. J. EEG Technol. **20:** 121-132.
5. DOYLE, J. C. & A. S. GEVINS. 1986. Spatial filters for event-related brain potentials. EEG Laboratory, Technical Report TR86-001.
6. BARLOW, J. S. 1986. Artifact processing (rejection and minimization) in EEG data processing. *In* Handbook of Electroencephalography and Clinical Neurophysiology, Vol. 2. F. H. Lopes da Silva, W. Storm van Leeuwen, A. Remond, Eds.: 15-65. Elsevier. Amsterdam.
7. GEVINS, A. S., G. M. ZEITLIN, J. C. DOYLE, C. D. YINGLING, R. E. SCHAFFER, E. CALLAWAY & C. L. YEAGER. 1979. Electroencephalogram correlates of higher cortical functions. Science **203:** 665-668.
8. GEVINS, A. S., G. M. ZEITLIN, C. D. YINGLING, J. C. DOYLE, M. F. DEDON, R. E. SCHAFFER, J. T. ROUMASSET & C. L. YEAGER. 1979. EEG patterns during "cognitive" tasks. I. Methodology and analysis of complex behaviors. Electroencephalogr. Clin. Neurophysiol. **47:** 693-703.
9. GEVINS, A. S., J. C. DOYLE, B. A. CUTILLO, R. F. SCHAFFER, R. L. TANNEHILL, J. H. GHANNAM, V. A. GILCREASE & C. L. YEAGER. 1981. Electrical potentials in human brain during cognition: New method reveals dynamic patterns of correlation. Science **213:** 918-922.
10. GEVINS, A. S. & S. L. BRESSLER. 1988. Functional topography of the human brain. *In* Functional Brain Imaging. G. Pfurtscheller, Ed.: 99-116. Hans Huber Publishers. Bern.
11. GEVINS, A. S., N. H. MORGAN, S. L. BRESSLER, J. C. DOYLE & B. A. CUTILLO. 1986. Improved event-related potential estimation using statistical pattern classification. EEG Clin. Neurophysiol. **6:** 177-186.

12. EFRON, B. 1982. The Jackknife, the Bootstrap, and Other Resampling Plans. Society for Industrial and Applied Mathematics. Philadelphia, PA.
13. GEVINS, A. S. 1987. Statistical pattern recognition. In Handbook of Electroencephalography and Clinical Neurophysiology. Vol 1. A. Gevins & A. Remond, Eds. Elsevier. Amsterdam.
14. GEVINS, A. S. & N. H. MORGAN. 1988. Applications of neural network (NN) signal processing in brain research. IEEE ASSP Trans., 36(7): 1152-1161.
15. GEVINS, A. S. 1980. Pattern recognition of brain electrical potentials. IEEE Trans. Patt. Anal. Mach. Intell. 2(5): 383-404.
16. GEVINS, A. S., N. H. MORGAN, S. L. BRESSLER, B. A. CUTILLO, R. M. WHITE, J. ILLES, D. S. GREER, J. C. DOYLE & G. M. ZEITLIN. 1987. Human neuroelectric patterns predict performance accuracy. Science 235: 580-585.
17. GEVINS, A. S., B. A. CUTILLO, S. L. BRESSLER, N. H. MORGAN, R. M. WHITE, J. ILLES & D. S. GREER. 1989. Event-related covariances during a bimanual visuomotor task. Part I: Methods & analysis of stimulus- and response-locked data. EEG Clin. Neurophysiol. 74(1): 58-75.
18. GEVINS, A. S., B. A. CUTILLO, S. L. BRESSLER, N. H. MORGAN, R. M. WHITE, J. ILLES & D. S. GREER. 1989. Event-related covariances during a bimanual visuomotor task. Part II: Preparation and feedback. EEG Clin. Neurophysiol. 74(2): 147-160.
19. TEUBER, H. L. 1964. In The Frontal Granular Cortex and Behavior. J. Warren & K. Akert, Eds. McGraw-Hill. New York, NY.
20. FUSTER, J. M. 1989. The Prefrontal Cortex: Anatomy, Physiology, and Neuropsychology of the Frontal Lobe. Raven Press. New York, NY.
21. GOLDMAN-RAKIC, P. S. 1988. Topography of cognition: Parallel distributed networks in primate association cortex. Annu. Rev. Neurosci. 11: 137-156.
22. GOLDMAN-RAKIC, P. S. 1988. Changing concepts of cortical connectivity: Parallel distributed cortical networks. In Neurobiology of Neocortex. P. Rakic and W. Singer, Eds.: 177-202. John Wiley. New York, NY.
23. STUSS, D. & D. F. BENSON. 1986. The Frontal Lobes. Raven Press. New York, NY.
24. GEVINS, A. S., S. L. BRESSLER, B. A. CUTILLO, J. ILLES & R. M. FOWLER-WHITE. 1989. Effects of prolonged mental work on functional brain topography. EEG Clin. Neurophysiol. 76: 339-350.
25. GARRETT, M. F. 1982. Production of speech: Observations from normal and pathological use. In Normality and Pathology in Cognitive Functions. A. W. Ellis, Ed., Vol. 9. Academic Press. New York, NY.

Computerized EEG Frequency Analysis and Topographic Brain Mapping in Alzheimer's Disease

CYRUS K. MODY,[a] HUGH B. McINTYRE,
BRUCE L. MILLER, KAREN ALTMAN, AND
STEPHEN READ

Clinical Neurophysiology Laboratory
Department of Neurology
Harbor-UCLA Medical Center
Torrance, California 90509

Dementia, a symptom complex, can be caused by more than 60 disorders.[1] Alzheimer's disease (AD) usually is estimated as causing about 50-60% of the cases and vascular disease about 10-20%; some patients have both disorders.[2-6] In perhaps as many as 5% of cases of dementia the cause remains unknown even after extensive postmortem studies.[7] The probability that a person who lives 85 years or more will develop severe dementia is about 20%.[8]

At present the clinical criteria for the diagnosis of AD, as defined by the National Institute of Neurological and Communicative Disorders and Stroke-Alzheimer's Disease and Related Disorders Association (NINCDS-ADRDA),[9] include an insidious onset and progressive impairment of memory and other cognitive functions. The diagnosis cannot presently be determined by laboratory tests. According to these criteria the diagnosis of probable Alzheimer's disease is supported by "a normal pattern or nonspecific changes in the EEG such as increased slow wave activity that may become more pronounced with progression of the disease."[9]

In this paper we describe findings of computerized EEG frequency analysis (CEEGFA) and topographic brain mapping (TBM) in 50 patients with AD and compare them to 46 normal elderly controls (NECs). The questions we set out to answer are as follows: Can quantitative EEG measure reliably differentiate between patients with AD and NECs? Can CEEGFA and TBM demonstrate dysfunction in regions of the brain where clinical dysfunction is observed in AD? Can the severity of dementia in AD patients as measured by certain validated clinical scales correlate with quantitative EEG measures?

---

[a] Address correspondence to Dr. Cyrus K. Mody, 8631 West Third Street, Suite 440E, Los Angeles, CA 90048.

MATERIALS AND METHODS

The study group included 45 patients with probable AD and 5 patients with definite AD (4 biopsy-proven and 1 autopsy-proven) as defined by NINCDS-ADRDA criteria.[9] The AD patients had a wide spectrum of severity of the disease and their Folstein Mini Mental Status Examination (MMSE)[10] scores ranged from 0 to 26 with a mean of 13.7 and a standard deviation of 8.6. The Clinical Dementia Rating (CDR)[11] in the patients ranged between 1 to 3 with a mean of 2.12 and a standard deviation of 0.75. The normal controls were 46 elderly subjects who had volunteered to participate in the study. They all had a normal general medical and neurological examination as performed by a neurologist. They were normal on neuropsychological testing as performed by a trained neuropsychologist. The neuropsychological test battery consisted of the Wechsler Adult Intelligence Scale-Revised (Satz-Mogel Format),[12] Wechsler Memory Scale,[13] Rey-Osterrieth Complex Figure Test,[14] Wisconsin Card Sort,[15] Stroop Test,[16] Consonant Trigrams,[17] Thurstone Controlled Oral Word Association Test,[18] and the Recognition Memory Test.[19] Also they were free of psychiatric disease as determined by the Structured Clinical Interview for DSM-III-R (SCID).[20] They uniformly scored 30 out of 30 points on the Folstein MMSE, and they all had a CDR of 0. They had a normal CBC, blood chemistry (M-300), and thyroid function tests, and a nonreactive serologic test for syphilis. They all had MRI scans of the brain which were read by a neuroradiologist and neurologist as normal.

All patients and normal subjects had 21 gold disc electrodes placed on the scalp according to the international 10-20 system. EEG data were acquired using both referential linked ears and nose montages utilizing a 20-channel QSI System 9000 instrument. The low-frequency filter was set at 0.5 Hz and the high-frequency filter at 30 Hz. The program is designed to collect 256 points per epoch. At least 3 min of raw EEG were acquired in the awake state with the eyes closed. All efforts were made to insure that the subjects and patients were awake. The EEG was visually analyzed in 2.5-sec epochs by two electroencephalographers, and epochs with any artifact were rejected from further analysis. The artifact-free EEG was then analyzed by fast Fourier transformation (FFT). The definition of the four frequency bands derived from the Fourier analysis is as follows: delta, 0.4-3.6 Hz; theta, 4.0-7.6 Hz; alpha, 8.0-13.6 Hz; beta, 14.0-24 Hz. The numerical data obtained by FFT analysis were analyzed for different trends, and topographic brain maps were constructed using the numerical data. Initial analysis of numerical data obtained by FFT and the topographic brain maps indicated that the most marked differences between the normal and AD groups were seen in the temporo-parieto-occipital (TPO) regions, and that the nose montage was the best montage to demonstrate these changes; thus we further analyzed the data from these areas. The mean delta, theta, alpha, and beta absolute power; the mean % delta, mean % theta, mean % delta + theta, mean % alpha, mean % beta, and mean % alpha + beta from channels T5-Nz, T6-Nz, P3-Nz, P4-Nz, 01-Nz, and 02-Nz were calculated for each AD patient and NEC. The mean peak frequency also was measured for each AD patient and NEC. The mean and standard deviation of each variable for the two groups are then calculated. Statistical analysis was performed using the Mann-Whitney test. Among the AD group the MMSE score and the CDR (which are indicators of the severity of dementia) were correlated, using the Pearson correlation, with all EEG quantitative variables to determine if any of these variables are indicative of the severity of AD.

Visual analysis alone of the raw EEG also was performed by an independent electroencephalographer, who was blinded to the patient's diagnosis, to compare with the computerized quantitative analysis in diagnosis of normality or AD, based on TPO dysfunction or generalized dysfunction plus TPO dysfunction.

RESULTS

A statistically significant difference between the ages of the AD patients and the NECs was found. To be certain that the age of a NEC did not influence any of the quantitative EEG measures, an analysis of variance was performed between age and all other variables, and it was determined that the age of a NEC was not a statistically significant variable. The AD patients and the NECs were comparable for gender (p < 0.35). The other results are presented in TABLE 1 and FIGURES 1-5.

The characteristic CEEGFA and TBM profiles of NECs (FIGS. 1 and 2) were that the predominant activity was in the alpha range and on an average made up 61% of the total activity. The mean % TPO delta + theta activity was on an average 26% and never exceeded 41%. The mean % TPO alpha + beta activity was on the average 74% and never less than 59% (FIG. 3).

The CEEGFAs and TBMs of the group of AD patients (FIGS. 1 and 2) showed that the predominant activity was in the delta range, comprising on the average 51% of the total activity. The mean % TPO delta + theta activity was on the average 79% and was greater than 46% in all but one patient with probable AD. The mean % TPO alpha + beta activity was on the average 20% and was less than 54% in all except in the one patient mentioned above (FIG. 3).

Thus, on CEEGFA and TBM a group of patients with AD differs from a group of NECs in the following manner:

1. In AD there is a loss of the normal predominant alpha activity, and the predominant rhythm is replaced with delta and/or theta activity.
2. In AD the mean % TPO delta + theta activity is usually greater than 46%, whereas it is always less than 41% in NEC.
3. In AD the mean % TPO alpha + beta activity is usually less than 54%, whereas it is always greater than 59% in NEC.

Using the above mentioned criteria, we correctly identified all NECs and all but one patient with probable AD. Thus CEEGFA and TBM have a sensitivity of 98% and a specificity of 100% when EEGs of NECs and AD patients are analyzed.

Independent visual analysis of the raw EEG revealed that all NECs could be correctly identified. Of the patients with AD, one EEG was read as normal and 49 as abnormal. Of the 49 abnormal EEGs, 38 (76%) were interpreted as showing a generalized abnormality, and eight (16%) were interpreted as showing posteriorly predominant dysfunction similar to the CEEGFA (TABLE 2). Thus visual analysis of raw EEG has a sensitivity of 16% and a specificity of 100% when EEGs of NEC and AD patients are analyzed.

The mean peak frequency of the NECs was 9.97 ± 1.07 Hz and that of the AD patients was 3.6 ± 2.7 Hz, the difference between the two groups being highly significant (p < 0.00001) (FIG. 5).

In patients with AD the MMSE score correlated significantly with the mean % alpha power ($r = 0.37$, $p = 0.0074$), the mean % alpha + beta power ($r = 0.34$, $p = 0.015$), the mean delta power ($r = -0.30$, $p = 0.037$), and the mean % delta power ($r = 0.29$, $p = 0.044$), indicating that as the degree of dementia increases, the amount of mean % alpha power and mean % alpha + beta power decreases, and the amount of mean delta power and mean % delta power increases.

In patients with AD the CDR also correlated significantly with the following quantitative EEG measures: mean delta power ($r = 0.37$, $p = 0.0087$), mean % alpha power ($r = -0.34$, $p = 0.0153$), mean % alpha + beta power ($r = -0.30$, $p = 0.0332$), and mean theta power ($r = 0.29$, $p = 0.0415$), which indicates that as the severity of dementia increases, the amount of mean delta and mean theta power increases, and the amount of mean % alpha and mean % alpha + beta power decreases.

DISCUSSION

The most powerful discriminators in distinguishing between the NEC group and the group of AD patients were the mean % alpha + beta power ($t = 21.41$, $p < 0.00001$) and the mean % delta + theta power ($t = 20.46$, $p < 0.00001$). The single measure that was the most powerful discriminator in distinguishing between the two groups was the mean % alpha power ($t = 18.35$, $p < 0.00001$). All the other measures also were highly statistically significant ($p < 0.00001$ for all variables, except for mean beta power where $p < 0.0002$).

Our finding of an increase in the amount of delta power in AD is in agreement with the studies performed by Penttila et al.[21] and Visser et al.[22] Duffy et al.,[23] Berg et al.,[24] and Coben et al.,[25] however, did not observe any increase in the amount of delta activity. This could be due to the fact that Coben et al.[25] and Berg et al.[24] studied power spectra of only occipital to Cz derivations which may have not adequately recorded the electrographic activity over the temporoparietal areas. This is the area where we observed the greatest amount of delta power. Our results also are contrary to those of Duffy et al.,[23] and this may be due to the fact that their patients had very mild disease whereas our patients exhibited a wider range in severity of disease. Another explanation for the difference is that Duffy et al. had a smaller sample, only 19 patients; a larger

FIGURE 1. Topographic brain maps of relative % power (percentage of total power in each frequency band at each electrode). Row D represents % delta; row T, % theta; row A, % alpha; row B, % beta. Column labeled NEC is from a 57-year-old female normal elderly control and demonstrates the predominant % alpha in the TPO regions. The % delta seen in the bifrontal regions is within normal limits and looks prominent on the map because of a small amount of other activity. Column labeled AD is from a 67-year-old female with Alzheimer's disease and demonstrates the predominant % delta in the TPO regions. A small amount of theta is seen in the central region. Column labeled NEC-AD is a map of the difference between the NEC and AD patient. The color scale used is labeled REL, and the lowest activity is color-coded white. As the % power increases the colors go through yellow, orange, red, and maroon.

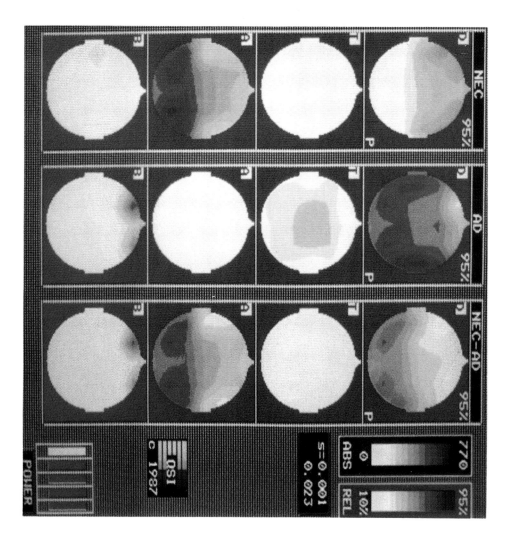

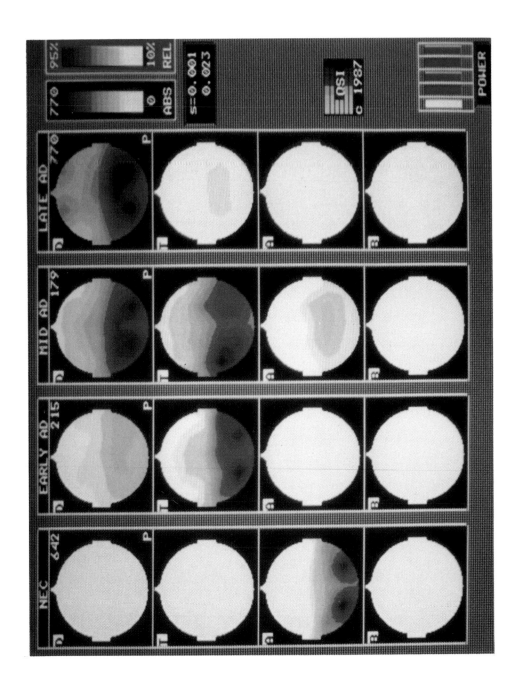

sample may have reached statistical significance. The third explanation is that a linked-ears reference was used which tends to attenuate activity in the TPO regions.

Our study showed a significant increase in the amount of theta activity in AD, measured as mean theta power and mean % theta power. This is in agreement with studies performed by others.[21-25]

In our AD patients the amount of alpha power was significantly decreased. This finding is similar to those of Coben *et al.*[25] and Visser *et al.*[22] However this finding is dissimilar to the findings of Penttila *et al.*,[21] Duffy *et al.*,[23] and Berg *et al.*[24] The fact that Duffy's patients had very early disease may explain this difference because in their stage of the disease they would not have had the time to develop a significant decrease in the amount of alpha activity. As mentioned previously, the problem with the studies performed by Berg *et al.* and Penttila *et al.* is the limitation of measuring power spectra using a single occipital-to-vertex derivation for each hemisphere.

When compared to controls, beta activity was significantly decreased in our patients with AD. This finding is in agreement with observations of Visser *et al.*,[22] Duffy *et al.*,[23] Berg *et al.*,[24] Coben *et al.*,[25] and Brenner *et al.*[26] The mean peak frequency in our AD patients was 3.6 Hz, which was significantly decreased compared to the normal elderly controls. This finding is in agreement with the studies performed by others.[21,22,24,25]

One of the potentially useful findings of this study is that the severity of dementia as measured with the MMSE and CDR correlates with electroencephalographic measures. The quantitative electroencephalographic measures that showed significant negative correlation with the MMSE score were mean delta power and mean % delta power. Those that showed significant positive correlation were mean % alpha power and mean % alpha + beta power. Our findings are in agreement with those of Brenner *et al.*[26] who also observed a significant Pearson correlation ($p < 0.001$) between the MMSE score and delta activity ($r = -0.51$). In our study quantitative EEG measures that showed significant positive correlation with CDR were mean delta power and mean theta power. Those that showed significant negative correlation were mean % alpha power and mean % alpha + beta power. To our knowledge, no investigators have correlated CDR with quantitative EEG measures. However, Berg *et al.*[24] have shown an inability to predict the CDR, 12 months after presentation, using electrographic power spectra derived from the left and right occipital-to-vertex derivations.

FIGURE 2. Topographic brain maps of absolute power measured in μV^2. Row D represents delta power; row T, theta power; row A, alpha power; row B, beta power. Column labeled NEC is from the same 57-year-old female normal elderly control shown in FIGURE 1 and demonstrates the predominant alpha (591 μV^2) in the TPO regions. Column labeled EARLY AD is from a 77-year-old male patient who had an MMSE score of 26 and demonstrates the predominant theta (171 μV^2) and less prominent delta (72 μV^2) in the TPO regions. Column labeled MID AD is from a 83-year-old female with AD of moderate severity who had an MMSE score of 24 and demonstrates an almost equal amount of delta (155 μV^2) and theta (151 μV^2) in the TPO regions. Column labeled LATE AD is from a 67-year-old male who had an MMSE score of 0 and demonstrates the predominant delta (747 μV^2) in the TPO regions. The three AD maps show markedly decreased alpha. The color scale used is labeled ABS, and the lowest activity is color-coded white. As the power increases the colors go through yellow, orange, red, and maroon. The scale maximum for NEC column is 642 μV^2; for EARLY AD, 215 μV^2; for MID AD, 179 μV^2; for LATE AD, 770 μV^2 (the only one labeled on the figure).

TABLE 1. EEG Frequency Analysis in Normal Controls and in Alzheimer's Disease

Group		Mean TPO (μV^2)				Mean %TPO					
		Delta	Theta	Alpha	Beta	Delta	Theta	Delta + Theta	Alpha	Beta	Alpha + Beta
NEC (N = 46)	Mean	34.2	25.1	204.7	35.2	16.3	9.6	25.9	61.1	12.9	74.1
	SD	14.4	21.3	203.1	33.9	6.9	5.4	9.1	12.1	7.3	9.1
	Min	15.2	5.3	33.7	3.2	4.8	2.5	8.2	31.5	3.8	58.8
	Max	95.5	97.3	1089.8	161.7	31.6	25.2	41.2	83.2	42.2	91.8
AD (N = 50)	Mean	228.5	111.9	57.8	17.8	50.7	29.5	79.4	14.9	4.9	19.7
	SD	192.7	80.7	76.9	17.3	18.2	12.6	15.4	12.5	5.0	14.8
	Min	20.5	19.3	8.2	0.5	7.7	11.7	29.0	3.0	0.3	4.3
	Max	849.5	364.0	427.8	75.0	80.0	70.3	96.0	67.0	25.7	71.2
p		< 0.00001	< 0.00001	< 0.00001	< 0.0002	< 0.00001	< 0.00001	< 0.00001	< 0.00001	< 0.00001	< 0.00001

CEEGFA and TBM demonstrate cerebral dysfunction in the temporo-parieto-occipital regions of the brain. These are the same regions where histology has shown higher plaque and tangle counts,[27] PET has shown decreased metabolism,[28] and SPECT has shown decreased blood flow.[29-31]

Some of the quantitative electroencephalographic measures correlate well with the clinical degree of severity of dementia as measured by the MMSE score and CDR. Thus, in the future, when therapeutic modalities become available for the treatment of AD, we may be able to quantitate objectively the improvement or rate of deterioration accompanying the treatment.

Our data indicate that when viewed in the clinical context CEEGFA and TBM can be useful adjuncts to the early and accurate diagnosis of AD and serve as a physiologic expression of the pathologic changes. However, further studies should be performed to validate this new technology of studying brain function. The specificity of the methodology in differentiating AD from other causes of slowly progressive dementia also will have to be studied.

ACKNOWLEDGMENTS

We thank our EEG technologists, Marianne Anderson, Sandy Bays, Myles West-brooks, and Larry Breeding, and our visiting EEG technologist Judy Nechanicky, for performing all the studies. We are also extremely grateful to Ms. Elizabeth Hill for her time and patience spent on the patients. We also thank Quantified Signal Imaging for providing technological help in performing these studies.

REFERENCES

1. HAASE, G. R. 1977. Diseases presenting as dementia. *In* Dementia. 2nd edit. C. E. Wells, Ed.: 27-67. F. A. Davis. Philadelphia, PA.
2. TOMLINSON, B. E., G. BLESSED & M. ROTH. 1970. Observations on the brains of demented old people. J. Neurol. Sci. **11:** 205-242.
3. JELLINGER, K. 1976. Neuropathological agents and dementia: Aspects of dementias resulting from abnormal blood and cerebrospinal fluid dynamics. Acta Neurol. Belg. **76:** 83-102.
4. SOURANDER, P. & H. SJOGREN. 1970. The concept of Alzheimer's disease and its clinical implications. *In* Alzheimer's disease and related conditions. G. E. W. Wolstenholm & M. O'Connor, Eds.: 11:36. Ciba Foundation Symposium. Churchill Livingstone. London.
5. WELLS, C. E. 1977. Diagnostic evaluation and treatment in dementia. *In* Dementia. 2nd edit. C. E. Wells, Ed.: 247-276. F. A. Davis. Philadelphia, PA.
6. SMITH, J. S. & L. G. KILOH. 1981. The investigation of dementia: Results in 200 consecutive admissions. Lancet **1:** 824-827.
7. KATZMAN, R. 1986. Alzheimer's Disease. N. Engl. J. Med. **314:** 964-973.
8. MORTIMER, J. A. 1983. Alzheimer's disease and senile dementia: Prevalence and incidence. *In* Alzheimer's Disease. B. Reisberg, Ed.: 141-148. The Free Press. New York, NY.
9. MCKHANN, G., D. DRACHMAN, M. FOLSTEIN, R. KATZMAN, D. PRICE & E. M. STADLAN. 1984. Clinical diagnosis of Alzheimer's disease: Report of the NINCDS-ADRDA work group under the auspices of Department of Health and Human Services taskforce on Alzheimer's disease. Neurology **34:** 939-944.

10. FOLSTEIN, M., S. FOLSTEIN & P. R. McHUGH. 1975. Mini Mental State: A practical method for grading the cognitive state of patients for the clinician. J. Psychiatr. Res. **12:** 189-198.

11. HUGHES, C. P., L. BERG, W. L. DANZIGER, L. A. COBEN & R. L. MARTIN. 1982. A new clinical scale for the staging of dementia. Br. J. Psychiatry **140:** 566-572.

12. ADAMS, R. L., J. SMIGIELSKI & R. L. JENKINS. 1984. Development of a Satz-Mogel short form of the WAIS-R. J. Consult. Clin. Psych. **52:** 908.

13. WECHSLER, D. A. & C. STONE. 1945. Wechsler Memory Scale. Psychological Corporation. New York, NY.

14. OSTERRIETH, P. A. 1944. Le test de copie d'une figure complexe. Arch. Psychol. **30:** 206-356.

15. BERG, E. A. 1948. A simple objective test for measuring flexibility in thinking. J. Gen. Psychol. **39:** 15-22.

16. STROOP, J. 1935. Studies of interference in serial verbal reactions. J. Exp. Psychol. **18:** 643-661.

17. STUSS, D. T., E. F. KAPLAN, D. F. BENSON, W. S. WEIR, S. CHIULLI & F. S. ARAZIR. 1982. Evidence for the involvement of orbitofrontal cortex in memory functions: An interference effect. J. Comp. Physiol. Psychol. **96:** 913-925.

18. BENTON, A. L., K. HAMSHER, Eds. 1976. Multilingual Aphasia Examination. University of Iowa. Iowa City, IA.

19. WARRINGTON, E. K. 1984. Recognition Memory Test. Nefr-Nelson. Windsor, England.

20. SPITZER, R. L., J. B. W. WILLIAMS & M. GIBBON. 1986. Structured Clinical Interview for DSM-III-R—Patient version (SCID-P, 8/1/86). New York State Psychiatric Institute. New York, NY.

21. PENTTILA, M., J. V. PARTANEN, H. SCININEN & P. J. RIEKKINEN. 1985. Quantitative analysis of occipital EEG in different stages of Alzheimer's disease. Electroencephalogr. Clin. Neurophysiol. **60:** 1-6.

22. VISSER, S. L., W. VAN TILBERG, C. HOOIJER, C. JONKER & W. DE RIJKE. 1985. Visual evoked potentials (VEPs) in senile dementia (Alzheimer type) and in non-organic behavioral disorders in the elderly; comparison with EEG parameters. Electroencephalogr. Clin. Neurophysiol. **60:** 115-121.

23. DUFFY, F. H., M. S. ALBERT & G. McANULTY. 1984. Brain electrical activity in patients with presenile and senile dementia of the Alzheimer type. Ann. Neurol. **16:** 439-448.

24. BERG, L., L. D. WARREN, M. STORANDT, L. COBEN, M. GADO, C. HUGHES, J. KNESEVICH & J. BOTWINICK. 1984. Predictive features in mild senile dementia of the Alzheimer's type. Neurology **34:** 563-569.

25. COBEN, L. A., W. L. DANZIGER & L. BERG. 1983. Frequency analysis of the resting awake EEG in mild senile dementia of the Alzheimer type. Electroencephalogr. Clin. Neurophysiol. **55:** 372-380.

26. BRENNER, R. P., R. F. ULRICH, D. G. SPIKER, R. J. SCLABASSI, C. F. RENOLDS, R. S. MARIN & F. BOLLER. 1986. Computerized EEG spectral analysis in elderly normal, demented and depressed subjects. Electroencephalogr. Clin. Neurophysiol. **64:** 483-492.

27. BRUN, A. & L. GUSTAFSON. 1976. Distribution of cerebral degeneration in Alzheimer's disease. A clinical pathologic study. Arch. Psychiatr. Nervenkr. **223:** 15-33.

28. BENSON, D. F., D. E. KUHL, R. A. HAWKINS, M. E. PHELPS, J. L. CUMMINGS & S. Y. TSAI. 1983. The fluorodeoxyglucose 18-F scan in Alzheimer's disease and multi-infarct dementia. Arch. Neurol. **40:** 711-713.

29. MODY, C. K., I. MENA, B. L. MILLER, H. B. McINTYRE, S. READ, K. GARRETT & M. A. GOLDBERG. 1988. Comparison of topographic brain mapping and EEG frequency analysis with SPECT in Alzheimer's disease. Neurology **38** (Suppl 1): 370.

30. JOHNSON, K. A., S. T. MUELLER, T. M. WALSHE, R. J. ENGLISH & B. L. HOLMAN. 1987. Cerebral perfusion imaging in Alzheimer's disease: Use of single photon computed tomography and iofetamine hydrochloride I-123. Arch. Neurol. **44:** 165-168.

31. JAGUST, W. J., T. F. BUDINGER & B. R. REED. 1987. The diagnosis of dementia with single photon emission computed tomography. Arch. Neurol. **44:** 258-262.

Quantitative Electroencephalography and Anatomoclinical Principles of Aphasia[a]

A Validation Study

TERESE FINITZO,[b,c] KENNETH D. POOL,[b] AND
SANDRA B. CHAPMAN [c]

[b]*Neuroscience Research Center*
Dallas, Texas 75220

[c]*Callier Center*
University of Texas at Dallas
Dallas, Texas 75235

INTRODUCTION

The neuroscience literature has abounded in recent years with descriptions of the effects of brain lesions on human behavior and performance. Consistent association of lesion site(s) with clinical deficits has contributed to the formulation of widely accepted "anatomoclinical principles." Historically, some of the best-recognized principles pertain to language. These principles originated in the mid-nineteenth century with the observations of Broca and Wernicke and were derived from postmortem study of the brain as it related to observed antemortem behavior.

Advances in neuroimaging provide diverse anatomic, metabolic, and electrophysiologic methods to detect and characterize brain lesions antemortem that may lead to the formation of new anatomoclinical principles. Electrophysiology is an alternative to metabolic neuroimaging because it offers an assessment of neuronal activity that preserves the dynamic and temporal nature of the system. However, in recent years, electroencephalography (EEG) and evoked potentials (EPs) have been surpassed in the arena of lesion identification. The reason is not because of the lack of information available from electrophysiology, but rather to the limited capacity of the researcher/clinician to utilize the overwhelming amount of information from purely visual inspection of the data.[1,2] The advent of quantitative electrophysiology offers the promise of effective access to this rich body of information.

It is an understatement to say that quantitative electrophysiology is controversial. One of the most contentious issues is the application of statistical methods to the data.[3-6] Three factors are of particular concern. First, data are, in general, not normally

[a]Supported, in part, by Grant No. NS 18276-06 from the National Institutes of Health.

distributed, precluding the use of many parametric statistical methods. Second, most quantitative electrophysiology studies involve a large number of comparisons requiring correction for multiple measures that may impede detection of "real" differences. Third, many measures are not independent. In fact they are strongly interrelated, although the relations are not well established. These issues have made it difficult to arrive at unequivocal conclusions from quantitative EEG (QEEG) and EP studies.

In spite of such controversies, it has been tempting to use QEEG to examine disorders whose neurologic substrates are not only unknown but may not even exist.[7-11] Theoretically, the intention of such research has been to further our knowledge of the neurophysiology of important clinical disorders. While we are not alone in such noble purposes, it rapidly becomes obvious that the technology's capability to provide "correct" answers must be validated using cases with established anatomoclinical principles.[12-15] Aphasia in stroke is an indisputable choice in order to examine the effectiveness of this new technology.

Thus, our purpose in this paper is to review our QEEG findings in stroke relative to language performance in order to validate this tool for investigation of brain function. We address three issues. First, can a population study using QEEG confirm well-known and accepted anatomoclinical principles? Second, can criteria be developed from QEEG that can predict behavior in an individual with complex and often multifocal lesions? Third, do the prediction criteria used in individual cases conform with the anatomoclinical principles—that is, do the results make sense?

To address the first issue, we review QEEG findings for 100 stroke subjects and relate the results to their language performance. This study is presented in detail in Chapman et al.[12] To address the second and third issues, individual subject data are examined to determine combinations of findings that most accurately classify the subject relative to his behavior. Statistical classification used was classification and regression trees (CART).[16] This method avoids the statistical difficulties referred to above by using a nonparametric approach. CART uses data to form prediction rules for one variable based on the values of other variables. This is done by a systematic analysis of possible rules which provide the most accurate prediction. These optimal rules are in the form of a classification or decision tree. Wong, Bencivenga, and Gregory[17] applied this methodology to EEG data in benign rolandic epilepsy. Bencivenga, Wong, Woo, and Jan[18] applied the approach to visual evoked potential data in cortical visual impairment. They concluded that CART was a valuable tool that could be used in problems involving multiple complex EEG and EP features with unknown distributions and interrelations. Their experience motivated us to evaluate this approach.

METHODS

Subjects

Subjects were 100 consecutive patients with the diagnosis of stroke admitted to the Dallas Rehabilitation Institute. Diagnosis was confirmed by neurologic examination on admission by one of the authors. Patients included 55 males and 45 females, aged 18 to 87 years (x = 57, SD = 14).

This population was heterogeneous as subjects were not selected by lesion site, presence, or type of aphasia. Patients with all combinations of unilateral or bilateral, left or right, and cortical or subcortical involvement were included. Homogeneity was present in terms of severity as all stroke subjects were admitted to a rehabilitation center.

Language Assessments

All subjects had a language assessment by a speech/language pathologist. The assessment included the Boston Diagnostic Aphasia Examination, Boston Naming Test, Reading Comprehension Battery for Aphasia, Selective Reminding Test, and the Token Test. As much of the above battery was administered as the patient's language deficits would allow. Two aphasiologists, blinded to QEEG results, independently and retrospectively reviewed results of the language exams. The subjects were classified as aphasic or non-aphasic, and behavior was rated for fluency and comprehension. The rating scale had four levels: normal, mildly impaired, moderately impaired, and severely impaired.

Quantitative Electroencephalography

Instrumentation. Gold cup electrodes were attached with collodion to each subject to achieve an impedance of less than 3K ohms. Electrodes were placed at Fp1, Fp2, F7, F3, FZ, F4, F8, A1, T3, C3, Cz, C4, T4, A2, T5, P3, Pz, P4, T6, O1, Oz, O2 by the international 10-20 standard with less than 3-mm error center to center. Additional electrodes were placed over the zygoma bilaterally, infraorbitally, and over the nuchal area to assist with artifact detection. The instrument used for quantitative electrocortical analysis was BEAM[*] (Nicolet Instrument Corporation, Madison, WI).

Data Analysis. Digitized EEG signals were saved on magnetic tape. EEG spectral analysis was achieved by fast Fourier transformation (FFT) of 2-sec segments of continuous EEG signals. Segments used for spectral analysis were selected by visual inspection. Careful attention was paid to exclude segments containing activity of noncerebral origin (i.e., eye movements, electrode artifacts, muscle artifact, etc.). Segments for analysis were inspected to insure that the desired arousal/attention state was represented. At least 30 two-sec segments were used in analysis. FFT was performed in 0.5-Hz steps from 0.5 to 32 Hz for each selected 2-sec segment. FFT curves for each of the segments were averaged. In addition to the mean, the standard deviation was calculated for each frequency. Total spectral amplitude (TSA) for all frequencies was also calculated. This value was used to calculate the percentage each frequency step contributes. A computer colorgraphic display of 9,216 pixels (96 $\times$ 96) was created. Values corresponding to electrode sites were represented by color on a rainbow colorscale. The intervening points were created by a 3-point linear interpolation. A complete description of QEEG methods can be found in Pool, Freeman, and Finitzo[8] and Finitzo and Freeman.[7]

Group Comparisons

Three group comparisons of the EEG delta frequency band are presented: (1) aphasic versus non-aphasic stroke subjects, (2) subjects with normal comprehension versus those with a severe comprehension deficit, and (3) subjects with normal fluency versus those with a severe fluency deficit.

Multiple-measure and small-sample corrected t tests were used to determine significant differences between groups. The t test values were selected to achieve $p < 0.01$ for each analysis, taking different sample sizes into account to achieve $p < 0.05$ for the entire study.

Classification and Regression Trees

One hundred and forty-four variables were entered for each subject. These consisted of age decade, presence or absence of aphasia, fluency rating, comprehension rating, and 140 QEEG values. The QEEG values were the absolute amplitude in delta (0.5-3.5 Hz), theta (4.0-7.5 Hz), and alpha (8.0-11.5 Hz) bands and total spectral amplitude (0.5-32.0 Hz), along with the percent of the total spectra (relative) present in the delta, theta, and alpha bands for each of the 20 cerebral recording electrodes.

For all CART runs, the Gini rule for constructing splits, a 1.0-SE rule for pruning, unitary misclassification costs, and a 10-fold cross-validation estimate of classification accuracy were used. For the analysis of aphasia, classification rules were based on the electrophysiologic variables, not the fluency and comprehension variables. Similarly, the aphasia and fluency variables for comprehension analysis and the comprehension and aphasia variables for fluency analysis were excluded. Five surrogate and five competing splitting criteria were reported.

RESULTS

Language Classifications

Forty-six of the 100 stroke subjects were behaviorally classified as aphasic by retrospective review of the language assessments. Thirty-six of the 100 stroke subjects were rated by the aphasiologists as having normal comprehension, 14 as mildly impaired, 17 as moderately impaired, and 33 as severely impaired. Fifty-nine of the 100 subjects were behaviorally rated as fluent, nine as mildly impaired, eight as moderately impaired, and 24 as severely non-fluent.

Group Comparisons

Can a population study using QEEG confirm well-known and accepted anato-moclinical principles?

The findings for all three comparisons were "correct" relative to the brain/language principles. Aphasic stroke subjects differed from non-aphasic stroke subjects, manifesting increased delta amplitude over the left hemisphere. In FIGURE 1, a left lateral view of the delta spectral amplitude for aphasic subjects (N = 46) is compared to non-aphasic stroke subjects (N = 54). The image on the far right is the *t*-test difference between the groups. As shown on the *t*-test map, the maximal delta amplitude difference between these groups is over the left perisylvian cortex.

The region of maximal difference between stroke subjects with severe comprehension deficits and those with normal comprehension was over the left posterior cortex. In FIGURE 2, delta spectral amplitude for subjects with severe comprehension deficits (N = 33) is compared to stroke subjects with normal comprehension (N = 36). While there was a global increase in delta amplitude over the left hemisphere with a severe comprehension deficit, the maximal difference, shown in FIGURE 2, is in left posterior temporoparietal cortex.

Severely non-fluent subjects (N = 24) exhibited a global increase in delta amplitude over left hemisphere when compared to stroke subjects with normal fluency (N = 59). The maximal difference between groups is just anterior to the difference noted for comprehension. As shown in FIGURE 3, this difference is over the left inferior frontal/anterior temporal cortex.

In an attempt to restrict the number of measures for statistical reasons, group analysis was limited to a single EEG frequency band (delta). We also reduced the number of recording electrodes to those overlying the left hemisphere thereby confining the spatial range of our examination. Such restrictions obviously precluded the detection of lesions that affect other frequencies or brain regions. Moreover, while the findings for the population study yield insights into the accuracy of lesion localization using quantitative electrophysiology, clinical utility requires unambiguous and accurate individual case classification. Clearly, one can often demonstrate statistical differences between groups even with substantial population overlap. Thus we are left with the question: Do group findings apply to individual subjects?

Individual Classification Analysis

The second question asked whether QEEG could be used to accurately predict the presence of aphasia and type of language impairment in stroke patients with complex and often multifocal lesions. The results of the CART analyses are shown in FIGURES 4, 5, and 6.

Aphasia

The structure of the optimal classification tree using QEEG is shown in FIGURE 4. The classification tree was 90% accurate in the identification of aphasia from QEEG

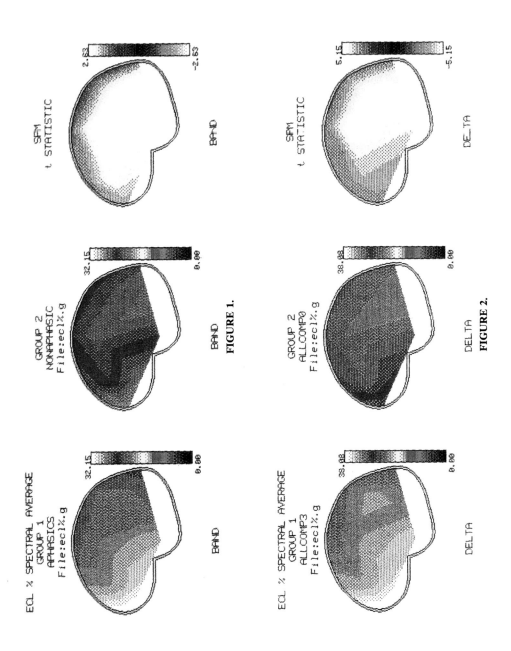

FIGURE 1.

FIGURE 2.

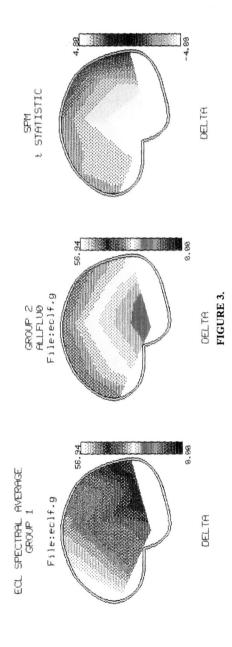

FIGURE 3.

FIGURE 1. Image at left: left lateral view of percent delta for aphasic stroke subjects; center, of non-aphasic stroke subjects. A small sample corrected *t* statistic on the right shows that the aphasic group has higher relative delta over the left perisylvian region of cortex.

FIGURE 2. Image at left shows percent delta for stroke subjects with severe comprehension deficits, compared to those with normal comprehension (*center*). The *t* statistic in right image shows that the region of maximal difference between the two groups is again the left perisylvian cortex, especially posterior temporoparietal.

FIGURE 3. Image at left is delta amplitude for stroke subjects with severe non-fluency compared to those with normal fluency (*center*). The *t* statistic in right image shows that the region of maximal difference between the two groups is in left lateral frontal/anterior temporal cortex.

data. Fifty-one of the 54 non-aphasics were correctly classified (94%), and 39 of the 46 aphasics were correctly classified (85%).

CART methodology established six rules (terminal nodes) for classifying a subject as aphasic.

1. If a subject had elevated relative delta (> 30.3%; normal in our lab, 21.7%) from left parietal area (P3) with preserved alpha (> 12.6%; normal in our lab, 27.9%) from right posterior temporal area (T6), the subject was classified as aphasic. Of 26 subjects meeting this criteria on CART, 25 (96%) were behaviorally classified as aphasic.

2. If there was elevated delta (over 30.3%) from the left parietal area (P3) but reduced alpha (< 12.6%) from the right posterior temporal area (T6), the subject was not predicted to be aphasic. All six subjects who met this criteria (100%) were non-aphasic. If alpha was not preserved over right hemisphere, the relative symmetry between hemispheres was interpreted by CART as evidence that a significant aphasia was not present.

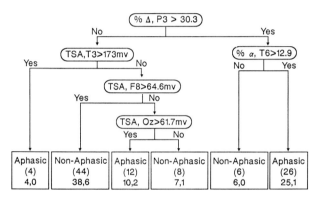

FIGURE 4. The optimal classification tree for predicting the presence of aphasia from QEEG (N = 100). There are five decision nodes, and hence six terminal nodes are shown here. The six terminal nodes represent the final QEEG classifications. The numbers in parentheses are the total number of subjects who were classified in that terminal node. The two numbers below this value are the correct and incorrect classifications respectively. % Δ = percent delta amplitude; TSA = total spectral amplitude; % α = percent alpha amplitude.

3. The next classification criterion was marked elevation of the total spectral amplitude (> 173 mV; normal, 95 mV) from left inferior frontal/anterior temporal cortex (T3). Even if relative delta from P3 was not elevated, if TSA at T3 was high, the subject was classified as aphasic. Four subjects (100%) meeting this criteria were aphasic.

4. If elevated left parietal (P3) relative delta and high left inferior frontal/anterior temporal (T3) TSA were not present, but normal or elevated TSA (> 64.6 mV; normal, 107 mV) from the right lateral frontal area (F8) was found, a subject was classified as non-aphasic. Forty-four subjects met these criteria; 38 were non-aphasic (86%).

5. If the subject was not classified by any of the foregoing rules and did have reduced TSA (< 61.7 mV; normal, 167 mV) at the occipital midline (Oz), the subject was classified as non-aphasic. Of eight subjects meeting these criteria, seven were non-aphasic (88%).

6. The remaining 12 subjects were classified as aphasic by default; ten (83%) were aphasic.

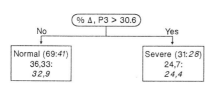

FIGURE 5. The optimal classification tree for predicting comprehension deficits from QEEG has one decision rule and two terminal nodes whether analysis includes all 100 subjects and four levels of comprehension, or 69 subjects and two levels of comprehension deficits. There are two numbers in each parentheses. The first number is the total number of subjects out of 100 who were classified in that node. The second number (in italics) is the total number of subjects in that node from the more limited analysis of two levels of comprehension. The two final pairs are the correct and incorrect classifications for four and two levels of comprehension, respectively.

Comprehension

The classification tree for comprehension is shown in FIGURE 5. Expected chance accuracy with four classes of severity would be 25% for an individual subject. Thirty-two of the 34 subjects (89%) with normal comprehension as defined by the behavioral evaluation were correctly classified by CART. As shown in the figure, the tree has only two terminal nodes and predicts only two levels of severity (normal and severe). The classification by these criteria correctly rated 56 subjects (56%). Since there was no prediction of mild or moderate comprehension deficits, these subjects were all incorrectly classified. All the mild subjects and 14 of the moderate subjects (82%) were classified as normal by CART. Twenty-four of 33 severe subjects (73%) were correctly classified.

The single rule for classifying a subject as having a severe comprehension deficit was elevated relative delta ($> 30.6\%$; normal, 21.7%) from the left parietal area (P3). Without this feature, the subject was classified as having normal comprehension. Twenty-four of 31 subjects (77%) who met this CART criterion were in fact behaviorally rated as severe. Thirty-two of the 69 subjects (46%) classified as normal by CART did demonstrate normal comprehension behaviorally.

That only two severity classes were predicted could be because of two factors. First, since we did not perform the original speech-language assessments, we had to rely on our retrospective review for the behavioral classifications. Second, the severity of language disruption is more likely to be a continuous rather than a discrete variable. In previous group analyses, these concerns prompted limiting comparisons to the two ends of the continuum—the "normal" and severely impaired groups. Differentiation between these two groups was significantly stronger than the intermediate classes of mildly and moderately impaired.

We therefore limited a second examination of the comprehension data to normal and severe classes. The random classification rate now would be 50%. We observed an

FIGURE 6. The optimal classification tree for predicting severe non-fluency from QEEG. There is one decision rule and two terminal nodes. Recall that CART could not identify a rule for predicting all degrees of fluency deficits. This tree was developed using only normal fluency and severe non-fluency ratings. (N = 83).

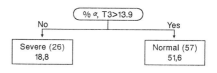

81% accuracy rate from the analysis of the 69 subjects with either normal or severe comprehension. This analysis produced the same tree as described above. Using this reduced data set, 24 of the 28 subjects (86%) classified as severe by CART were behaviorally classified as severe, and 32 of the 41 (78%) classified as normal by CART were behaviorally normal.

Fluency

No classification tree for the analysis of all 100 subjects predicted fluency significantly better than classifying all subjects as normal. This occurred because 59% did have normal fluency. A second analysis restricted to the 83 subjects with either normal fluency or severe non-fluency was performed following the rationale used above. A single rule for classification was determined. If the subject demonstrated reduced relative alpha (< 13.9%; normal, 21.5%) from the left inferior frontal/anterior temporal area (T3), then the subject was classified as severely non-fluent; otherwise the subject was classified as normal. This criterion classified 26 subjects as severely non-fluent, of whom 18 (69%) were behaviorally classified non-fluent, and 57 subjects as normal, of whom 51 (89%) were normal behaviorally. The overall classification accuracy was 83%. This tree is shown in FIGURE 6.

Are the Classification Rules Reasonable?

One of the goals of the CART analysis is not only to determine the tree structure that can best separate subjects, but to do so with the simplest structure possible. The third question asked whether such a structure and the rules that were developed were consistent with the established anatomoclinical principles of stroke and aphasia. In other words, did the rules make sense?

Aphasia

To begin, an elevation in the percent of delta activity at the P3 electrode is highly compatible with the presence of aphasia. Indeed, Metter *et al.* [19] recently proposed that involvement of the left temporoparietal cortex may be the common substrate for all aphasia. Interestingly, the presence of left hemispheric dysfunction is combined with a measure of right hemispheric function (preserved alpha at T6). This ensures that the right hemisphere is relatively "intact" in contrast to the left hemisphere. If this asymmetry is not seen, the relative symmetry (elevated relative delta over the left and reduced relative alpha over the right) is interpreted by CART as evidence that a significant aphasia is not present. The CART rule requiring significant interhemispheric asymmetry is likely specific to stroke. Although subjects with bihemispheric lesions were not excluded, interhemispheric asymmetry is more common in stroke than in other disorders such as dementias or even aneurysms with vasospasm.

In stroke, elevation of total spectral amplitude would not be unexpected; thus, this decision rule based on the TSA at T3 is also reasonable. In contrast, the physiologic basis for elevated right lateral frontal total spectral amplitude is initially less evident than the preceding rules. We interpret this rule as follows. Elevated right lateral frontal TSA may reflect injury from stroke. Evidence of right hemispheric injury without the preceding confirmation of left hemispheric infarction would argue for an isolated right hemispheric infarction. Right hemispheric involvement in isolation would not be consistent with aphasia. If the TSA over F8 is normal without meeting the above criteria of left hemispheric infarction, then the possibility that the infarction is isolated to the subcortex is strengthened.[20] Aphasia is also less likely in this setting. Although other interpretations can be proposed, this one is congruent with our knowledge of aphasia and EEG changes in stroke.

The final rule in aphasia classification used TSA at the Oz electrode and may be interpreted in a manner similar to the preceding one. This rule combined with the absence of the elevated relative delta over P3, absence of elevated TSA at T3, and the presence of a low TSA at F8 is consistent with a low voltage record with no clear evidence of cortical damage in the left hemisphere. The absence of an aphasia in this setting would not be unexpected.

Comprehension

The selection of relative (percent) delta amplitude at P3 as the discriminating feature in identifying comprehension impairments and the proximity of this electrode to Wernicke's area (auditory comprehension) make this an "appropriate" solution. The simplicity of this classification is in contrast to the complexity of the decision rules needed to encompass all of the physiologic subtypes of aphasia. Auditory comprehension, as measured by the instruments routinely used here, is more homogeneous than aphasia. Such greater homogeneity is reflected in the far simpler classification scheme.

Fluency

The selection of relative alpha at T3 as the discriminating feature in identifying fluency impairment is certainly plausible. This one variable may be reduced if there is either a loss of "normal" alpha activity or an increase in "pathologic" delta or theta activity. The selection of relative alpha reflects the CART bias to separate subjects using the simplest structure possible.

The expected region of maximal difference between fluent stroke subjects and those who were severely non-fluent was the left inferior frontal cortex. The F7 electrode most closely overlies this area and could have been expected to be the electrode with the greatest difference.[21] However, the electrode with the greatest between-group difference on the group analysis was also T3. T3 is immediately adjacent to F7 and in our data appears to consistently reflect altered function of the inferior frontal cortex. Finally, this localization is anterior to the localization rule developed for predicting comprehension deficits—another suitable solution.

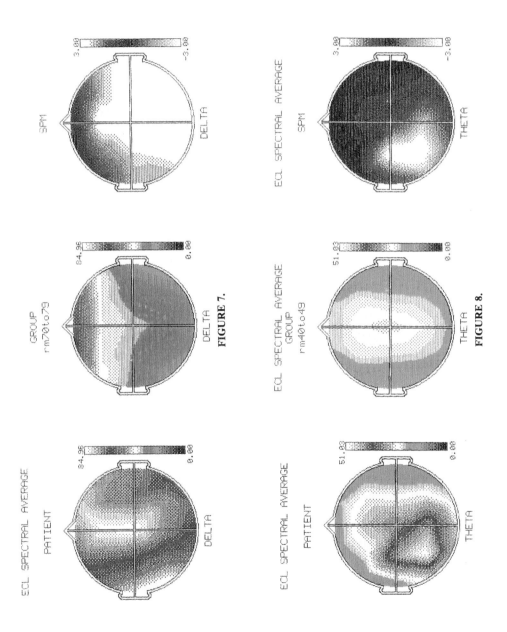

FIGURE 7.

FIGURE 8.

DISCUSSION

Limitations in Study

Several limitations in the current study design need to be acknowledged. First, this was a retrospective study. The specific aphasia instruments were not universally applied and the expertise of the examiners varied. Second, this was an exploratory effort to determine classification criteria to predict language behavior in stroke. As such, it needs to be replicated with the addition of other patient populations to determine the specificity as well as the sensitivity of the approach. Third, we restricted our evaluation to criteria that were dependent only on one variable at a time. The use of linear combinations might improve prediction accuracy, but it would have complicated physiologic interpretation. Since this effort was not intended to develop the best method of prediction, but rather to see if the methods of prediction were consistent with anatomoclinical principles, we chose not to include linear combinations in this analysis. Fourth, we used eyes-closed, resting EEG spectra only. Had we considered EEG spectra in other conditions, the change in EEG spectra between conditions, and evoked potential data, the sensitivity and specificity of these predictions might have been improved. Finally, this study did not examine changing language performance over time, and therefore no conclusions may be drawn regarding prognosis.

Individual Case Misclassification

Aphasia

The decision rules for classifying the presence of aphasia were 90% accurate. Only ten subjects were misclassified by these CART criteria. One subject had a mixed transcortical aphasia. Two others were clinical "surprises" as well as classification errors. One had a right hemispheric infarction and was aphasic (FIG. 7). The other had a left middle cerebral artery infarction but was not aphasic. Both of the two subjects were right-handed. The fourth error case demonstrated focal elevated relative theta, rather than delta, from the P3 electrode (FIG. 8). Two additional subjects were classified

---

FIGURE 7. The behavioral classification for this patient was aphasic. CART classified the patient as non-aphasic. Note the increased delta amplitude in the right posterior quadrant and in left occipital when compared to the age-matched normal controls resident in the system. This subject had suffered a right hemispheric infarction with a left hemiparesis. There was agreement between the speech/language pathologist and the neurologist on the diagnosis of aphasia.

FIGURE 8. The behavioral classification for this subject was aphasic. CART classified the subject as non-aphasic. Note the focal theta at P3 when compared to the age-matched normal controls. CART did not use theta in its decision rules to predict aphasia, although the region of increased theta was the same as that used by CART. Center and right images are abnormal due to increased amplitude in the left parietal central area.

as having normal fluency and comprehension by CART, but were nonetheless classified as aphasic by default on the last decision criterion. Another subject was included in error because he had a ruptured left anterior cerebral artery aneurysm, rather than a stroke. For three subjects, data entry errors occurred regarding the behavioral classification of aphasia. Thus, these last four of the ten errors are easily corrected, which would produce an accuracy of 94% on the aphasia classification.

Comprehension

For the 13 subjects with normal or severely impaired comprehension who were misclassified by CART, six were described above and included the two clinical "surprises," the mixed transcortical aphasic, and the three subjects whose data were miscoded. One subject's stroke was due to rare bilateral occipital infarctions secondary to herniation from idiopathic hydrocephalus. Three subjects were erroneously predicted to have severe comprehension deficits. All three were correctly predicted not to be aphasic. These obviously conflicting predictions would have been avoided had the prediction of aphasia been a criterion of severe comprehension deficit. Thus, as many as six of the 13 errors could be corrected with little modification in the approach.

Fluency

The 14 subjects with normal or severely impaired fluency who were misclassified included the clinical "surprises" and the three subjects with miscoded data. Six of the false positive predictions of severe non-fluency were correctly predicted not to be aphasic, producing conflicts as above. In this case, nine of the 14 errors are easily remedied.

SUMMARY

No single technology in isolation can provide a full view of the anatomoclinical principles evident in the clinical populations we study. The dynamic nature of quantitative electrophysiology makes it an ideal complement to anatomic and metabolic imaging. The statistical conundrum it has presented may be resolved by the approach incorporated in CART. The intent of this study was to examine QEEG and CART in the evaluation of the neurologic bases of a well-defined behavioral disorder like aphasia. The combined power of QEEG and CART yielded objective electrophysiologic methods to predict aphasia that rival the reliability of the language examination. Such success is unprecedented. This success allows us to incorporate QEEG and CART into our technological armamentarium and to return to the evaluation of less well-understood disorders with confidence in both our findings and anatomoclinical principles we derive from them.

ACKNOWLEDGMENTS

We express our appreciation to Dr. Frank Morrison of the Dallas Rehabilitation Institute (DRI) for the referral of the patients and the Speech Pathology Department at DRI for the language evaluations. Laurie Linenberger's contribution as the second aphasiologist was invaluable. Our students, Jackie Clark, Alan Rampy, Susan Rampy, and Beth Wallace, assisted us with manuscript preparation. Reidun Pickett completed EEG data collection and preparation in her usual meticulous way. We are especially indebted to Dr. Peter Wong for his statistical suggestions.

REFERENCES

1. DUFFY, F. H. 1988. Issues facing the clinical use of brain electrical activity mapping. *In* Functional Brain Imaging. G. Pfurtscheller & F. H. Lopes da Silva, Eds.: 149-160. Hans Huber. Stuttgart.

2. FINITZO, T. & K. D. POOL. 1987. Brain electrical activity mapping: A future for audiologists or simply a future conflict? ASHA. June: 21-25.

3. OKEN, B. S. & K. H. CHIAPPA. 1986. Statistical issues concerning computerized analysis of brainwave topography. Ann. Neurol. 19(5): 493-494.

4. DUFFY, F. H., P. H. BARTELS & R. NEFF. 1986. A response to Oken and Chiappa. Ann. Neurol. 19(5): 494-497.

5. WALTER, D. O., P. ETEVENON, B. PIDOUX, D. TORTRAT & S. GUILLOU. 1984. Computerized topo-EEG spectral maps: Difficulties and perspectives. Neuropsychobiology 11: 264-272.

6. FISCH, B. J. & T. A. PEDLEY. 1989. The role of quantitative topographic mapping of 'Neurometrics' in the diagnosis of psychiatric and neurological disorders: The cons. Electroencephalogr. Clin. Neurophysiol. 75: 5-9.

7. FINITZO, T., F. J. FREEMAN & DALLAS CENTER FOR VOCAL MOTOR CONTROL. 1989. Spasmodic dysphonia, whether and where: Results of seven years of research. J. Speech Hearing Res. 32: 541-555.

8. POOL, K., F. J. FREEMAN & T. FINITZO. 1987. Brain electrical activity mapping: Applications to vocal motor control disorders. *In* Speech Motor Dynamics in Stuttering. H. F. M. Peters & W. Hulstijn, Eds.: 151-160. Springer-Verlag. Vienna.

9. DUFFY, F. H., M. B. DENCKLA, P. BARTELS, G. SANDINI & L. KEISSLING. 1980. Dyslexia: Automated diagnosis by computerized classification of brain electrical activity. Ann. Neurol. 7: 421-428.

10. JOHN, E. R., B. Z. KARMEL, W. C. CORNING, P. EASTON, D. BROWN, H. AHN, T. JOHN, T. HARMONY, L. PRICHEP, A. TORO, I. GERSON, F. BARTLETT, R. THATCHER, H. KAYE, P. VALDES & E. SCHWARTZ. 1977. Neurometrics. Science 196: 1393-1410.

11. YINGLING, C. D., D. GALIN, G. FEIN, D. PELTZMAN & L. P. DAVENPORT. 1986. Neurometrics does not detect 'pure' dylexics. Electroencephalogr. Clin. Neurophysiol. 63: 426-430.

12. CHAPMAN, S. B., K. D. POOL, T. FINITZO & C. T. HONG. 1989. Comparison of language profiles and electrocortical dysfunction in aphasia. *In* Clinical Aphasiology. T. Prescott, Ed.: 41-60. College-Hill Press. Boston, MA.

13. POOL, K. D., T. FINITZO, C. T. HONG, J. ROGERS & R. B. PICKETT. 1989. Infarction of the superior temporal gyrus: A description of auditory evoked potential latency and amplitude topology. Ear Hear 10: 144-152.

14. HONG, C. T., K. D. POOL & T. FINITZO. 1988. Topographic, quantitative electrophysiologic patterns in right middle cerebral artery territory infarction (abstract). Ann. Neurol. 24: 1.

15. JONKMAN, E. J., D. C. J. POORTVLIET, M. M. VEERING, A. W. DE WEERD & E. R. JOHN. 1985. The use of neurometrics in the study of patients with cerebral ischaemia. Electroencephalogr. Clin. Neurophysiol. **61:** 333-341.

16. BREIMAN, L., G. H. FRIEDMAN, R. A. OLSHEN & C. J. STONE. 1984. Classification and Regression Trees. Wadsworth Int. Belmont, CA.

17. WONG, P.K.H., R. BENCIVENGA & D. GREGORY. 1988. Statistical classification of spikes in benign rolandic epilepsy. Brain Topogr. **1:** 123-129.

18. BENCIVENGA, R., P. K. H. WONG, S. WOO & J. E. JAN. 1989. Quantitative VEP analysis in children with cortical visual impairment. Brain Topogr. **1(3):** 193-198.

19. METTER, E. J., W. HANSON, C. JACKSON, D. KEMPLER & D. LANCKER. 1989. Temporoparietal cortex: The common substrate for aphasia. *In* Clinical Aphasiology. T. Prescott, Ed. College Hill Press. Boston, MA.

20. MACDONNELL, R. A. L., G. A. DONNAN, P. F. BLADIN, S. F. BERKOVIC & C. H. R. WRIEDT. 1988. The electroencephalogram and acute ischemic stroke: Distinguishing cortical from lacunar infarction. Arch. Neurol. **45:** 520-524.

21. HOMAN, R. W., J. HERMAN & P. PURDY. 1987. Cerebral location of international 10-20 system of electrode placement. Electroencephalogr. Clin. Neurophysiol. **66:** 376-380.

Late Auditory Evoked Potentials in Alcoholics

Identifying Those with a History of Epileptic Seizures during Withdrawal

JACK NEIMAN,[a,b,c] NANCY E. NOLDY,[a,d]

BARBARA EL-NESR,[a] MICHAEL McDONOUGH,[a]

AND PETER L. CARLEN [a]

[a]Addiction Research Foundation
Toronto, Ontario, Canada M5S 2S1

[b]Department of Clinical Alcohol and Drug Addiction Research
Karolinska Institutet
S-104 01 Stockholm, Sweden

INTRODUCTION

Alcohol has frequently been implicated as an etiologic agent for convulsive seizures[1-3] and status epilepticus.[4] Although some alcoholics may develop convulsions while they are still drinking,[5,6] seizures are more common in the 24-48 hours after cessation of alcohol use.[1-3,7,8]

In the past, various electrophysiological techniques have been used to detect changes in the function of the central nervous system (CNS) associated with alcoholism. It has been found that many alcoholics have abnormal electroencephalograms (EEG)[9] with less alpha,[10] but more beta and theta activity.[11] Moreover, some alcoholics occasionally develop convulsive or myoclonic response to photic stimulation.[8]

Chronic alcoholics with only subtle mental impairment may have decreased latencies of some event-related potential components.[12,13] Recently, event-related potential abnormalities in nonalcoholic individuals with a positive family history for alcoholism have been reported.[14,15] Furthermore, changes in latencies and peak amplitudes of several types of evoked potentials (EPs) have been described in alcoholics.[16-18] Interest-

[c]Supported by travel grants from the Swedish Medical Research Council and the Swedish Epilepsy Society.

[d]Address correspondence to Dr. Nancy E. Noldy, Addiction Research Foundation, Neurology Program, 33 Russell Street, Toronto, Canada M5S 2S1.

73

ingly, some investigators have found brainstem auditory EPs particularly impaired in alcoholics with epileptic seizures.[19]

Seizures are probably a physical expression of enhanced neuronal excitability. According to a previous study, the recovery cycle of somatosensory EPs was shortened in alcoholics during experimental alcoholization, and the recovery was most enhanced on the first day of ethanol withdrawal.[20] These findings were interpreted as increased cerebral excitability during and immediately after cessation of alcohol consumption.

The present study was designed to assess whether the changes in the N_1-P_2 component of auditory EPs could be used to detect changes in cerebral function during the detoxification period in chronic alcoholics. Comparisons were made among alcoholics with and without seizure history and healthy, nonalcoholic volunteers.

PATIENTS AND METHODS

The study included 19 alcoholics, 16 male and 3 female, aged 31 to 72 yr (mean, 52 yr). All alcoholics were admitted to a ward specializing in the treatment of alcoholism and drug abuse. The patients had abused alcohol for 2-40 yr (mean, 23 yr). Five of them were binge drinkers. The mean alcohol consumption before admission to the Institute was 3.3 g (range, 1.3-5.5 g) of ethanol per kg of body weight per day. The last drinking period before the admission had lasted from 4 days to several years, with a median of 6 yr. Fourteen subjects used hard liquor, three subjects were beer drinkers, and two others drank wine or fortified wine.

Patients were excluded if they had clinically evident liver disease, mental disease, or a systemic illness that required extensive medication. Also the patients with a history of severe head trauma, stroke, or epileptic seizures other than those attributed to alcohol withdrawal were excluded.

The assessment included physical examination and routine laboratory work-up. Withdrawal symptoms were monitored by recording the Clinical Institute Withdrawal Assessment of Alcohol (CIWA-A) scale.[21] This is a graded rating system which includes 15 common objective and subjective signs and symptoms of ethanol withdrawal.

After admission, the alcoholics were investigated by a neurologist and interviewed, using a specially designed seizure history questionnaire. Five of the alcoholics had a reliable history of withdrawal epilepsy, although none of these patients had a seizure during the withdrawal associated with this study. Their seizures were described by a witness and were characterized by a sudden loss of consciousness, generalized convulsions, urinary or fecal incontinence, laceration of the tongue, and postictal confusion. The seizures had occurred within 24-72 h after the last drink. The total number of seizures varied from 1 to 10, but none of the patients had more than one seizure on any one occasion. None of the alcoholics was taking antiepileptic medication on a regular basis. In addition, available previous medical records, EEG, and computerized tomography (CT-scan) reports were reviewed. None of the patients had focal abnormalities on CT-scan, and all patients with seizures had repeated EEGs without epileptiform abnormalities.

All alcoholics smoked at least 20 cigarettes per day. No changes were made in their smoking habits during the withdrawal period. They were put on a regular hospital diet and received 100 mg of thiamine and various doses of diazepam (range, 15-80 mg), according to the technique described in detail elsewhere.[22] Briefly, during the day of admission, withdrawal symptoms were monitored by the CIWA-A score and the tranquilizer was given until the score did not exceed 10 points. For detoxification of alcoholics with seizure history, diazepam was given according to a schedule for prophylactic treatment of withdrawal epilepsy.[23]

The control group consisted of eight healthy, nonalcoholic volunteers (5 females and 3 males), 29-62 yr of age (mean, 50 yr). The control subjects were occasional drinkers and had abstained from alcoholic beverages at least 5 days before participating in the study. One of them was a current smoker.

All subjects denied taking tranquilizers or illicit drugs, and none of the alcoholics had positive drug screening tests on admission. The subjects were aware of the experimental nature of the study and a written informed consent was obtained from each. Permission for the study was granted by the Addiction Research Foundation Ethics Committee.

Auditory EPs were recorded at 1 and 5 days after cessation of drinking. Electroencephalographic (EEG) activity was recorded from Ag-AgCl electrodes at Fz and Cz. The right mastoid served as reference, and the shoulder as ground. Electro-occular activity was recorded from the supra-orbital ridge of the right eye and the infra-orbital ridge of the left eye. Impedance was less than 10 K ohms on all channels. The high frequency filter was set at 70 Hz and the time constant at 0.3 s. Recording epochs began 167 ms prior to stimulus onset to establish a prestimulus baseline and continued for 333 ms poststimulus. Waveforms were averaged on-line by an IBM-AT-based system which also controlled stimulus presentation, artifact rejection, and scoring of the resulting averaged waveforms. Trials on which EEG exceeded $\pm$ 50 μV were rejected before averaging and were replaced by artifact-free trials. N_1 was defined as the largest negative peak between 75 and 120 ms, and P_2 as the largest positive peak between 150 and 240 ms.

A series of 1000-Hz 70-dB tones of 50 ms duration were presented monaurally through headphones. The interval preceding each tone was either 600, 1600, or 2600 ms in duration. These ISIs (interstimulus intervals) were presented in a random sequence. The first trial of each session was discarded. Two blocks of 32 artifact-free trials were averaged for each ISI to ensure replicability.

All the results are expressed as mean $\pm$ SEM. Differences of the N_1-P_2 voltage and of the latency of N_1 and P_2 within and between the groups of research subjects were calculated using Student's *t* test for paired and unpaired observations. The effect of benzodiazepine treatment was tested with the aid of analysis of covariance (ANCOVA) from a statistical package (SPSS-X).

RESULTS

Eighteen of the 19 alcoholics included in the study exhibited changes in biological markers of alcoholism, i.e., elevation of serum transaminases and mean red cell corpuscular volume. Thrombocytopenia, slight elevation of blood sugar, and small changes in serum electrolytes were also occasionally seen on admission. Only one alcoholic, who had had a short binge prior to admission, had normal laboratory results. There was no difference in these indices between those alcoholics with and without a seizure history.

No difference was found regarding average alcohol intake prior to admission between the patients with generalized seizures (3.3 $\pm$ 0.5 g/kg/day) and those without seizures (3.3 ± 0.3 g/kg/day). The patients with a seizure history were younger (41.8 ± 4.9 yr) than the alcoholics without seizures (56 ± 2.8 yr) (p < 0.05).

One day after the patients stopped drinking, the CIWA-A scores were not significantly different in the alcoholics who had a seizure history (8.3 ± 1.0 points) when compared with the alcoholics without seizures (11.2 ± 0.9 points). A somewhat higher total dose of diazepam was prophylactically given to the patients with a reliable seizure history (56.6 ± 3.4 mg) than to the nonseizure patients (45.8 ± 5.9 mg), but the difference was not statistically significant. Within 5 days, the withdrawal symptoms disappeared and CIWA-A scores were measured at zero in both patient groups.

Consistent with the recovery process of EPs,[24] the amplitude of the N_1-P_2 increased as ISIs were prolonged (FIGS. 1 and 2). The amplitude was almost always significantly (p < 0.05, 0.01, or 0.001) higher at 1600 and 2600 ms when compared with those at 600 ms.

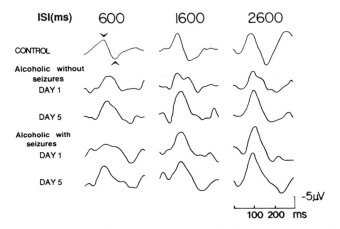

FIGURE 1. Representative waveforms of N_1-P_2 in a nonalcoholic control subject, in a patient without history of withdrawal seizures, and in a patient with history of withdrawal seizures, as indicated. The arrows indicate the peaks of N_1 and P_2, respectively. Notice the increase of the N_1-P_2 amplitude as ISI is prolonged and augmented amplitudes at Day 5 compared to Day 1.

N_1 and P_2 peak latencies were slightly but consistently delayed for the alcoholics compared to controls. This effect was statistically significant for P_2 at 1600 ms ISI on Day 1 (TABLE 1). There was no clear-cut difference between the alcoholics with and without seizure history. By Day 5 of withdrawal, the latencies frequently shortened from the initial values in both patient groups. Occasionally the change was statistically significant and reached the range of values of the control subjects.

One day after alcohol withdrawal, the N_1-P_2 amplitude was significantly reduced in the alcoholics, compared to controls. However, N_1-P_2 amplitude was significantly enhanced in alcoholics with a seizure history compared to alcoholics without seizures (FIG. 2).

Five days after their last drink when withdrawal symptoms had subsided, the N_1-P_2 amplitude of the alcoholic patient groups always increased from the admission values, and the differences were significant across several ISIs. By that time, the alcoholics with a reliable withdrawal seizure history had significantly higher amplitudes

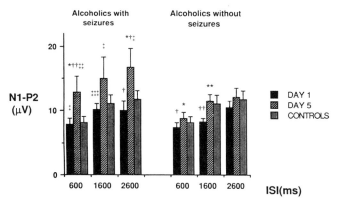

FIGURE 2. Mean ± SEM of N_1-P_2 amplitude in 19 alcoholics, 6 of whom had a history of withdrawal seizures. Eight healthy nonalcoholic volunteers were used as controls. Key to symbols: * $p < 0.05$ and ** $p < 0.01$ indicate differences within the patient groups comparing Day 1 with Day 5. † $p < p\ 0.05$ and †† $p < 0.01$ indicate differences between nonalcoholic controls and the patient groups. ‡ $p < 0.05$, ‡‡ $p < 0.01$, and ‡‡‡ $p < 0.001$ indicate differences between the alcoholics with and without seizure history.

at all ISIs than did the alcoholics without seizures and also exceeded those of control subjects at the 600 and 2600 ms ISIs. Although the recovery function of the N_1-P_2 amplitude varied between recording occasions and groups of research subjects, the increase of N_1-P_2 amplitude occurred across all ISIs, study groups, and recording occasions, yielding no appreciable difference in the recovery function of EPs between subject groups.

TABLE 1. Latencies of N_1 and P_2 in Alcoholics during Withdrawal and in Nonalcoholic Volunteers[a]

| | Alcoholic Patients | | | | |
| | With Seizures | | Without Seizures | | |
ISI	Day 1	Day 5	Day 1	Day 5	Controls
N_1					
600 ms	102.0 ± 3.0	93.7 ± 4.0	104.6 ± 3.8	99.6 ± 2.8	98.9 ± 3.4
1600 ms	102.5 ± 3.4	99.2 ± 2.9	101.5 ± 3.0	99.2 ± 2.9	95.0 ± 2.1
2600 ms	94.5 ± 5.7	95.0 ± 2.2	103.5 ± 2.7	99.5 ± 3.0	96.3 ± 4.0
P_2					
600 ms	194.7 ± 16.8	207.0 ± 8.5	209.0 ± 4.9	208.6 ± 4.7	201.4 ± 7.0
1600 ms	215.7 ± 5.0†	201.7 ± 4.6*	202.5 ± 4.2	205.2 ± 5.4	190.0 ± 6.5
2600 ms	217.2 ± 5.0	216.2 ± 5.4	207.2 ± 5.8	200.8 ± 6.2	195.0 ± 7.1

[a] Values are mean ± SEM of 19 alcoholics, 6 of whom had a history of withdrawal seizures. Eight nonalcoholic subjects were used as controls. * $p < 0.05$ indicates differences within each patient group, i.e., alcoholics with or without seizure history comparing Day 1 with Day 5. † $p < 0.05$ indicates differences between nonalcoholic controls and each patient group.

DISCUSSION

In the present study, the recording of late auditory EPs was employed to monitor alcohol withdrawal in alcoholics. In this method, the amplitude and latency of the N_1-P_2 complex to tones presented randomly at three different ISIs were investigated. Our previous experiments have shown that the method has a low intra-individual variability, is less time-consuming and less invasive than somatosensory stimulation,[39] and is safer than visual EPs in alcoholics who might have a low seizure threshold.[8]

Our results indicate that one day after alcohol withdrawal the N_1-P_2 amplitude is reduced in alcoholics, compared to control subjects. At the same time, alcoholics with a seizure history had higher N_1-P_2 amplitude compared to those without seizures. These results are in agreement with some earlier studies showing that N_1-P_2 has generally lower amplitude in human volunteers on the first day of alcohol withdrawal than in controls.[25] Depression of visual EPs has also been observed in experimental animals during alcohol withdrawal by some investigators,[26] but not by others.[27] According to a previous study, the recovery cycle of somatosensory EPs reached a peak on the first day of withdrawal after 5 days of experimental alcoholization of sober alcoholics.[20] It is possible that the different patient population, the long period of alcohol abuse in our patients prior to withdrawal, and the use of different (auditory) stimulation in our study may account for different results.

How late auditory EPs behave after a detoxification period when the clinical symptoms of withdrawal have subsided has not been previously investigated. In our study, the amplitude of N_1-P_2 always increased from the admission values. After 5 days of abstinence, the alcoholics with withdrawal seizures had significantly higher amplitudes than the alcoholics without seizures or the nonalcoholic volunteers. Excitatory abnormalities in the CNS tend to increase the size of EP components.[28] Consequently, our findings might suggest that the excitability of the brain is increased in alcoholics, particularly in those with a previous seizure history.

The latencies of N_1 and P_2, which were generally slightly prolonged for our patients, shortened within the detoxification period and almost attained the values of the controls, presumably indicating a partial recovery of neuronal transmission. These results agree with previous data from animal experiments, showing that the visual EP latencies rapidly recover after alcohol withdrawal.[26] Interestingly, in the same study the EP voltages remained elevated at least 7 days after alcohol withdrawal, whereafter they started to decline.

The duration of the changes in the EP amplitudes, following alcohol withdrawal in alcoholics, is not entirely known. Four of our patients, two of them belonging to the seizure group, were reinvestigated 10-21 days after discontinuance of alcohol intake. By that time, the N_1-P_2 amplitude had increased by 23-41% from the previous recording (recorded 5 days postwithdrawal), suggesting a continuous enhancement of cerebral excitability. No appreciable difference was observed between the patients with and without seizure history. These findings support some previous reports, suggesting that the state of CNS hyperexcitability may persist long after removal of alcohol in human subjects[29] and experimental animals.[30] However, the relationship between enhanced cerebral activity, measured as increased voltage of N_1-P_2, and epileptic seizures may not be straightforward. Convulsive seizures commonly occur during the 24-48 h after cessation of drinking.[1-3,7,8] During that period the voltage of N_1-P_2 was low in our patients. Moreover, none of our patients with a history of epileptic seizures developed convulsions, in spite of increased N_1-P_2 voltage by the end of detoxification.

It cannot entirely be excluded that changes in EP voltages were influenced, at least in part, by benzodiazepines, which were used for detoxification purposes. However, it may not be considered ethical to investigate patients with serious withdrawal symptoms without offering them drug therapy. Withdrawal from benzodiazepines after long-term high-dose use is associated, in some cases, with convulsions.[31] However, no significant changes in the latency or amplitude of several types of EPs were seen after intravenous administration of moderate doses of diazepam.[32] Our previous experiments on healthy volunteers suggest that the administration of benzodiazepines may reduce N_1-P_2 voltage, but the amplitude returns to the pretreatment level within 2 days without overshoot.[39] Moreover, in our current study, no significant effect of diazepam on N_1-P_2 voltage was seen when the dose of the drug was used as a covariate in the statistical calculations. It is therefore unlikely that the tranquilizer had a major effect on the increased amplitude of N_1-P_2 in our patients.

Cerebral processes underlying the generation of the N_1-P_2 wave of auditory EPs have recently been reviewed elsewhere,[33] but the neuronal mechanisms whereby the EP voltage is increased in alcoholics with a seizure history during withdrawal are not yet understood. The effects of ethanol and its withdrawal are manifold and probably specific for particular brain regions. Moreover, the extent of the changes caused by the substance may vary among different individuals. Ethanol withdrawal may alter noradrenergic,[34] cholinergic,[35] dopaminergic,[36] and GABA-mediated neurotransmission[37] in alcoholics. Several of these factors may be determinants of withdrawal symptoms and/or be involved in generation of enhanced CNS activity, either by interfering with inhibitory mechanisms through direct excitatory action on the cerebrum or by boosting arousal mechanisms. Interestingly, ethanol withdrawal in brain slices has been shown to cause hyperexcitable neuronal activity from drug-naive or ethanol-fed animals, along with reduced inhibitory postsynaptic potentials and postspike train afterhyperpolarizations.[38]

SUMMARY

The N_1-P_2 wave of the auditory evoked potential was studied in 19 alcoholics, six of whom had withdrawal seizures on previous admissions. The recordings were made at 1 and 5 days after cessation of drinking. Eight nonalcoholic volunteers were used as controls. The latencies of N_1 and P_2 were slightly prolonged in alcoholics, but during the detoxification period they frequently shortened ($p < 0.05$), occasionally attaining the values of the controls. One day after withdrawal, the amplitude of N_1-P_2 was consistently reduced in the alcoholics compared to the controls ($p < 0.05$ and $p < 0.01$), but higher in alcoholics with a seizure history compared to alcoholics without seizures ($p < 0.05$ and $p < 0.001$). Five days after cessation of drinking, the amplitude in the alcoholic groups always increased from the admission values ($p < 0.05$ and $p < 0.01$). By that time, the alcoholics with a history of withdrawal seizures had significantly ($p < 0.05$ and $p < 0.01$) higher amplitudes than those of the controls or the alcoholics without seizures. Large N_1-P_2 amplitude during alcohol withdrawal may reflect increased cerebral excitability and contribute to the identification of alcoholics with high risk for withdrawal seizures.

ACKNOWLEDGMENTS

The authors are grateful to Dr. Howard Kaplan for excellent technical assistance, to the nurses of the Clinical Institute for research assistance, to Dr. Wen-Jenn Sheu for help with statistical calculations, and to Mrs. Yvonne Bedford for typing the manuscript.

REFERENCES

1. VICTOR, M. & R. D. ADAMS. 1953. The effect of alcohol on the nervous system. Res. Publ. Assoc. Res. Nerv. Ment. Dis. 32: 526-573.
2. EARNEST, M. P. & P. R. YARNELL. 1967. Seizure admission to a city hospital: The role of alcohol. Epilepsia 17: 387-393.
3. HILLBOM, M. E. 1980. Occurrence of cerebral seizures provoked by alcohol abuse. Epilepsia 21: 459-466.
4. PILKE, A., M. PARTANEN & J. KOVANEN. 1984. Status epilepticus and alcohol abuse: An analysis of 82 status epilepticus admissions. Acta Neurol. Scand. 70: 443-450.
5. DEVETAG, F. G., G. ZAIOTTI & G. G. TOFFLO. 1983. Alcoholic epilepsy: Review of a series and proposed classification and ethiopathogenesis. Ital. J. Neurol. Sci. 3: 275-284.
6. NG, S. K. C., W. A. HAUSER, J. C. M. BRUST & M. SUSSER. 1988. Alcohol consumption and withdrawal in new-onset seizures. N. Engl. J. Med. 319: 666-673.
7. ISBELL, H., H. F. FRAZER, A. WIKLER, R. E. BELLEVILLE & A. J. EISENMAN. 1955. An experimental study of the etiology of "rum-fits" and delirium tremens. Q. J. Stud. Alcohol 16: 1-33.
8. VICTOR, M. & C. BRAUSCH. 1967. The role of abstinence in the genesis of alcoholic epilepsy. Epilepsia 8: 1-20.
9. JOHANNESSON, G., M. J. BERGLUND & D. H. INGVAR. 1982. EEG abnormalities in chronic alcoholism related to age. Acta Psychiatr. Scand. 65: 148-157.
10. GERSON, I. M. & S. KARABELL. 1979. The use of electroencephalogram in patients admitted for alcohol abuse and seizures. Clin. Electroencephalogr. 10: 40-49.
11. PROPPING, P., J. KRÜGER & N. MARK. 1981. Genetic disposition of alcoholism: An EEG study in alcoholics and their relatives. Hum. Genet. 59: 51-59.
12. PORJESZ, B., H. BEGLEITER, B. BIHARI & B. KISSIN. 1987. The N_2 component of the event-related potential in abstinent alcoholics. Electroencephalogr. Clin. Neurophysiol. 66: 121-131.
13. EMMERSON, R. Y., R. E. DUSTMAN, D. E. SHEARER & H. M. CHAMBERLIN. 1987. EEG, visual and event related potentials in young abstinent alcoholics. Alcohol 4: 241-248.
14. BEGLEITER, H., B. PORJESZ, B. BIHARI & B. KISSIN. 1984. Event-related potentials in children with high risk for alcoholism. Science 225: 1493-1496.
15. BEGLEITER, H., B. PORJESZ, R. RAWLINGS & M. ECKARDT. 1987. Auditory recovery function and P_3 in boys with a high risk for alcoholism. Alcohol 4: 315-321.
16. ROSENHAMER, H. J. & B. SILVERSKIÖLD. 1980. Slow tremor and delayed brainstem auditory evoked responses in alcoholics. Arch. Neurol. 37: 293-296.
17. SPITZER, J. B. & C. W. NEWMAN. 1987. Brainstem auditory evoked potentials in newly detoxified alcoholics. J. Stud. Alcohol 48: 9-13.
18. LEVY, L. J. & M. S. LOSOWSKY. 1987. Visual evoked potentials and alcohol-induced brain damage. Alcohol Alcohol. 22: 355-357.
19. TOUCHON, J., G. RONDOUIN, C. DE LUSTRAC, M. BILLIARD, M. BALDI-MOULINER & J. CADILHAC. 1984. Potentiels evoques auditifs du tronc cerebral dans l'epilepsie ethylique. Rev. EEG Neurophysiol. 14: 133-137.
20. BEGLEITER, H., B. PORJESZ & C. YERRE-GRUBSTEIN. 1974. Excitability cycle of somatosensory evoked potentials during experimental alcoholization and withdrawal. Psychopharmacologica 37: 15-21.
21. SHAW, J. M., G. S. KOLESAR, E. M. SELLERS, H. KAPLAN & P. SANDOR. 1981. Development of optimal treatment tactics for alcohol withdrawal: I. Assessment of effectiveness of supportive care. J. Clin. Psychopharmacol. 1: 382-389.
22. SELLERS, E. M., C. A. NARANJO, M. HARRISON, P. DEVENYI, C. ROACH & K. SYKORA. 1983. Diazepam loading: Simplified treatment of alcohol withdrawal. Clin. Pharmacol. Ther. 34: 822-826.

23. DEVENYI, P. & M. L. HARRISON. 1985. Prevention of alcohol withdrawal seizures with oral diazepam loading. Can. Med. Assoc. J. **134:** 798-800.
24. DAVIS, H., T. MAST, N. YOSHIE & S. ZERLIN. 1966. The slow response of the human cortex to auditory stimuli. Recovery process. Electroencephalogr. Clin. Neurophysiol. **21:** 105-113.
25. JÄRVILEHTO, T., M. L. LAAKSO & V. VIRSU. 1975. Human auditory evoked responses during hangover. Psychopharmacologica **42:** 173-177.
26. BIERLEY, R. A., D. S. CANNON, C. K. WEHL & R. E. DUSTMAN. 1980. Effects of alcohol on visual evoked responses in rats during addiction and withdrawal. Pharmacol. Biochem. Behav. **12:** 909-915.
27. BEGLEITER, H. & M. COLTERA. 1975. Evoked potential changes during ethanol withdrawal in rats. Am. J. Drug Alcohol Abuse **2:** 263-268.
28. PICTON, T. W. & R. F. HINK. 1984. Evoked potentials: How? what? and why? J. Electrophysiol. Technol. **10:** 5-43.
29. BEGLEITER, H. & B. PORJESZ. 1979. Persistence of "subacute withdrawal syndrome" following chronic ethanol intake. Drug Alcohol Depend. **4:** 353-357.
30. BEGLEITER, H., B. PORJESZ & R. YOUDIN. 1978. Protracted brain hyperexcitability after withdrawal from ethanol in rats. Alcohol. Clin. Exp. Res. **2:** 192.
31. OWEN, R. T. & P. TYRER. 1983. Benzodiazepine dependence. A review of evidence. Drugs **25:** 387-389.
32. LOUGHAN, B. L., P. S. SEBEL, D. THOMAS, C. F. RUTHERFORD & H. ROGERS. 1987. Evoked potentials following diazepam and fentanyl. Anaesthesia **42:** 195-198.
33. NÄÄTÄNEN, R. & T. PICTON. 1987. The N$_1$ wave of the human electric and magnetic response to sound: A review and an analysis of the component structure. Psychophysiology **24:** 375-425.
34. BORG, S., A. CZARNECKA, H. KVANDE, D. MOSSBERG & G. SEDVALL. 1983. Clinical conditions and concentration of MOPEG in the cerebrospinal fluid and urine in male alcoholics during withdrawal. Alcohol. Clin. Exp. Res. **7:** 411-415.
35. NORDBERG, A., C. LARSSON & E. PERDAHL. 1983. Changes in cholinergic activity in human hippocampus following chronic alcohol abuse. Pharmacol. Biochem. Behav. **18**(Suppl 1): 397-400.
36. ROOS, B. E. & B. P. SILVERSKIÖLD. 1973. Homovanillic acid in cerebrospinal fluid in alcoholics. N. Engl. J. Med. **288:** 1358-1359.
37. GOLDMAN, C. D., L. VOLICER, B. I. GOLD & R. H. ROTH. 1981. Cerebrospinal fluid GABA and cyclic nucleotides in alcoholics with and without seizures. Alcohol. Clin. Exp. Res. **5:** 431-434.
38. CARLEN, P. L., I. ROUGIER-NAQUET & J. N. REYNOLDS. 1990. Alterations of neuronal calcium and potassium ionic currents during alcohol administration and withdrawal. *In* Alcohol and Seizures: Basic Mechanisms and Clinical Concepts. R. J. Porter, R. H. Mattson & I. Diamond, Eds.: 68-78. F. A. Davis Co. Philadelphia, PA.
39. NOLDY, N. E., J. NEIMAN, B. EL-NESR & P. L. CARLEN. 1990. Late auditory evoked potentials: A method for monitoring drug effects on the central nervous system. Neuropsychobiology **23:** 48-52.

Comprehensive Predictions of Outcome in Closed Head-Injured Patients

The Development of Prognostic Equations

R. W. THATCHER,[a,b,c] D. S. CANTOR,[a,c]
R. McALASTER,[c] F. GEISLER,[c] AND P. KRAUSE[c]

[a] Applied Neuroscience Research Institute
University of Maryland Eastern Shore
Princess Anne, Maryland

[c] Applied Neuroscience Laboratory
Maryland Institute for Emergency Medical Services Systems
Baltimore, Maryland

INTRODUCTION

Accurate prognostic evaluation of patients with severe head injury is of importance for acute patient management, the establishment of appropriate long-term treatment and rehabilitation, as well as in family counseling. It is critical to obtain diagnostic and prognostic information as soon as possible after injury in order to optimize therapeutic approaches.[1,2] There are two major categories of prognostic information that are needed: (1) acute prognostics for the immediate physical/physiological evaluation and (2) long-term prognostics for the purposes of physical and/or occupational rehabilitation and family counseling. Obtaining the information has been attempted using single measures[3-11] such as the CT-scan,[12,13] EEG,[14-17] or evoked potentials.[18-21] Other studies have utilized a multimodal approach to acute prognostic evaluation by combining diverse measures such as some of the indicants listed above.[22-25] An emphasis on comprehensive or multimodal evaluations has recently arisen because it has been shown that combined measures are more reliable and accurate than any single measure alone.[25] These latter studies have focused primarily on acute prognostic indices that help determine the probability of survival and gross morbidity. In contrast, very few comprehensive or multimodal studies have been conducted to establish long-term prognostic indices, for example, at one year following injury.[25]

Most prognostic studies of patients with head trauma have concentrated on the ability to predict membership in diagnostic categories of the Glasgow Coma Score

[b] Address correspondence to Dr. Robert W. Thatcher, 193 Inverness Avenue, Severna Park, MD 21146.

(GCS)[3,26] or a variation of it which lumps the entire spectrum of outcome into two-to-four outcome categories such as complete recovery versus death or vegetative state, etc. In contrast, few studies have utilized multiple regression statistical procedures to predict the quality of function in patients whose outcome is intermediate between complete recovery versus death or disability.[27] The latter is important because an increasing proportion of trauma victims survive, and thereby exhibit survival instead of death. Accordingly, a multimodal prognostic index for a wide range of disability needs to be developed. For these reasons the purpose of the present paper is twofold: (1) to compare the ability of single and multimodal measures obtained shortly after injury to predict outcome at one year following injury, and (2) to begin the development of a heuristic regression equation capable of accurately predicting a wide range of outcome measures. The first step toward this goal will involve the evaluation of two different prognostic prediction techniques in two different categories of patients: (1) in patients in the two extremes of complete recovery versus death and (2) in patients in the intermediate range between the extremes of complete recovery and/or death.

METHODS

Patient Population

A total of 162 patients were included in the study. All of the patients were admitted to the Neurotrauma Service of the Maryland Institute for Emergency Medical Services Systems (MIEMSS). Patients with gunshot wounds to the head or primary anoxia brain injury or who fulfilled the criteria of brain death were not included in the study. All of the patients had initial care by emergency medical system paramedics at the scene of the accident and transportation to MIEMSS within 24 hours. Although the majority of patients arrived directly from the scene of the accident by helicopter, some were stabilized at a local facility before transfer to MIEMSS several hours after the accident. Of the 162 patients 60% were motor-vehicle accident victims, another 10% were pedestrians, and the remainder were victims of industrial or home accidents, or violent crime. All of the patients were diagnosed as having a closed head injury.

Patient Management

Approximately 70% of the patients arrived at the Shock Trauma Center by helicopter. The patient was met at the MIEMSS heliport by an anesthesiologist, general surgeon, and specially trained admitting nurses. Acute respiratory insufficiency was treated with intubation and manual ventilation on the heliport prior to transporting the patients. Patients with a GCS less than or equal to eight received an endotracheal tube and mechanical ventilation after a neurologic evaluation or earlier if required by ventilatory status. If the patient required specific central nervous system studies, such as a CT-scan or angiogram, then these were performed after initial protocol admission workup, which included cervical spine and chest X-rays. Patients were not transferred for CT-scan of the head until cardiopulmonary stability had been obtained in the admitting area. A carotid stick angiogram was performed occasionally in the resuscitation area when the patient was not transferable because of cardiopulmonary instability.

Patients with a GCS less than or equal to eight had a subarachnoid bolt or intraventricular catheter inserted to monitor the intracranial pressure; approximately 31% in this study had initial intercranial monitoring. If a patient was spastic or restless on a ventilator, sedation was used to calm him. Narcotics were used as the principal sedatives during the initial respiratory management phase of medical care because their action can be reversed for neurologic and clinical evaluation.

The first computerized EEG and evoked potential tests were obtained at the patient's bed in one of the intensive care units or subacute step-down units at MIEMSS depending on the patient's status. Electrophysiologic testing occurred within 1 to 21 days following injury (mean, 7.5 days; SD, 7.6 days).

CT-scan Measures

The CT-scan data for each patient was collected using a modified version of the Traumatic Coma Data Bank (version 2).[11] According to this scheme, lesions were classified by location as extracerebral or intracerebral. Extracerebral lesions were further classified as right, left, midline, or posterior fossa (left or right). Intracerebral lesions were placed in subcategories by region as frontal, temporal, central, parietal, occipital, cerebellum, basal ganglia (all the above noted as left or right hemisphere), and brainstem. Extracerebral and intracerebral lesions were classified as 0 (none), 1 (low density), 2 (isodense), 3 (high density), 4 (mixed density [mottled]), 5 (distinct high and low areas), or 6 (not visible or unknown). All lesions were rated by approximate size in millimeters.

In addition, data were collected on the presence or absence of bone lesion, intraventricular blood, diffuse brain atrophy, intracranial air, and subarachnoid hemorrhage. The ventricular system was rated according to a scale of 0 (normal), 1 (enlarged), 2 (small), and 3 (absent). The ventricular system was also rated as either 0 (symmetric) or 1 (asymmetric). Midline structures were rated as 0 (normal), 1 (< 5), 2 (5-10), or 3 (> 15). Brainstem cisterns were rated as 0 (absent), 1 (present), or 2 (compressed). Posterior fossa were rated as 0 (normal), 1 (left-to-right infratentorial shift), or 2 (right-to-left infratentorial shift). Missing or unknown data for the above categories were classified as 9. In addition to the above information, lesions were classified as subdural, epidural, or neither.

Several CT-scans were read by the trauma surgeons for each patient. The CT-scan which correlated most closely with the date of the electrophysiologic test was used for the analysis. TABLE 1 shows the number of patients in the various categories of CT-scan classification.

Electroencephalographic Measures

Silver disk electrodes (Grass Instrument Co., Quincy, MA) were applied to the 19 scalp sites of the international 10/20 system.[28] A transorbital eye channel (electrooculogram [EOG]) was used to measure eye movements, and all scalp recordings were referenced to linked ear lobes. Impedance measures for all channels were generally less than 5,000 ohms. Amplifier bandwidths were normally 0.5-30.0 Hz, the outputs being 3 dB down at these frequencies. The EEG activity was digitized on-line by a PDP 11/03 data acquisition system. An on-line artifact rejection routine was used which excluded segments of EEG if the voltage in any channel exceeded a preset limit determined at the beginning of each session to be typical of the subject's resting EEG and EOG.

One minute of artifact-free EEG was obtained at a digitization rate of 100.0 Hz. The EEG segments were analyzed off-line by a PDP 11/70 computer and plotted by a Versatec printer/plotter. Each subject's EEG was then visually examined and edited to eliminate any artifacts that may have passed through the on-line artifact rejection process.

A second-order recursive digital filter analysis was used to compute the auto- and cross-spectral power density[29] for each channel. This procedure is essentially identical to the fast Fourier transform (FFT) method of computing power spectral density. The advantage of using the recursive digital filter when a limited number of bands are analyzed is increased computational efficiency and a simpler design, since the recursive filters provide a natural form of windowing and leakage suppression. The procedure involved using a first-difference, prewhitening filter and a two-stage (four-pole) Butterworth band-pass filter.[29] Frequency bands, including the center frequencies and one half of power B values were as follows: delta (0.5-3.5 Hz; fc = 2.0 Hz, and B = 2.0 Hz), theta (3.5-7.0 Hz; fc = 4.25 Hz, and B = 3.5 Hz), alpha (7.0-13.0 Hz; fc = 9.0 Hz, and B = 6.0 Hz); beta (13.0-22.0 Hz; fc = 19.0 Hz, and B = 14.0 Hz). Degrees of freedom = $2 \times$ BwT, where Bw = the bandwidth and T = the length of the record (e.g., for 20 sec of EEG there are 160° of freedom) and the start-up and trail-off periods of the filter are in seconds, 2/BW (e.g., 0.5 sec for a 4.0 Hz bandwidth). The artifact rejection routines precluded EEG segments less than 0.8 sec in length and the range of total EEG length/subject varied from 16-60 sec (mean, 34.37; SD, 13.34).

Coherence and phase were computed for all pairwise combinations of electrodes.[29,30] Coherence is analogous to a cross-correlation in the frequency domain and reflects the number and strength of connections between spatially distant generators.[29,31] Measures of phase provide estimates of lead- and lag-times between spatially separate but connected systems of generators, as well as measures of frequency dispersion and conduction velocity.[30-32] Mathematical equations describing the method of computing coherence and phase are provided elsewhere.[29,30,32]

In order to reduce the coherence and phase measure set, three different categories of electrode combinations were employed: (1) left intrahemispheric combinations, (2) right intrahemispheric combinations, and (3) homologous interhemispheric combinations.

EEG Amplitude Differences

Because the recursive filter analysis was performed over specific frequency bands, the absolute power of the EEG was computed in μV^2 for each frequency band. Differences in absolute amplitude were computed between the same pairs of electrodes as in coherence described in the previous section (i.e., left and right intrahemispheric and interhemispheric electrode combinations). The formula for amplitude differences was (left − right) for the interhemisphere comparison and (anterior derivation − posterior derivation) for intrahemisphere comparisons.

Brainstem Auditory Evoked Potentials

Auditory click stimuli 100 μsec in duration were delivered through air-conducting tubes from piezoelectric transducers (Motorola #KSM20004A) at 10 clicks/sec. The stimulus intensity was 90 dB SPL to each ear. The vertex signal was led to an amplifier with a gain of 100,000, a noise level of 4 μV peak-to-peak; a common mode rejection ratio of 200 dB, and a bandwidth from 100.0-2.9 Hz at −4 dB points. The prefiltered analog signal was digitized at a rate of 10,000 samples/sec with 12-bit resolution. Digital data were collected for a set of 10 "trials" or subaverages. Each such trial consisted of the average of 200 evoked potentials using an analysis epoch of 12 msec and a sampling interval of 200 msec. Averages of brainstem evoked potentials were thus based upon 1,000 responses.

Brainstem auditory evoked response (BAER) peak detection first involved spectral analyzing each trial using a 512-point fast Fourier transform (FFT) and computing the mean amplitude of each spectral component across all 20 trials. In order to enhance the signal-to-noise ratio the BAERs were digitally filtered with frequency components outside of 440-2400 Hz band set to zero.[32] The enhancement of the BAER signal by digital filtering permitted reliable peak detection by locating the zero crossing of the first derivative. The standard deviation, amplitude, and latency of waves 1 through 5, as well as the interpeak latencies of waves 1-3, waves 3-5, and waves 1-5 for each ear were calculated. Only analyses using the absolute and interpeak latencies were used in order to maintain a high subject:variable ratio for multivariate regression analyses.

Since it was possible to have some peaks missing while others could be present, it was not desirable to code the absolute latency of a particular wave as a "0" latency. This would bias the mean severely. Additionally, we did not want to code absent waves as missing data because the absence of a wave (e.g., wave 3) in the presence of clearly discernible waves (e.g., waves 1 and 5) indicated likely neuropathy for the corresponding brain region. Thus, in order to code absent waves as indicators of pathology, all absolute latencies were Z-score transformed using the standard Z-score equation

$$Y_z = \frac{X - M}{SD_x}$$

where X is the absolute latency for a given wave and M and SD_x are the means and standard deviations derived from a normative study.[33] Abnormality was considered to be increasingly more severe with increasing Z-score values.

Glasgow Coma Score

Two different GCS scores[34] were obtained: one at the time of admission (GCS-A) and a second at the time of computerized EEG and evoked potential testing (GCS-T). The mean time between injury and GCS-T was 7.5 days and the standard deviation was 7.6 days.

The distribution of GCSs at the time of admission for the patients in this study is shown in FIGURE 1.

Disability Outcome Measures

TABLE 1 shows the Rappaport Disability Rating Scale (DRS),[35] which measures disability in six different diagnostic categories of (1) eye opening, (2) best verbal response, (3) best motor response, (4) self-care abilities, (5) level of daily functioning, and (6) employability. TABLE 1 shows the categories and items used for assessing functional outcome. Studies have demonstrated reliability and validity in the DRS and good interrater reliability.[35]

TABLE 1. Rappaport Disability Rating Scale

Eye Opening		Best Verbal Response	
Spontaneous	0	Oriented	0
To speech	1	Confused	1
To pain	2	Inappropriate	2
None	3	Incomprehensive	3
		None	4
Best Motor Response		Self Care Items	
Obeying	0	Complete	0
Localizing	1	Partial	1
Withdrawing	2	Minimal	2
Flexing	3	None	3
Extending	4		
None	5		
Level of Functioning			
Completely independent		0	
Independent in special environment		1	
Mildly dependent		2	
Moderately dependent		3	
Markedly dependent		4	
Totally dependent		5	
Employability			
Not restricted		0	
Selective jobs, competitive		1	
Sheltered workshops, noncompetitive		2	
Nonemployable		3	

The method of scoring and exact definitions of each of the six items are discussed in detail by Rappaport *et al.*[20,21,35] Scores range from 0 (for complete recovery) to 30 (for death). These evaluations were obtained through telephone interviews with the guardians or caretakers of the patients. To minimize errors in the estimates of patient status, the interviews with guardians and parents were structured so as to obtain both yes and no answers to specific questions as well as to provide descriptions of the patient's behavior and progress within a given category. Reliability of the Rappaport scores was obtained by both the simple nature of the score and the accuracy by which it separated functional and independent patients from nonindependent patients.

STATISTICAL METHODS

Data Screening and Transforms

Data analyses involved first double-checking all scores before and after entry into the PDP 11/70 computer files. Each measure category was then screened for extreme values (outliers) and for normality of distribution (BMDP-P7D; P2D).[36] All univariate and multivariate statistical analyses utilized the BMDP Biomedical Computer Programs.[36] Previous work with EEG and evoked potential measures have resulted in the use of standard transforms[7,37] to insure Gaussian normality. For relative power and

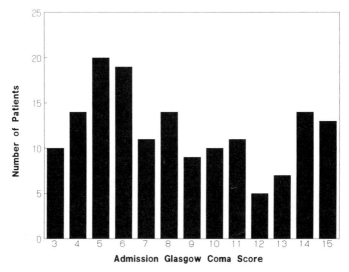

FIGURE 1. Distribution of Glasgow Coma Scores obtained at time of admission (GCS-A).

coherence variables, the transforms were $\log_{10} \dfrac{(X)}{(100-X)}$. For the amplitude asymmetry variables, the transform was $\log_{10} \dfrac{(200 + X)}{(200 - X)}$. After applying the appropriate transforms, all variables approximated the normal distribution.

Discriminant Analyses

Stepwise discriminant analyses with a leave-one-out (for jackknife) replication (BMDP = 7M) were used to determine the ability of individual variables as well as groups of variables to categorize patients into the two extreme categories of (1) complete recovery (i.e., DRS = 0) or (2) a vegetative state and/or death (i.e., DRS = 30) at one year following injury. Of the 162 patients in the study there was a total of 77 with DRS outcome scores of 0 or 30. Fifty-seven patients had DRS scores of 0, and 20 patients had DRS scores of 30. Initially, each diagnostic measure was evaluated individually (i.e., CT-scan, BSAEP, EEG, GCS, etc). Once the best discriminating variables from each independent variable category were identified, then these variables were combined into a final analysis in order to derive an optimal discriminant function based upon a multimodal analysis.

Multivariate Regression Analysis

The ability of the various diagnostic measures to predict outcome at one-year postinjury in patients with an intermediate Rappaport DRS (i.e., between 1 and 29) was evaluated using multivariate regression analyses (BMDP-2R). Of the 162 patients in the study, a total of 85 patients had DRS scores from 2 to 29. The multiple regression analyses involved first conducting separate analyses of each variable category in order to compare the predictive ability of each independent variable category. Once the best predictor variables from each independent variable category were determined, then these variables were entered into a combined or multimodal stepwise regression analysis. The final analysis adjusted for the intercorrelations between the variables and resulted in a regression equation that contained the strongest predictor variables from the previous analyses.

Prediction Accuracy of Multivariate Analyses

A primary concern is determining how well the discriminant and regression analyses from a sample of patients predict outcome in the population at large. Large sample sizes and multiple cross-validation are necessary to accurately measure prediction accuracy. However, if only a small sample size is available, then constraints must be placed on the ratio of subjects to variables. Recently, Sawyer[38] showed that when a prediction equation is based on a sample from a multivariate normal population, the mean absolute error of prediction can be closely approximated by a simple function of the number of predictor variables and the base sample size. The mean absolute error (MAE) of prediction is equal to the product of $\sigma\sqrt{(2/\pi)}$ and an inflation factor $K = \dfrac{(n + 1)\,(n - 2)}{[n(n - p - 2)]}$ that is greater than 1. In other words, the inflation factor is a linear function of N and the number of predictor variables p. With this formulation it is possible to estimate the prediction accuracy of a given base sample using a limited number of predictor variables. In all of the discriminant and regression analyses, care was taken to limit the number of predictor variables entered into the discriminant and regression equation to a prediction accuracy of greater than 90%. Thus, in the analyses to follow, the subject:variable ratios were determined by the sample size capable of yielding greater than 90% prediction accuracy.

RESULTS

Discriminant Analyses of Extreme DRS Scores

Individual Discriminant Analyses

TABLE 2 shows the discriminant accuracy of the different independent variable categories to classify patients into the two ends of the Rappaport DRS (good outcomes versus death). The best overall discriminant was provided by EEG phase with 90.2% leave-one-out replication accuracy, and the worst discriminant was provided by EEG relative and total power with 67.1% jackknife accuracy. The order of accuracy of the leave-one-out replicated discriminant (i.e., evaluating both false positives and false negatives) was EEG phase > BSAEP > GCS-T > EEG coherence = amplitude asymmetry > CT-scan > GCS-A > EEG relative and total power. The peak latency of waves 1, 3, 5 and the interpeak latencies between waves 1-3 and 3-5 were the best discriminating variables from the brainstem auditory evoked potential. For CT-scan the best discriminating variables were cerebral atrophy and intraventricular bleeding. For the EEG variables the left and right hemisphere were equally represented with most of the significant variables involving the frontal, central, and temporal leads. The subject:variable ratios of the discriminant analyses ranged from 6:1 for EEG phase to 40:1 for GCS-A and GCS-T.

Combined Discriminant Analyses

The results of the jackknife discriminant analyses using various combinations of independent variables is shown in TABLE 3. Because of listwise deletion in the BMDP analyses, the number of subjects was relatively small in many of the combined analyses and, therefore, the subject:variable ratio was unfavorable (e.g., N = 36 for BSAEP + GCS-T in TABLE 3). However, a relatively large sample size (N = 48) was available in the combined EEG + GCS-T analyses, which yielded the most reliable leave-one-out replicated discriminant (e.g., the subject:variable ratio was 6:1) with a total jackknife discriminant accuracy of 95.8% (TABLE 3).

Regression Analyses of Intermediate DRS Scores

Age

Age ranged from 12.49 to 97.44 yr with a mean of 30.07 and a standard deviation of 17.95. The distribution of age was not skewed; however, it was somewhat kurtotic (e.g., kurtosis = 5.69) with the majority of patients being less than 25 yr of age. A direct relationship was noted between age and the intermediate range of the disability

TABLE 2. Individual Discriminant Analyses

Variable	Predicted Good			Predicted Poor			Total Actual Outcome		
	% Correct	Actual Good (N)	Actual Poor (N)	% Correct	Actual Good (N)	Actual Poor (N)	% Correct	Good (N)	Poor (N)
GCS-A	68.6	35	16	76.5	4	13	70.6	39	29
GCS-T	80.6	29	7	78.6	3	11	80.0	31	28
CT-scan	86.1	31	5	47.1	9	8	73.6	40	13
BSAEP	94.3	50	3	53.8	6	7	86.4	56	10
EEG relative power	69.4	43	19	60.0	8	12	67.1	51	31
EEG amplitude asymmetry	83.0	52	10	65.0	7	13	79.3	59	23
EEG coherence	79.0	49	13	80.0	4	16	79.3	53	29
EEG phase	91.9	57	5	85.0	3	17	90.2	60	22

TABLE 3. Combined Discriminant Analyses

Variables	Predicted Good			Predicted Poor			Total Actual Outcome		
	% Correct	Actual Good (N)	Actual Poor (N)	% Correct	Actual Good (N)	Actual Poor (N)	% Correct	Good (N)	Poor (N)
EEG + GCS-T	94.4	34	2	100.0	0	12	95.8	34	14
BSAEP + GCS-T	100.0	28	0	87.5	1	7	97.2	29	7
CT-scan + GCS-T	94.7	18	1	70.0	3	7	86.2	21	8
EEG + BSAEP	98.1	52	1	92.3	1	12	97.0	53	13
CT-scan + BSAEP	93.5	29	2	70.0	3	7	87.8	32	9
EEG + CT-scan	92.3	34	2	66.7	2	4	87.5	26	6

rating scale. At 12 months postinjury, age was correlated with the Rappaport DRS at .3812, and it accounted for 14.53% of the variance. Examination of residual scatter plots showed that age was a relatively poor predictor of outcome with a large number of both overly optimistic and overly pessimistic predictions. To control for the severity of injury, the regression analyses were repeated with the severity of injury equated across age by forcing the GCS-T into the regression equation at the first step. The results of this analysis showed that age was correlated at .513 and accounted for 26.32% of the variance. The results indicate that the major determiner of outcome is the severity of injury; however, if severity of injury is held constant, then the older an individual the poorer the prognosis.

GCS

As can be seen in FIGURE 2, GCS-A correlated with the intermediate range of the DRS at .5013 and accounted for 25.13% of the variance, while GCS-T correlated with the intermediate range of the DRS at .5907 and accounted for 34.89% of the variance.

CT-scan Measures

As described previously, the CT-scan measures were grouped into three gross anatomic categories: cortical, subcortical, and diffuse. The comparative ability of the different categories of CT-scan measures to predict intermediate outcome scores at 12 months postinjury is shown in FIGURE 3. None of the univariate analyses of subcortical measures was significantly related to outcome. However, there was a significant mutlivariate F in which the multiple R = 0.2637 and the R^2 = 6.95%. Of the cortical measures only lesions of the parietal lobes were statistically significant. The multivariate R was 0.4017 and the R^2 was 16.13%. The most significant univariate CT-scan measure was obtained from the diffuse category in which diffuse cortical atrophy was highly significant (R = 0.5113, R^2 = 26.14%). Multivariate analyses of the diffuse category yielded an R = 0.6897 and R^2 = 47.57%.

Brainstem Auditory Evoked Potential

FIGURE 4 shows the ability of the brainstem auditory evoked potential peak latency and amplitude measures to predict intermediate outcome DRS scores. Peak latency measures exhibited a multiple R = 0.5209 and accounted for 27.13% latency and amplitude measures to predict intermediate DRS scores. Peak amplitude measures exhibited a multiple R = 0.3891 and accounted for 15.14% of the variance. The variance of peak amplitude was not significantly predictive of outcome. Of the peak latency measures, the interpeak latency between waves 3 and 5 and the latency between waves 1 and 5 accounted for the most variance. Of the peak amplitude measures, the

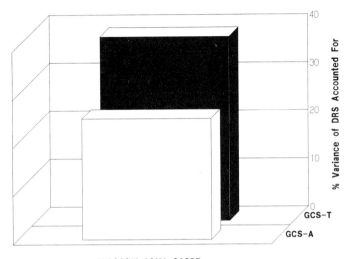

GLASGOW COMA SCORE

FIGURE 2. Percent variance of the intermediate range of Rappaport Disability Rating Scores (DRS) accounted for by Glasgow Coma Scores obtained at admission (GCS-A) and at the time of computerized EEG and evoked potential testing (GCS-T).

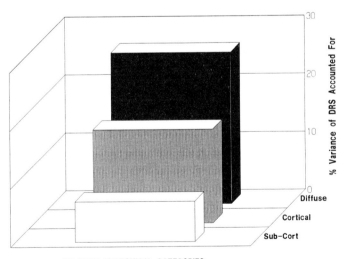

CT-SCAN ANATOMICAL CATEGORIES

FIGURE 3. Percent variance of the intermediate range of Rappaport DRS accounted for by CT-scan measures. The CT-scan measures were divided into subcortical damage, cortical damage, and diffuse damage (*see* METHODS for details).

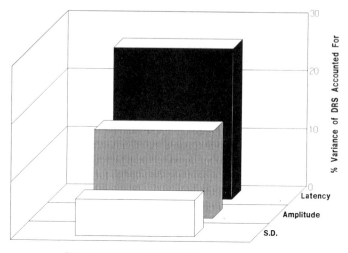

BSAEP MEASUREMENT CATEGORIES

FIGURE 4. Percent variance of the intermediate range of Rappaport DRS accounted for by brainstem auditory evoked potential measures. Amplitude represents the baseline to peak μV amplitude value of waves 1, 2, and 3, while latency represents the absolute latency of waves 1, 3, and 5 as well as interpeak latencies between waves 1-3, 1-5, and 3-5.

absolute amplitude of peaks 2 and 5 accounted for the most variance. The direction of the partial correlations indicate an inverse relationship between peak latency and outcome, that is, the longer the latency the worse the prognosis. Similarly, for peak amplitude, the lower the peak amplitude the worse the prognosis.

Computerized EEG

The ability of the EEG to predict outcome was assessed in separate regressions of five different categories of EEG variables: (1) relative power, (2) total power, (3) amplitude asymmetry, (4) EEG coherence, and (5) EEG phase.

FIGURE 5 shows the ability of the various EEG measures to predict intermediate outcome scores at one year postinjury. It can be seen that the best predictor was EEG phase which had an R = 0.664 and accounted for 44.21% of the variance of the disability rating scale, while the least predictive was absolute power with R = 0.437 and an R^2 = 19.14%. When the statistically significant EEG variables obtained from the individual analyses were combined into a final EEG analysis, then the multiple R equaled 0.725 and accounted for 52.56% of the variance of the disability rating scores. In the final multivariate regression analysis none of the relative power or total power variables were entered into the regression equation, because these variables were weaker predictors than the amplitude asymmetries, coherence, and phase measures.

Ability of Combined Measures to Predict Outcome

FIGURE 6 shows the comparative strength of predictability of intermediate DRS scores for the various clinical measures. It can be seen that the best predictor of intermediate outcome was the EEG, the second strongest predictor was GCS, the third was brainstem far-field evoked potentials, the fourth strongest was CT-scan measures, and the least predictive was patient age. The final multiple regression analyses were performed on various combinations of the statistically significant variables obtained from the individual analyses shown in FIGURE 6. TABLE 4 shows the results of the combined analyses. It can be seen that the best predictor of outcome was the combination of EEG and GCS-T with R = 0.864 and accounted for 74.65% of the variance of the intermediate range of the Rappaport DRS. The second best combination of variables were from the EEG and brainstem auditory evoked potentials with a multiple R = 0.839 and accounted for 70.53% of the variance. The addition of age, CT-scan, and GCS did not significantly improve predictability.

DISCUSSION

The results of the present study support the view that multimodal measures are more predictive of functional outcome in neurotrauma patients than any one measure set alone.[14–16,29] The results also indicated that EEG measures of cerebral symmetry

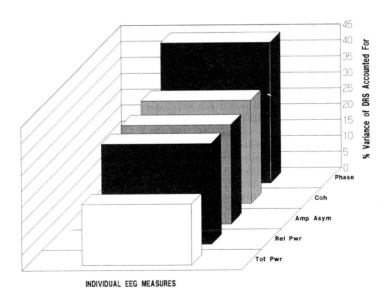

FIGURE 5. Percent variance of the Rappaport DRS accounted for by individual EEG measures. The measures were total EEG power (μv^2), relative power, amplitude asymmetries, coherence, and phase.

(i.e., coherence, phase, and amplitude symmetry) were the best predictors of outcome whether a discriminant analysis of extreme outcome scores was used or a multiple regression analysis of the mid-range of outcome scores was employed. This represents a cross-validation in that entirely different subjects were used in the two different multivariate analyses. The best combination of variables was EEG and GCS, which accounted for 74.65% of the variance with a multiple $R = 0.864$ and which also exhibited a discriminant accuracy between good outcome and death of 95.8% (TABLE 3).

One difficulty in establishing and evaluating long-term prognostic indices is the fact that many nonneurologic factors, such as associated somatic injuries, sepsis, and medical complications, influence a patient's course and outcome. These factors tend to increase false-positive predictions or errors on the side of overoptimism. The opposite category of error is the false-negative error or the error of overpessimism. Although both categories of error are undesirable, their consequences are different depending on their direction and whether they influence acute management or long-term rehabilitation planning or both. For example, false-positive predictions due to nonneurologic causes have only minimal adverse implications with regard to treatment for recovery of cognitive function. More serious consequences of false-positive predictions occur when they are due to inaccurate measurements of neurologic status.[25] On the other hand, false-negative predictions or errors due to undue pessimism have a bearing on patient outcome if the prediction is for vegetative state or death. A major objective of any program of patient prognostication is to evaluate the consequences of errors and, where possible, to minimize both false positives and false negatives by improving the reliability of measures.

Since different patients with different outcomes were used in the two different analyses, the reliability of the predictor measures can be evaluated by comparing the

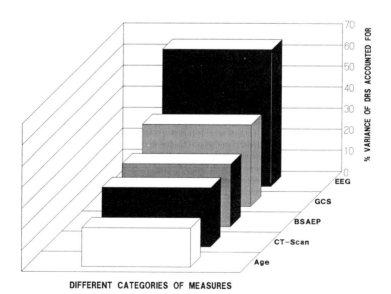

DIFFERENT CATEGORIES OF MEASURES

FIGURE 6. Comparison of percent variance of the Rappaport DRS accounted for by various measures. In this figure, measures from each category were combined into a single multiple regression analysis.

TABLE 4. Percent Variance of Rappaport Disability Rating Scale Accounted for by Combined Analyses

Variables	N* (p)**	% Variance
EEG + GCS	129 (12)	74.65
EEG + BSAEP	107 (11)	70.53
EEG + Age	129 (12)	66.82
EEG + CT-scan	80 (7)	60.96
EEG + GCS + Age	129 (12)	74.65
EEG + BSAEP + Age	107 (11)	70.53
EEG + BSAEP + CT-scan	65 (5)	66.09
EEG + Age + CT-scan	80 (7)	61.87
EEG + BSAEP + GCS + Age	88 (7)	72.59
EEG + BSAEP + CT-scan + Age	64 (5)	71.98
EEG + GCS + CT-scan + Age	68 (6)	66.57
EEG + BSAEP + CT-scan + Age + GCS	54 (5)	71.67

* N = Number of subjects; ** p (in parentheses) = Number of variable predictors.

measures that were entered into the final discriminant analysis to the measures that were entered into the final regression analysis. Examination of the variable lists revealed relatively good replication of the measures for the two groups of patients. In particular, the same EEG phase, coherence, and amplitude asymmetry variables exhibited the highest F values in the discriminant analyses and the highest R^2 values in the multiple regression analyses, thus indicating that these measures are reliable and relatively robust in their ability to predict outcome over the entire range of Rappaport DRS. Further, the gradient of prognostic strength from EEG phase > EEG coherence and amplitude asymmetry > CT-scan > EEG relative and total power was also replicated. The reliability and predictive strength of the EEG measures were further demonstrated by the observation of no statistically significant correlation between the date of injury and the date of EEG test (e.g., R = −0.052). Thus, the EEG coherence and phase measures appear to be relatively independent of changes in brain edema and other acute injury dynamics.

Diffuse Axonal Injury

Several studies have shown that a predominant pattern of injury in cerebral trauma is of a diffuse and nonspecific nature,[39–41] with the most common substrate for the diffuse effects being diffuse axonal injury (DAI). DAI is the consequence of the shear-strain forces on brain tissue that result from rapid acceleration and deceleration which accompany high velocity impact.[42] The shear-strain forces result in torn axonal fibers, damage to supportive structures (e.g., glia and vascular), and degeneration of neuronal fibers that are often distal to the point of impact.[43] Severe DAI can sometimes be imaged on CT or magnetic resonance imagery (MRI)[43] as a collection of 2.0- to 5.0-mm lesions in deep white matter, brainstem, or basal ganglia. However, CT and MRI do not reliably image mild DAI and hence cannot provide quantitative measures of the neurophysiologic consequences of DAI. In contrast, EEG coherence and phase have been shown to reflect the topographic patterning of human corticocortical fiber bundles.[30-32] Based upon these studies, the most concise explanation of the consistently strong prognostic measures of EEG phase and coherence on the one hand and the latency of brainstem auditory evoked potentials on the other hand is that these measures reflect, to some extent, the magnitude of diffuse axonal injury in the cerebral cortex and brainstem.

Topography of EEG Features

The most significant EEG predictors of outcome were from frontal scalp leads. This is consistent with the features of the skull-brain interface, which place the frontal lobes at risk for injury in high velocity accidents.[43] For example, of the scalp variables that were entered into the final regression analysis, 41.4% involved the frontal leads, 20.6% involved the central leads, 13.7% involved the temporal leads, and 10.3% involved the occipital leads. In all cases there was an approximately equal distribution for the left and right hemispheres. Of the EEG features that were most predictive of outcome, EEG phase exhibited the highest discriminant accuracy (TABLE 2) as well as being the most frequently entered variable in the final regression analysis (e.g., 50%). Coherence was the next most frequently entered variable in the final regression analysis (e.g., 35%), amplitude asymmetry the next (e.g., 10%), and EEG relative and total power were the least represented (0.5% for relative power and 0% for total power). The relatively weak prognostic value of relative and total power is consistent with the fact that these variables tend to reflect the effects of medication as well as global variables such as cerebral swelling. Relative and total power are strongly influenced by the general level of cortical excitability,[31] which is nearly always attenuated following severe-to-moderate closed head injuries, and thus relative and total power have limited ability to discriminate and predict outcome in closed head-injured patients. On the other hand, EEG phase and coherence appear to be relatively insensitive to global cerebral phenomena such as swelling and medication and tend to reflect more accurately the magnitude of structural damage, including damage to the white matter.[30,31]

SUMMARY

A comprehensive diagnostic evaluation was administered to 162 closed head-injured patients within 1 to 21 days (mean, 7.5 days) after injury. Each evaluation consisted of (1) power spectral analyses of electroencephalogram (EEG) recorded from 19 scalp locations referenced to age-matched norms, (2) brainstem auditory evoked potentials, (3) computed tomography (CT)-scan, and (4) Glasgow Coma Score (GCS) at time of admission (GCS-A) and at time of EEG test (GCS-T). Functional outcome at one year following injury was assessed using the Rappaport Disability Rating Scale (DRS), which measures the level of disability in the six diagnostic categories of (1) eye opening, (2) best verbal response, (3) best motor response, (4) self-care ability for feeding, grooming, and toileting, (5) level of cognitive functioning, and (6) employability. The ability of the different diagnostic measures to predict outcome at one year following injury was assessed using stepwise discriminant analyses to identify patients in the extreme outcome categories of complete recovery versus death and multivariate regression analyses to predict patients with intermediate outcome scores. The best combination of predictor variables was EEG and GCS-T, which accounted for 74.6% of the variance in the multivariate regression analysis of intermediate outcome scores and 95.8% discriminant accuracy between good outcome and death. The best single predictors of outcome in both the discriminant analyses and the regression analyses were EEG coherence and phase. A gradient of prognostic strength of diagnostic measures was EEG phase > EEG coherence > GCS-T > CT-scan > EEG relative power. The value of EEG coherence and phase in the assessment of diffuse axonal injury was discussed.

ACKNOWLEDGMENTS

We would like to acknowledge the assistance of Bill Cantor, Deloris Onersty, and Sonia Cantor for the diligent collection of the EEGs at MIEMSS. The MIEMSS patient data was collected while Dr. Thatcher was Principal Investigator and Scientific Director of the Neurometrics Clinical Service and Dr. Geisler was Chief of MIEMSS Neurotrauma and Supervisory Physician of the Neurometrics Clinical Service.

REFERENCES

1. KNOBLICH, O. E. & M. GAAB. 1979. Prognostic information from EEG and ICP monitoring after severe closed head injuries in the early post-traumatic phase. Acta Neurochir. Suppl. **28:** 58-62.
2. LANGFITT, T. W. & T. A. GENNARELLI. 1982. Can the outcome from head injury be improved? J. Neurosurg. **56:** 19-25.
3. AVEZAAT, C. J., H. J. VAN DEN BERG & R. BRAAKMAN. 1979. Eye movements as a prognostic factor. Acta Neurochir. Suppl. **28:** 26-28.
4. BRAAKMAN, R., G. J. GELPKE, J. D. E. HABBEMA, A. R. MAAS & J. M. MINDERHOUD. 1980. Systematic selection of prognostic features in patients with severe head injury. Neurosurgery **6:** 362-370.
5. GENNARELLI, T. A., G. M. SPIELMAN, T. W. LANGFITT, P. L. GILDENBER, T. HARRINGTON, J. A. JANE, L. F. MARSHALL, J. D. MILLER & L. H. PITTS. 1982. Influence of the type of intracranial lesion on outcome from severe head injury. J. Neurosurg. **56:** 26-32.
6. HABBEMA, J., R. BRAAKMAN & C. AVEZAAT. 1979. Prognosis of the individual patient with severe head injury. Acta Neurochir. Suppl. **28:** 158-160.
7. JENNETT, B., G. TEASDALE, R. BRAAKMAN, J. MINDERHOUD & R. KNILL-JONES. 1976. Predicting outcome in individual patients after severe head injury. Lancet **1:** 1031-1034.
8. MILLER, J.D. 1979. Barbiturates and raised intracranial pressure. Ann. Neurol. **6:** 189-193.
9. OVERGAARD, J., S. CHRISTENSEN, O. HVID-HANSEN, *et al.* 1973. Prognosis after head injury based on early clinical examination. Lancet **2:** 631-635.
10. ROBERSON, F. C., P. R. KISHORE, J. D. MILLER, *et al.* 1979. The value of serial computerized tomography in the management of severe head injury. Surg. Neurol. **12:** 161-167.
11. TABADDOR, K., A. DANZIGER & H. WISOFF. 1982. Estimation of intracranial pressure by CT scan in closed head trauma. Surg. Neurol. **18:** 212-215.
12. CLIFTON, G. L., R. G. GROSSMAN, M. E. MAKELA, M. E. MINER, S. HANDEL & V. SADHU. 1980. Neurological course and correlated computerized tomography findings after severe closed head injury. J. Neurosurg. **52:** 611-624.

13. LOBATO, R., F. CORDOBES, J. RIVAS, M. DE LA FUENTE, A. MONTERO, A. BARCENA, C. PEREZ, A. CABERA & E. LAMAS. 1983. Outcome from severe head injury related to the type of intracranial lesion. J. Neurosurg. **59:** 762-774.
14. NAU, H.E., E. B. BONGARTZ, W. J. BOCK & C. WEICHERT. 1979. Computerized tomography (CT), electroencephalography (EEG), and clinical symptoms in severe cranio-cerebral injuries. Acta Neurochir. **45:** 209-216.
15. COOPER, R. & A. HUYLME. 1969. Changes of the EEG, intracranial pressure and other variables during sleep in patients with intracranial lesions. Electroencephalogr. Clin. Neurophysiol. **27:** 12-22.
16. ASKENAZY, J. J., L. SAZBON, P. HACKETT & T. NAJENSON. 1980. The value of electroencephalography in prolonged coma: a comparative EEG-computed axial tomography study of two patients one year after trauma. Resuscitation **9:** 181-194.
17. JOHN, E. R., B. KARMEL, W. CORNING, P. EASTON, D. BROWN, H. AHN, M. JOHN, T. HARMONY, L. PRICHEP, A. TORO, I. GERSON, F. BARTLETT, R. THATCHER, H. KAYE, P. VALDES & E. SCHWARTZ. 1977. Neurometrics: Numerical taxonomy identifies different profiles of brain functions within groups of behaviorally similar people. Science **196:** 1393-1410.
18. CURRY, S. H. 1980. Event-related potentials as indicants of structural and functional damage in closed head injury. Prog. Brain Res. **54:** 507-515.
19. FEINSOD, M. 1976. Electrophysiological correlates of traumatic visual damage. *In* Head Injuries. Proceedings of the Second Symposium on Neural Trauma. R. L. McLaurin, Ed.: 95-100. Grune and Stratton. New York, NY.
20. RAPPAPORT, M., K. HALL, H. K. HOPKINS & T. BELLEZA 1977. Evoked brain potentials and disability in brain-damaged patients. Arch. Phys. Med. Rehabil. **58:** 333-338.
21. RAPPAPORT, M., K. HALL, H. K. HOPKINS & T. BELLEZA. 1981. Evoked potentials and head injury: I. rating of evoked potential abnormality. Clin. Electroencephalogr. **12:** 154-156.
22. NARAYAN, R., R. GREENBERG, J. MILLER, G. ENAS, S. CHOI, P. KISHORE, J. SELHORST, H. LUTZ & D. BECKER. 1981. Improved confidence of outcome prediction in severe head injury. J. Neurosurg. **54:** 751-762.
23. GREENBERG, R. P., D. J. MAYER, D. P. BECKER & J. D. MILLER. 1977. Evaluation of brain function in severe human head trauma with multimodality evoked potentials. Part 1: Evoked brain-injury potentials, methods, and analysis. Post-traumatic neurological conditions. J. Neurosurg. **47:** 150-162.
24. GREENBERG, R. P., D. P. BECKER, J. D. MILLER & D. J. MAYER. 1977. Evaluation of brain function in severe human head trauma with multimodality evoked potentials. Part 2: Localization of brain dysfunction and correlation with posttraumatic neurological conditions. J. Neurosurg. **47:** 163-177.
25. GREENBERG, R. P., P. G. NEWLON, M. S. HYATT, R. K. NARAYAN & D. P. BECKER. 1981. Prognostic implications of early multimodality evoked potentials in severely head-injured patients. J. Neurosurg. **55:** 227-236.
26. JENNETT, B. 1986. Head Trauma. *In* Diseases of the Nervous System. A. K. Asbury, G. M. McKhaan & W. I. McDonald, Eds.: 1282-1291. W. B. Saunders. Philadelphia, PA.
27. WILLIAMS, J. M., F. GONES, O. W. DRUDGE & M. KESSLER. 1984. Predicting outcome from closed head injury by early assessment of trauma severity. J. Neurosurg. **61:** 581-585.
28. JASPER, H. H. 1958. The ten-twenty electrode system of the International Federation. Electroencephalogr. Clin. Neurophysiol. **10:** 371-375.
29. OTNES, R. K. & L. ENOCHSON. 1972. Digital Time Series Analysis. John Wiley. New York, NY.
30. THATCHER, R. W., P. KRAUSE & M. HRYBYK. 1986. Corticocortical associations and EEG coherence: A two-compartmental model. EEG Clin. Neurophysiol. **64:** 123-143.
31. NUNEZ, P. 1981. Electrical Fields of the Brain: the Neurophysics of EEG. Oxford University Press. New York, NY.
32. THATCHER, R. W., R. A. WALKER & S. GIUDICE. 1987. Human cerebral hemispheres develop at different rates and ages. Science **236:** 1110-1113.
33. STARR, A. & L. J. ACHOR. 1975. Auditory brainstem responses in neurological disease. Arch. Neurol. **32:** 761-768.

34. JENNETT, B. & M. BOND. 1975. Assessment of outcome after severe brain damage. A practical scale. Lancet **1:** 480-487.

35. RAPPAPORT, M., K. M. HALL, K. HOPKINS, B. S. BELLEZA & D. N. COPE. 1982. Disability rating scale for severe head trauma: Coma to community. Arch. Phys. Med. Rehabil. **63:** 118-123.

36. DIXON, W. & M. BROWN. 1979. Biomedical Computer Programs P-Series. University of California Press. Los Angeles, CA.

37. THATCHER, R. W., R. MCALASTER, M. L. LESTER, R. L. HORST & D. S. CANTOR. 1983. Hemispheric EEG asymmetries related to cognitive functioning in children. *In* Cognitive Processing in the Right Hemisphere. A. Perecman, Ed: 125-146. Academic Press. New York, NY.

38. SAWYER, R. 1982. Sample size and the accuracy of predictions made from multiple regression equations. J. Ed. Stat. **7:** 91-104.

39. ADAMS, J. H., D. J. GRAHAM & T. A. GENNEARELLI. 1985. Contemporary neuropathological considerations regarding brain damage in head injury. *In* Central Nervous System Trauma Status Report—1985. D. P. Becker & J. T. Povlishack, Eds. National Institutes of Health National Institute for Neurological and Communicative Disorders and Stroke. Washington, D.C.

40. AUERBACH, S. H. 1986. Neuroanatomical correlates of attention and memory disorders in traumatic brain injury: An application of neurobehavioral subtypes. J. Head Trauma Rehabil. **1:** 1-12.

41. JANE, J. A., O. STEWARD & T. GENNARELLI. 1985. Axonal degeneration induced by experimental noninvasive minor head injury. J. Neurosurg. **62:** 96-100.

42. STRICH, S. J. 1961. Shearing of nerve fibres as a cause of brain damage due to head injury. A pathological study of twenty cases. Lancet **2:** 443-448.

43. BIGLER, E. D. 1987. Neuropathology of acquired cerebral trauma. J. Learn. Disabil. **20:** 458-473.

Magnetoencephalography in the Study of Human Auditory Information Processing[a]

MIKKO SAMS[b] AND RIITTA HARI

Low Temperature Laboratory
Helsinki University of Technology
02150 Espoo, Finland

NONINVASIVE METHODS TO STUDY NEURAL MECHANISMS OF AUDITORY INFORMATION PROCESSING IN HUMANS

Recent advances in the methods for brain research have provided keys to unlock some of the classical "black boxes" that have long been the basic elements in the analysis of human information processing. In the auditory system, for example, the flow charts describing the hypothetical stages in processing can now be paralleled and even replaced by hypotheses about the actual neural events in different structures of the auditory system, bringing psychological description of auditory behavior and its neural mechanisms closer together. Whereas animal experiments have been the main source of information about neural mechanisms of behavior until recently, we today have methods to attack directly the neural mechanisms of human cerebral activity.

The most useful noninvasive tools to study brain activity in healthy humans, while performing some well-controlled tasks, are electroencephalography (EEG) and magnetoencephalography (MEG). In a typical experiment, the subject is presented with a set of sensory stimuli and the weak responses, time-locked to these, are extracted by averaging. Both EEG and MEG have a good time resolution, allowing studies of the flow of information and its transformations in different brain structures. The good spatial resolution of MEG makes it superior to EEG in locating active cortical areas. Although auditory processing is strongly distributed and parallel, and although the interaction between various neuroanatomical structures is the basis of auditory perceptions, the specific roles of different brain areas in this processing can be studied with MEG.

[a] Supported by the Academy of Finland and by the Körber-Foundation (Hamburg).

[b] Address correspondence to Dr. Mikko Sams at the Low Temperature Laboratory, Helsinki University of Technology, Otakaari 3A, 02150 Espoo, Finland.

BASICS OF MAGNETOENCEPHALOGRAPHY

Biomagnetic Fields and Their Detection

Electric currents in the human brain produce a magnetic field outside the head, in addition to potential distribution on the scalp. Cerebral magnetic fields evoked by sensory stimuli are very small—on the order of 50-500 femtotesla (fT $= 10^{-15}$ Tesla) in magnitude, i.e., roughly 10^{-8} times the earth's steady magnetic field. The only method sensitive enough for the detection of these small fields is based on SQUID (Superconducting QUantum Interference Device) sensors. Effective shielding against magnetic artefacts produced by electrical equipment, power lines, vehicles, etc., can be provided by making the measurements within a chamber constructed of mu-metal and aluminum.[1] The first recordings, done with one-channel magnetometers, were truly heroic deeds since signals from 40-70 locations were needed for a detailed description of the magnetic field pattern. During long recordings the subject's vigilance varies greatly, causing variance to the measured responses. Fortunately, the development has led quickly in 4-, 5-, 7-, 24-, and even 37-sensor arrays,[2-6] which allow more rapid and accurate field measurements.

An important concept used in locating active brain areas with MEG recordings is the current dipole, which refers to current concentrated to a point. The dipole has location, orientation, and strength (i.e., dipole moment: unit $=$ ampere $\cdot$ meter). The magnetic field generated around the dipole follows the right-hand rule: When the thumb of the right hand points to the direction of the current, the fingers show the direction of the field lines. FIGURE 1 shows current dipoles of different orientations in a conducting sphere and the isopotential and isofield contours in the vicinity of them. The dipole is located in the center of the magnetic field pattern, and its depth determines the distance between the field extrema.

Only tangential currents produce magnetic fields outside a sphere (FIG. 1). If the current dipole is tilted in respect to the surface, the sensors measure the field generated by its tangential component. For example, a dipole deviating 60° from the tangential orientation produces a field that has still 50% of the strength of that of a purely tangential source of the same size. This is sometimes a useful difference with respect to electric recordings that "see" sources of any orientation. Since MEG detects the tangential currents, it is mainly sensitive to fissural activity. In some cases,[7] an important contribution can come from tilted sources in the convexial cortex. A powerful approach is to measure simultaneously both the magnetic and electric fields. From the magnetic data one first estimates the tangential sources and calculates their contribution to the electric field. What cannot be explained by these sources is due to radial or deep cortical currents.[8,9]

Because of their orientation, neural currents in the human supratemporal auditory cortex generate magnetic fields that can be detected outside the head. Therefore, MEG can be used to study the role of the human auditory cortex in the processing of different types of sounds; this can be done separately for both hemispheres.

Neural Sources of Magnetic Fields

Pyramidal neurons are the main cell category of cerebral cortex. These elongated neurons have their cell bodies in different cortical layers and their long dendrites pass

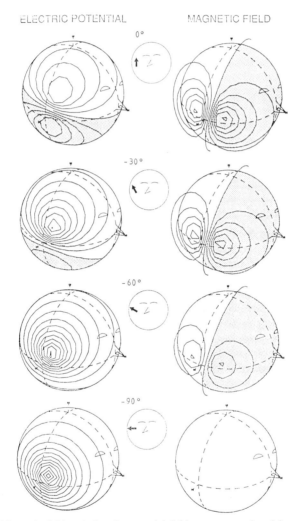

FIGURE 1. Magnetic field and electric potential field patterns produced by a current dipole (strength 20 nA·m) 20 mm below the surface of a sphere simulating the head. The dipole is assumed to be located in the supratemporal auditory cortex. The sphere contains four concentric layers with different electric conductivities. The outside radii (r) and conductivities (s) of the different layers are for brain: r = 92 mm, s = 0.33 1/Ωm; for cerebrospinal fluid: r = 94 mm, s = 1.40 1/Ωm; for skull: r = 102 mm, s = 0.006 1/Ωm; and for scalp: r = 106 mm, s = 0.28 1/Ωm. The current dipole is progressively tilted from the purely tangential (0°) to the purely radial (−90°) orientation, as indicated in the small schematic heads. The isocontour lines are separated by 0.5 μV for the electric potential and by 80 fT for the magnetic field patterns. The areas with positive electric potential and magnetic flux coming out of the head are shadowed.

several cortical laminae. When, for example, thalamic afferents synapse with apical dendrites of cortical pyramidal cells, transmitters change the permeability of the post-synaptic membrane creating a transmembrane current that is the "battery" of both the axial intracellular current and the extracellular return currents. These currents form a closed circuit, all parts of which create a magnetic field. However, the field outside the sphere is determined directly by the net intracellular current flow which thus can be considered the "current dipole."[8]

It would be impossible to record the magnetic field associated with the activity of any single cell outside the head. A sound always activates thousands of cortical cells in concert. Seen a few centimeters away this is equivalent to a current dipole at the center of gravity of the activated cells. Therefore, synchronous firing of neurons in a cortical area of less than a few square centimeters can be described by an equivalent current dipole (ECD).

In a single neuron, intracellular current directed towards deep cortical layers is caused either by excitatory synaptic activity in the superficial cortical layers or by inhibitory activity within deep layers. Current source density analysis[10] suggests that inhibitory postsynaptic potentials produce considerably smaller currents than excitatory ones, thus implying their smaller role in the generation of external magnetic fields as well. Therefore, dipoles of opposite directions can be considered to mainly reflect excitatory currents in superficial and deep cortical layers, respectively, or at opposite walls of a fissure.

Experimental Situation and Data Analysis

FIGURE 2 shows an example of the measurement of auditory evoked magnetic fields in the Low Temperature Laboratory.[11] The subject is lying comfortably on a bed and auditory stimuli are brought to his ear through a plastic tube and an earpiece. The magnetic field outside the head is detected by a 7-channel first-order SQUID-gradiometer[4], or, more recently, with a 24-channel planar gradiometer.[5] The pickup coils are situated on a hexagonal grid at the concave bottom of the dewar. The dewar, also containing the SQUIDs, is filled with liquid helium (temperature 4.2 K, −269° C). The magnetic field passing through the superconducting pickup coils is detected by the SQUIDs; their output is monitored by electronic devices at room temperature.

FIGURE 3 shows a set of seven simultaneously measured magnetic responses to short auditory stimuli over the right temporal area. The large signal at 120 ms (N100m) has opposite polarities at channels 2 and 5, suggesting a dipolar source somewhere in between, most probably at the supratemporal auditory cortex. However, to make reliable inferences about the source, the whole field pattern must be determined by recording responses from tens of locations. FIGURE 4 shows such a map during the peak of N100m. The equivalent current dipole that best explains the pattern is found by a least-squares fit; in this case the dipole explains 92% of the field variance. The "calculated field" in the figure would be produced by the equivalent current dipole in the absence of experimental noise. The "residual field" shows the pattern obtained when the calculated field is subtracted from the measured one. If a single dipole does not satisfactorily explain the measured field pattern, the residual field contains systematic features or exceeds in amplitude the experimental noise.

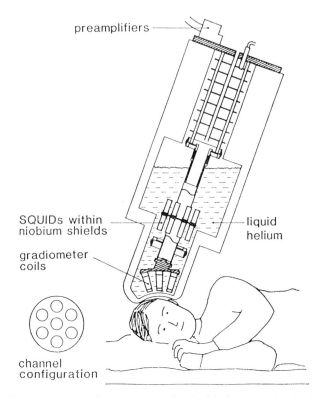

FIGURE 2. The measurement of neuromagnetic signals of the human brain with SQUID sensors. The top portion shows a dipolar current source located in auditory cortex and the magnetic field generated by it. From Hari and Lounasmaa.[11]

SPATIAL AND TEMPORAL RESOLUTION OF MAGNETOENCEPHALOGRAPHY

A convenient feature of magnetic fields is that the intervening cerebral and extracerebral tissues are practically transparent to them, whereas electric recordings are often smeared by electric inhomogeneities of the cerebrospinal fluid, the skull, and the scalp.[8] This feature is especially useful in investigating two simultaneously active but anatomically separate brain areas. For example, with MEG it is possible to separate activities generated at the first and second somatosensory cortices.[12,13]

Even with MEG it is difficult to estimate the functional anatomical areas where the source currents are generated. This is partly due to the large inter-individual anatomical differences with respect to landmarks on the head. Further, several brain areas may be active at the same time. For example, the auditory association "belt" area is probably activated simultaneously with the auditory koniocortex, and it is not easy to estimate the contribution of single areas to the response. However, the reliability of the location of the ECD can be very good, as is shown both by recording fields generated by an artificial current dipole within a plastic skull[14] and by theoretical calculations using the spherical model.[15] In optimal conditions, MEG recordings can differentiate between two nonsimultaneous sources a few millimeters away. Spatial resolution is best for superficial and strong sources.

The problems encountered in the absolute localization can be partly circumvented by manipulating stimulus parameters and studying the effect of these on the relative source locations. For example, the sites of N100m-sources have been shown to depend on the stimulus frequency[14,16]—the depth of the source increases when the frequency of the tone increases. This result agrees with the known tonotopical organization of monkey's auditory cortex.[17]

The time resolution of MEG is limited only by the recording passband. Perhaps the most fascinating feature of MEG and EEG recordings is that they allow a "semi-online" analysis of cortical information processing from the preparation to analyze the forthcoming stimulus up to the time of the decision processes and behavioral responses needed. This, in principle, enables us to tackle directly questions concerning such processes or stages that were previously only hypothetical, as illustrated by the research on different brain structures involved in selective attention.[18,19] The evoked response recordings are especially advantageous when the researcher is interested in the processing of stimuli which are not consciously analyzed, such as nonattended sounds in dichotic listening tasks.

MAGNETOENCEPHALOGRAPHY STUDIES OF HUMAN AUDITORY FUNCTIONS

The results obtained by MEG measurements in studies of human auditory functions have been recently summarized in several reviews,[8,9,20] and we give here only a brief description about the main results.

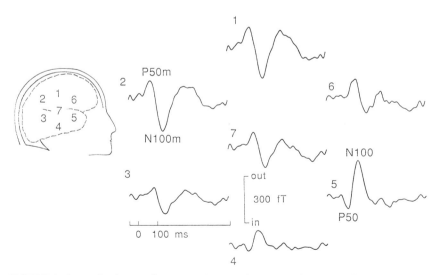

FIGURE 3. Seven simultaneously measured averaged responses (N = 500) from the locations indicated in the schematic head. The P50m and N100m responses are of opposite polarities at channels 2 and 5, suggesting a dipolar source between these sites in the underlying cortex. The stimuli were 1000-Hz sinusoids (90 dB SPL, 100 ms) repeated once every 510 ms.

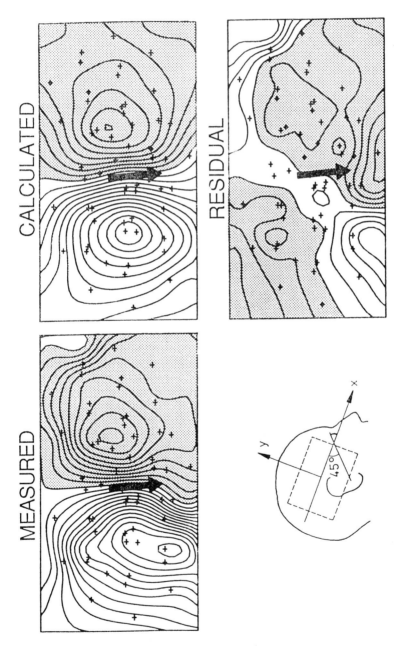

FIGURE 4. Field maps during the peak of N100m. The "measured" field represents the real measurement. Schematic head shows the approximate measurement area on the scalp surface. The areas where the flux is coming out of the head are shadowed.

The first magnetic cortical response after a click peaks at 19 ms, and thereafter the activity continues around the supratemporal auditory cortex for at least 200 ms. The source areas of different deflections differ slightly from each other. Although any abrupt change in the acoustic environment triggers an evoked response complex, the neural generators of these apparently similar responses are stimulus-specific. For example, responses evoked by noise and square-wave bursts or stimuli presented to different ears interact less than responses to similar stimuli or to sounds presented to the same ear.[21]

Interstimulus interval (ISI) is one important factor in determining the response amplitude. When the ISI increases, the response amplitudes also increase; N100m reaches a saturation level at ISIs of 8-10 s.[22,23] However, if sounds are presented in pairs, with interpair intervals of 1.2-1.4 s, the response to the second stimulus of the pair can be enhanced with respect to that of the first sound, when the sound onset asynchrony is less than 300 ms.[24] This type of behavior cannot be explained by the known recovery cycles of the responses but is probably based on changed properties of the neural network underlying the responses. Offsets of stimuli evoke "off-responses" that depend on sound duration in a very similar way as onset-responses depend on the ISI.[23,25]

Attention to tones presented randomly to either ear changes the MEG responses from 150 to 250 ms after the stimulus onset.[19] The field distributions suggest that this enhancement is due to a change of activity at the supratemporal auditory cortex. When tones are repeated at about 3 Hz, the attention effect may be seen already in the latency range of N100m,[26] whereas in a word-categorization task the effect is seen as an increase of the sustained field occurring during the word.[19]

Recordings of AEFs have also been used to study the integrity of sensory pathways, from periphery to cortex, in deaf patients with cochlear prostheses and in aphasic patients with cerebral infarctions.[27-29] Most probably, the same method could be used to monitor activity in children during the maturation of auditory pathways.

"MISMATCH" RESPONSES TO CHANGES IN MONOTONOUS SOUND SEQUENCES

Examples of Mismatch Fields

In the following, we discuss a MEG response called the mismatch field (MMF) to illustrate one interesting approach to human auditory information processing. An infrequent "deviant" sound, embedded in repetitive "standard" stimuli, elicits a vertex-negative evoked potential deflection about 200 ms from the stimulus. Näätänen et al.[30] named this deflection the mismatch negativity (MMN) and proposed that it is generated by a mismatch between the neural representation of the standard stimulus and an afferent inflow caused by the deviant stimulus. Subsequently, MMN-type responses have been recorded to deviations in frequency, intensity, apparent and real location of an auditory stimulus, changes in otherwise invariant interstimulus interval, violation in a repetitive alternating pattern of two stimuli (...ABABAABABA...), and deviations in phonetic stimuli.[30-35] The electric recordings have not resolved the generation site of the mismatch process.

Some years ago we recorded the mismatch field to frequency deviants of 1030 Hz presented among standard tones of 1000 Hz.[36,37] MMF peaked at about 200 ms and was of opposite polarity at the anterior and posterior ends of the Sylvian fissure. These studies showed that the mismatch process is generated either in the supratemporal auditory cortex or in auditory relay centers directly projecting to these areas.

Previous EEG studies had suggested that MMN might be independent of attention, but this has been difficult to show conclusively because in active discrimination tasks MMN is overlapped by another deflection, N2b.[38] Further, the response amplitude, per se, does not tell the source strength unless source depth is also known. We compared the dipole moments for MMFs when the subject either read a book ignoring the auditory stimuli or paid attention to them by counting the number of shorter-duration deviant tones. MMF did not increase during attention, and there was even a trend towards smaller dipole moments for MMF during attended than nonattended condition.[39] This might be due to an overlap by the following deflection of opposite polarity.

Sams et al.[40] recently compared the locations of equivalent dipoles for MMFs to deviations in frequency, intensity, and duration. The standard stimuli were 100-ms sinusoids, 1000 Hz in frequency, and 90 dB SPL in intensity. Each deviant differed from standards in one dimension only: in frequency (1500 Hz), intensity (57 dB), or duration (50 ms). All deviants elicited a MMF (FIG. 5). The locations of the corresponding equivalent dipoles did not differ systematically from each other, but were always more anterior than the equivalent dipole for N100m to standards. Similarly, the source of MMF elicited by a change in the second tone of a tone pair is also clearly more anterior than that of N100m.[41]

This experiment with multiple stimulus deviations might mean that the underlying neural network is not selective to physical stimulus features, per se, but that it is activated by any change in the ongoing stimulation. This suggestion has received support from a recent experiment[42] about the additivity of MMFs. Three subjects were presented with 100-ms, 1000-Hz standard stimuli. Among the standards there were frequency deviants of 1500 Hz, duration deviants of 50 ms, and deviants that differed from the standards both in frequency and duration. If the neural sources of different MMF were totally separate, the MMF elicited by the last-mentioned deviants should be the sum of the MMF elicited by the frequency and duration deviants alone. However, the 1500-Hz, 50-ms deviants elicited a MMF that was of approximately the same magnitude as that of MMFs to the single frequency and duration deviations (FIG. 6). This result suggests that the sources of different MMFs are, at least in part, the same.

Functional Significance of Mismatch Fields

The above results suggest the existence of two different subpopulations of neurons in the supratemporal auditory cortex: one underlying N100m and the other MMF. Our finding that N100m and MMFs to different deviants are generated in slightly different areas suggests that they have different functional roles in auditory signal processing. The occurrence of standards is a necessary condition for the elicitation of MMF: identical stimuli presented at long interstimulus intervals produce no MMF-type signal.[37] MMF, like MMN, therefore seems to be a specific response to a change in a monotonous sound sequence. On the other hand, N100m reflects more intimately the processing of the physical parameters of an auditory stimulus.

We propose that the neural networks underlying N100m analyze the physical stimulus features (feature extraction) and those underlying MMF detect changes in stimulation (change extraction). The main part of N100m might therefore be generated by neurons tuned to different physical features of auditory stimuli; such neurons have

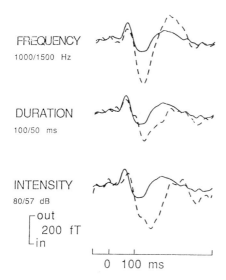

FREQUENCY
1000/1500 Hz

DURATION
100/50 ms

INTENSITY
80/57 dB

out
200 fT
in

0 100 ms

FIGURE 5. MEG responses to standards (*continuous lines*) and to deviants (*broken lines*) differing in frequency, duration, or intensity from the standards. The recordings are from the posterior temporal area in one subject.

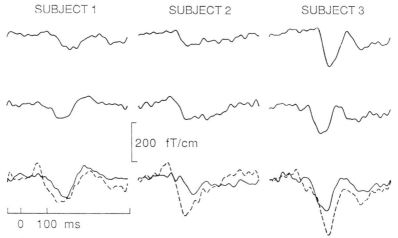

SUBJECT 1   SUBJECT 2   SUBJECT 3

200 fT/cm

0 100 ms

FIGURE 6. Difference waveforms (responses to standards subtracted from the responses to deviants) from three subjects to duration (*top panel*) and frequency (*middle panel*) deviants as well as their combination (*bottom panel*). The broken lines in bottom waveforms show the calculated sum of frequency and duration MMFs. The recordings were made with a planar gradiometer.[5]

been observed in the auditory cortex of primates.[17] On the other hand, there is no experimental evidence of "change" or "novelty" neurons outside hippocampus.[43] Sokolov[44] has presented a model for a neural network which might perform novelty detection. In his model, repetitive stimuli (standards) establish a cerebral neuronal model that registers the properties of the applied stimulus and stores them for a short time. A different afferent input, due to a change in the stimulus (deviant), causes a mismatch with the neuronal model and results in an orienting response. The formation of the neuronal model involves detectors tuned to different physical features of the stimulus. Their activation then converges on novelty neurons where the matrix of potentiated synapses (due to their repeated activation) is the neural model of the stimulus.

The output of the novelty neurons declines during repeated presentation. When some property of the stimulus is suddenly changed, their output is restored due to activation of a new set of feature detectors. Such a system can be thought of as a device which compares the stimulus with the history of stimulation, restored in the "neuronal model." This type of novelty or rather change neurons might underlie MMF in humans.

The model assumes the existence of a detector map for different stimulus features as a prerequisite for the generation of the mismatch process. If this assumption is correct, MMF measurements may give evidence of the organization of the detector maps in human auditory cortex. Interpreted within this framework the MEG results obtained so far suggest that the human auditory cortex contains detector maps for frequency, intensity, and duration of an auditory stimulus. Animal data obtained using the same stimulus paradigm would be of much interest.

Based on his studies on mustached bats, Suga[45,46] has developed an elegant neuro-ethological theory of auditory information processing. He suggests that the auditory cortex contains neural maps which are formed according to information-bearing parameters (IBPs) of auditory stimuli. IBPs have a specific role in the natural acoustic environment of a species. In mustached bats, the biosonar echolocation system is a species-specific form of auditory behavior according to which the auditory system has developed. In humans, speech communication might be a specific type of behavior which has had an important role in the formation of feature maps in our auditory cortex. Most IBP-maps are computational in the sense that they do not have a correspondence in the periphery, in contrast to the "epithelial" tonotopical map. An example is the auditory space map which is based on the computation of inter-aural phase and intensity differences.[47] Our MMF to duration changes might reflect the existence of a computational cortical map for stimulus duration.[39] Accurate discrimination of short time intervals is important, for example, for the differentiation of voiced versus voiceless consonants. Therefore, sound duration may be an IBP for humans.

MMF seems to be nearly as sensitive to a change in stimulus duration as psychophysical performance of subjects.[39] The same is true for the frequency MMN.[38] Because MMFs, like MMNs, can be recorded when the subject does not pay attention to the stimuli, these measurements provide a possibility for "objective psychophysics," which would be especially useful in the study of the integrative auditory functions in infants and in noncooperative adults.

Memory as a Prerequisite for the Mismatch Process

Some kind of neural trace, formed according to the features of the standard stimuli and active up to the presentation of the deviant tone, seems to be inherently involved in the MMF generation. This trace can be regarded as a memory that stores the physical features of the stimulus. In our model of the MMF generation, the synaptic contacts between the neurons in feature maps and the hypothetical change neurons can be regarded as an adaptive filter which is constantly updated according to the incoming stimuli. Short-term history of the stimulation affects the properties of this filter.

MMF recordings suggest that this trace is located in the supratemporal auditory cortex, although in a more frontal location than the feature maps whose activation probably underlie N100m generation. This finding is well in accord with lesion studies showing that although the auditory cortex is not necessary for conventional auditory discrimination, it is important in tasks demanding delayed discrimination based on the memory of previous stimuli.[48] Interestingly, the two features of the trace revealed by the mismatch response—independence of attention and accurate representation of the physical stimulus features—are the main determinants of the short-duration auditory memory often called the echoic memory.[49] Sensory auditory memory and the trace probed by MMF share common properties: passiveness, specificity to auditory stimulus features, and modality specificity. Therefore, the trace reflected by MMF generation might serve as the neural basis for auditory sensory memory.[50]

Mäntysalo and Näätänen[51] attempted to estimate the duration of the memory trace underlying MMN by varying the ISI. A significant MMN was elicited by 1150 Hz deviants (standards 950 Hz) with ISIs up to 2 s but not with longer ISIs. However, Näätänen et al.[52] were able to record a significant frequency MMN (standard 600 Hz, deviant 625 Hz) with an ISI of 4 s. We have recorded MMF with much longer ISIs. FIGURE 7 shows the responses to standards and deviants, as well as the corresponding difference waveforms. Standard stimuli were pairs of identical tones (1000 Hz, 50 ms, 80 dB SPL), separated by 25 ms. In the deviant pairs, the second tone was of 1200 Hz. The deviants elicited a conspicuous MMF at every ISI. After an initial drop in amplitude from 0.75 to 3 s by about 30%, the amplitude remained at a rather constant level. Interestingly, a MMF was elicited even at the ISI of 12 s. In our recent study with frequency deviants, we recorded a significant MMF at 9-s ISI.[53] These results suggest that the duration of the passive sensory auditory memory is about 10 s. Previous estimates, based on behavioral experiments, have ranged from a few hundred milliseconds up to tens of seconds.[54] The discrepancy between our estimate and that of Mäntysalo and Näätänen[51] might be due to the stimulus types used; it is reasonable to assume that the duration of the sensory memory is dependent on the stimulus material.

CONCLUSIONS AND FUTURE PERSPECTIVES

The reviewed results show that MEG can serve as an effective tool in the study of neural mechanisms of human auditory information processing and can be used in building a bridge between the behavioral description of auditory performance and its neural basis. Although we are still far from understanding the detailed neural events underlying the MEG and EEG responses, it is already time to realize that the neural events underlying these responses, not peaks and bumps of the waveforms, are to be correlated with performance.

The new branch of neuroscience, neural computing, seems to be promising in providing us with tools to study the activity in neural networks (see, for example, Kohonen[55]). While the last few decades were full of enthusiasm about the perspectives provided by single-unit recordings in brain research, it is now broadly accepted that the spatially organized maps of neurons are probably more relevant analysis units of cortical organization than single neurons.[45,55] The concept of a neural network is especially useful in describing activity underlying such mass responses as MEG.

The strongest feature of MEG is its ability to locate accurately and noninvasively brain activity under rather normal circumstances. It would be challenging to study the role and sequential activation of different cortical areas under performance which

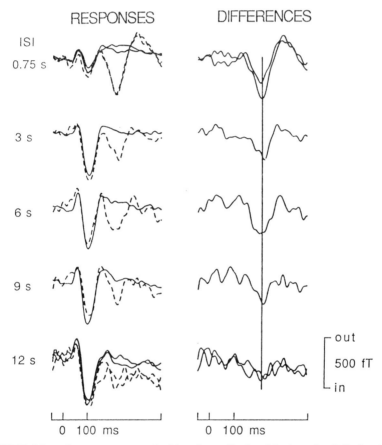

FIGURE 7. Magnetic responses to standard (*continuous lines*) and deviant stimuli (*broken lines*) and the corresponding difference waveforms (deviant or standard) at different ISIs. Recordings are from posterior temporal area in one subject. The responses from two experiments at the ISIs of 0.75 and 12 s show the replicability of our data. MMF peaking at about 220 ms is elicited at every ISI.

demands, for example, processing of both auditory and visual information. This type of experiments will surely become possible with the development of multichannel instruments with 100-200 detectors in a helmet covering the whole scalp. It is our conviction that MEG studies of healthy, alert subjects will significantly contribute to the understanding of the neural basis of human mental activity.

ACKNOWLEDGMENTS

We thank Dr. Lea Leinonen and Prof. Olli V. Lounasmaa for comments on the manuscript.

REFERENCES

1. KELHÄ, V. O., J. M. PUKKI, R. S. PELTONEN, A. J. PENTTINEN, R. J. ILMONIEMI & J. J. HEINO. 1982. Design, construction, and performance of a large volume magnetic shield. IEEE Trans. Magn. **18:** 260-270.
2. ILMONIEMI, R., R. HARI & K. REINIKAINEN. 1984. A four-channel SQUID magnetometer for brain research. Electroencephalogr. Clin. Neurophysiol. **58:** 467-473.
3. WILLIAMSON, S. J., M. PELIZZONE, Y. OKADA, D. B. KAUFMAN & J. R. MARSDEN. 1985. Five channel SQUID installation for unshielded neuromagnetic measurements. *In* Biomagnetism: Applications & Theory. H. Weinberg, G. Stroink & T. Katila, Eds.: 46-51. Pergamon. New York, NY.
4. KNUUTILA, J., S. AHLFORS, A. AHONEN, J. HÄLLSTRÖM, M. KAJOLA, O. V. LOUNASMAA, C. TESCHE & V. VILKMAN. 1987. A large-area low-noise seven-channel DC SQUID magnetometer for brain research. Rev. Sci. Instrum. **58:** 2145-2156.
5. KAJOLA, M., S. AHLFORS, G. J. EHNHOLM, J. HÄLLSTRÖM, M. S. HÄMÄLÄINEN, R. J. ILMONIEMI, M. KIVIRANTA, J. KNUUTILA, O. V. LOUNASMAA, C. D. TESCHE & V. VILKMAN. 1989. A 24-channel magnetometer for brain research. *In* Advances in Biomagnetism. S. J. Williamson, M. Hoke, G. Stroink & M. Kotani, Eds.: 673-676. Plenum Press. New York, NY.
6. GUDDEN, F., E. HOENIG, H. REICHENBERGER, R. SCHITTENHELM & S. SCHNEIDER. 1989. A multi-channel system for use in biomagnetic diagnosis in neurology and cardiology: Principle, method and initial results. Electromedica **57:** 2-7.
7. TIIHONEN, J., R. HARI & M. HÄMÄLÄINEN. 1989. Early deflections of cerebral magnetic responses to median nerve stimulation. Electroencephalogr. Clin. Neurophysiol. **74:** 270-276.
8. HARI, R. & R. J. ILMONIEMI. 1986. Cerebral magnetic fields. CRC Crit. Rev. Biomed. Eng. **14:** 93-126.
9. HARI, R. 1990. The neuromagnetic method in the study of the human auditory cortex. *In* Auditory Evoked Magnetic Fields and Potentials, Advances in Audiology. F. Grandori, M. Hoke & G. L. Romani, Eds.: 222-282. Karger. Basel.
10. MITZDORF, U. 1985. Current source-density method and application in cat cerebral cortex: Investigation of evoked potentials and EEG phenomena. Physiol. Rev. **65:** 37-100.
11. HARI, R. & O. V. LOUNASMAA. 1989. Recording and interpretation of cerebral magnetic fields. Science **244:** 432-436.
12. HARI, R., K. REINIKAINEN, E. KAUKORANTA, M. HÄMÄLÄINEN, R. ILMONIEMI, A. PENTTINEN, J. SALMINEN & D. TESZNER. 1984. Somatosensory evoked magnetic fields from SI and SII in man. Electroencephalogr. Clin. Neurophysiol. **57:** 254-263.
13. HARI, R., H. HÄMÄLÄINEN, M. HÄMÄLÄINEN, J. KEKONI, M. SAMS & J. TIIHONEN. 1990. Separate finger representations at the human second somatosensory cortex. Neuroscience **37:** 245-249.
14. YAMAMOTO, T., S. J. WILLIAMSON, L. KAUFMAN, C. NICHOLSON & R. LLINAS. 1988. Magnetic localization of neuronal activity in the human brain. Proc. Natl. Acad. Sci. USA **85:** 8732-8736.
15. HARI, R., S. L. JOUTSINIEMI & J. SARVAS. 1988. Spatial resolution of neuromagnetic records: Theoretical calculations in a spherical model. Electroencephalogr. Clin. Neurophysiol. **71:** 64-72.
16. PANTEV, C., M. HOKE, K. LEHNERTZ, B. LÜTKENHÖNER, G. ANOGIANAKIS & W. WITTKOWSKI. 1988. Tonotopic organization of the human auditory cortex revealed by transient

auditory evoked magnetic fields. Electroencephalogr. Clin. Neurophysiol. 69: 160-170.

17. BRUGGE, J. F. & R. A. REALE. 1985. Auditory cortex. In Cerebral Cortex. Vol. 4. Association and Auditory Cortices. A. Peters & E. G. Jones, Eds.: 229-271. Plenum Press. New York, NY.

18. NÄÄTÄNEN, R. 1988. Implications of ERP data to psychological theories of attention. Biol. Psychol. 26: 117-163.

19. HARI, R., M. HÄMÄLÄINEN, E. KAUKORANTA, J. MÄKELÄ, S. L. JOUTSINIEMI & J. TIIHONEN. 1989. Selective listening modifies activity of the human auditory cortex. Exp. Brain Res. 74: 463-470.

20. MÄKELÄ, J. & R. HARI. 1990. Long-latency auditory evoked magnetic fields. In Magnetoencephalography: Clinical Applications and Comparison of EEG. S. Sato, Ed. Raven Press. New York, NY.

21. MÄKELÄ, J. 1988. Contra- and ipsilateral auditory stimuli produce different activation patterns at the human auditory cortex. A neuromagnetic study. Pflügers Arch. 412: 12-16.

22. HARI, R., K. KAILA, T. KATILA, T. TUOMISTO & T. VARPULA. 1982. Interstimulus-interval dependence of the auditory vertex response and its magnetic counterpart: Implications for their neural generation. Electroencephalogr. Clin. Neurophysiol. 54: 561-569.

23. HARI, R., M. PELIZZONE, J. P. MÄKELÄ, J. HÄLLSTRÖM, L. LEINONEN & O. V. LOUNASMAA. 1987. Neuromagnetic responses of the human auditory cortex to on- and offsets of noise bursts. Audiology 25: 31-43.

24. LOVELESS, N., R. HARI, M. HÄMÄLÄINEN & J. TIIHONEN. 1989. Evoked responses of human auditory cortex may be enhanced by preceding stimuli. Electroencephalogr. Clin. Neurophysiol. 74: 217-227.

25. JOUTSINIEMI, S., R. HARI & V. VILKMAN. 1989. Cerebral magnetic responses to noise bursts and pauses of different durations. Audiology 28: 325-333.

26. CURTIS, S., L. KAUFMAN & S. WILLIAMSON. 1987. Divided attention revised: Selection based on location and pitch. In Biomagnetism '87. M. Kotani, S. Ueno, T. Katila & S. J. Williamson, Eds.: 138-141. University Press, Tokyo.

27. PELIZZONE, M., R. HARI, J. MÄKELÄ, E. KAUKORANTA & P. MONTANDON. 1986. Activation of the auditory cortex by cochlear stimulation in a deaf patient. Neurosci. Lett. 68: 192-196.

28. HARI, R., M. PELIZZONE, J. MÄKELÄ, J. HÄLLSTRÖM, J. HUTTUNEN & J. KNUUTILA. 1988. Neuromagnetic responses from a deaf subject to stimuli presented through a multichannel cochlear prosthesis. Ear Hear. 9: 148-152.

29. LEINONEN, L. & S. JOUTSINIEMI. 1989. Auditory evoked potentials and magnetic fields in patients with lesions of the auditory cortex. Acta Neurol. Scand. 79: 316-325.

30. NÄÄTÄNEN, R., A. W. K. GAILLARD & S. MÄNTYSALO. 1978. Early selective attention effect reinterpreted. Acta Psychol. 42: 313-329.

31. NÄÄTÄNEN, R., P. PAAVILAINEN, K. REINIKAINEN & M. SAMS. 1987. The mismatch negativity to intensity changes in an auditory stimulus sequence. Electroencephalogr. Clin. Neurophysiol. Suppl. 40: 125-131.

32. NORDBY, H., W. T. ROTH & A. PFEFFERBAUM. 1988. Event-related potentials to time-deviant and pitch-deviant tones. Psychophysiology 25: 249-261.

33. NORDBY, H., T. W. ROTH & A. PFEFFERBAUM. 1988. Event-related potentials to breaks in sequences of alternating pitches or interstimulus intervals. Psychophysiology 25: 262-268.

34. PAAVILAINEN, P., M. KARLSSON, K. REINIKAINEN & R. NÄÄTÄNEN. 1989. Mismatch negativity to changes in the spatial location of an auditory stimulus. Electroencephalogr. Clin. Neurophysiol. 73: 129-141.

35. AALTONEN, O., P. NIEMI, T. NYRKE & M. TUHKANEN. 1987. Event-related brain potentials and the perception of a phonetic continuum. Biol. Psychol. 24: 197-207.

36. HARI, R., M. HÄMÄLÄINEN, R. ILMONIEMI, E. KAUKORANTA, K. REINIKAINEN, J. SALMINEN, K. ALHO, R. NÄÄTÄNEN & M. SAMS. 1984. Responses of the primary auditory cortex to pitch changes of tone pips: Neuromagnetic recordings in man. Neurosci. Lett. 50: 127-132.

37. SAMS, M., M. HÄMÄLÄINEN, A. ANTERVO, E. KAUKORANTA, K. REINIKAINEN & R. HARI. 1985. Cerebral neuromagnetic responses evoked by short auditory stimuli. Electroencephalogr. Clin. Neurophysiol. 61: 254-266.

38. SAMS, M., P. PAAVILAINEN, K. ALHO & R. NÄÄTÄNEN. 1985. Auditory frequency discrimination and event-related potentials. Electroencephalogr. Clin. Neurophysiol. **62:** 437-448.
39. KAUKORANTA, E., M. SAMS, R. HARI, M. HÄMÄLÄINEN & R. NÄÄTÄNEN. 1989. Reactions of human auditory cortex to changes in tone duration. Hearing Res. **41:** 15-22.
40. SAMS, M., E. KAUKORANTA, R. NÄÄTÄNEN & M. HÄMÄLÄINEN. 1991. Cortical activity elicited by changes in auditory stimuli: Different sources for the magnetic N100m and mismatch responses. Psychophysiology. In press.
41. HARI, R., J. RIF, J. TIIHONEN, S. T. LU & M. SAMS. 1990. Effects of infrequent changes of spectral and periodicity pitch on the activity of human auditory cortex. Submitted.
42. SAMS, M. & J. KNUUTILA. 1989. Unpublished observations.
43. VINOGRADOVA, O. S. 1975. The hippocampus and the orienting reflex. In Neuronal Mechanisms of the Orienting Reflex. E. N. Sokolov & O. S. Vinogradova, Eds.: 128-154. Lawrence Erlbaum. Hillsdale, NJ.
44. SOKOLOV, E. N. 1975. The neural mechanisms of the orienting reflex. In Neuronal Mechanisms of the Orienting Reflex. E. N. Sokolov & O. S. Vinogradova, Eds.: 217-235. Lawrence Erlbaum. Hillsdale, NJ.
45. SUGA, N. 1988. Auditory neuroethology and speech processing: Complex-sound processing by combination-sensitive neurons. In Auditory Function: Neurobiological Basis of Hearing. G. M. Edelman, W. E. Gall & W. M. Cowan, Eds.: 679-720. John Wiley. New York, NY.
46. SUGA, N. 1988. What does single-unit analysis in the auditory cortex tell us about information processing in the auditory system. In Neurobiology of Neocortex. P. Rakic & W. Singer, Eds.: 331-350. John Wiley. New York, NY.
47. KONISHI, M., T. T. TAKAHASHI, H. WAGNER, W. E. SULLIVAN & C. E. CARR. 1988. Neurophysiological and anatomical substrates of sound localization in the owl. In Auditory Function. Neurobiological Bases of Hearing. G. M. Edelman, W. E. Gall & W. M. Cowan, Eds.: 721-745. John Wiley. New York, NY.
48. WHITFIELD, I. C. 1985. The role of auditory cortex in behavior. In Cerebral Cortex. Vol. 4. Association and Auditory Cortices. A. Peters & E. G. Jones, Eds.: 329-349. Plenum Press. New York, NY.
49. CROWDER, R. G. 1976. Principles of Learning and Memory. Lawrence Erlbaum. Hillsdale, NJ.
50. NÄÄTÄNEN, R. 1984. In search for short-duration memory trace of a stimulus in the human brain. In Human Action and Personality. L. Pulkkinen & P. Lyytinen, Eds.: 22-36. University of Jyväskylä. Jyväskylä, Finland.
51. MÄNTYSALO, S. & R. NÄÄTÄNEN. 1987. Duration of a neuronal trace of an auditory stimulus as indicated by event-related potentials. Biol. Psychol. **24:** 183-195.
52. NÄÄTÄNEN, R., P. PAAVILAINEN, K. ALHO, K. REINIKAINEN & M. SAMS. 1987. Interstimulus interval and the mismatch negativity. In Evoked Potentials III. C. Barber & T. Blum, Eds.: 392-397. Butterworths. London.
53. SAMS, M., R. HARI, J. RIF & J. KNUUTILA. 1991. The human auditory sensory memory trace persists about 10 s: Neuromagnetic evidence. Submitted.
54. COWAN, N. 1984. On short and long auditory stores. Psychol. Bull. **96:** 341-370.
55. KOHONEN, T. 1988. Self-organization and Associative Memory. Springer. Berlin.

Applications of Magnetoencephalography to the Study of Cognition[a]

ANDREW C. PAPANICOLAOU,[b]
ROBERT L. ROGERS, AND STEPHEN B. BAUMANN

Division of Neurosurgery
The University of Texas Medical Branch
Galveston, Texas 77550

INTRODUCTION

Relating or reducing cognitive operations to various aspects of cerebral physiology has been an abiding aspiration and preoccupation of psychology throughout its history. Specific hypotheses relating cognitive processes to variations in cerebral blood supply, temperature, or metabolism and utilization of particular substances such as phosphorus were vigorously pursued since the last century in European laboratories. William James has summarized in his *Principles* these early endeavors that constitute testimonials to human ingenuity grappling with problems beyond the reach of the then available technology.[1]

In our times we have witnessed the arrival of a host of technologies that have gradually unveiled many facets of the previously occult workings of the cerebral machinery: electrophysiology (EEG) and evoked potentials (EPs), regional cerebral blood flow (rCBF), single photon emission computed tomography (SPECT), positron emission tomography (PET) and, more recently, magnetoencephalography (MEG). The availability of these procedures has certainly reinvigorated the long-standing aspirations and has suggested even more specific queries regarding the dependence of cognitive operations on neurophysiological processes. These queries, however varied and numerous, address, nevertheless, the following smaller set of basic and general issues:

1. Are there any indices of brain activity that can disambiguate and constrain abstract cognitive models—indices, that is, that would help specify what component operations intervene between presentation of a cognitive challenge and execution of the overt responses that constitute its resolution?
2. What brain regions are engaged in a particular cognitive operation or a set of operations required for the adequate handling of specific cognitive tasks, and in what order?

[a] Supported by a grant from the Moody Foundation and a grant from the Mobility Foundation.
[b] To whom correspondence should be sent.

3. Of what precisely does the "engagement" of particular areas to particular cognitive operations consist? Or, in other terms, to what aspect of cerebral physiology do the abstractly conceived cognitive operations correspond?
4. Can such indices of cognitive, operation-specific cerebral engagement be used to assess independently levels of performance? Or, can they be used to assess physiologic limitations of cognitive processing capacity?
5. Can such indices be used for accurate diagnosis of specific cognitive deficits— to reveal, that is, a breakdown of specific component operations that accounts for deficient overt performance in complex and multifaceted tasks such as reading or finding directions in a map?

Adequate treatment of these interrelated questions depends, in part, on the availability of adequate models of cognition, but it also requires that functional imaging procedures possess certain characteristics. Three such characteristics are indispensable in view of what is presently known about cognitive processes on the one hand and neurophysiological processes on the other:

1. Given the rapidity of information processing as testified by overt performance and by the speed with which events in the nervous system transpire, it is necessary that the functional imaging procedures have high temporal resolution.
2. Given the high probability that a number of functional units in the brain, whether adjacent or distant, are successively, simultaneously or quasi-simultaneously activated during a given cognitive operation or set of operations, the imaging procedures must possess considerable spatial resolution if they are to distinguish the contributions of the various functional cerebral units in the operation or operations at hand.
3. It is also desirable, from a pragmatic point of view, that the imaging procedures interfere minimally with either cerebral physiology and structure or with the conduct of the cognitive task. That is, the procedures must be as noninvasive as possible, both in the sense of not impacting injury and in the sense of not compromising the ecological validity of the experimental setting.

None of the existing functional imaging procedures meets all three requirements equally. Electrophysiological procedures that possess the highest temporal resolution are quite limited in terms of spatial detail. Metabolic imaging procedures, on the other hand, are quite satisfactory in terms of spatial resolution, but they lack in temporal resolution and are quite cumbersome, if not invasive, in their application.

MEG, however, appears to offer a good compromise between EEG and metabolic imaging procedures. It equals electrophysiology in temporal resolution and, under certain circumstances, approaches and even surpasses the spatial resolution of the metabolic imaging procedures. As for ease of application, it is at present somewhat more demanding than electrophysiology, yet not as cumbersome as PET, SPECT, or rCBF.

The advantages and limitations of MEG have been described in some detail elsewhere in this volume; therefore, they need not be reiterated here. At this point suffice it to say that MEG is a procedure that meets all three requirements listed above to a degree sufficient to warrant its utilization in studies of cognition.

Yet such studies are still very rare in the literature. Their relative scarcity, however, does not reflect the limits of the potential usefulness of MEG. Rather, it appears to reflect temporary limitations imposed by the following logistic factors. First, there are few MEG laboratories worldwide. Second, most of those laboratories have been established very recently. Third, as with most new technologies and procedures in physiology and medicine, the bulk of initial research efforts is directed towards (1) improving the measuring instruments, (2) establishing normative data bases regarding the nature of the main dependent measure (in this case spontaneous fields or sensory evoked fields, which are the counterparts of the EEG and of EPs, respectively), and (3) exploring the clinical utility of the new technology (in this case mainly the efficacy of MEG in estimating the locus of epileptogenic foci).

SPONTANEOUS MAGNETOENCEPHALOGRAPHY

The few MEG studies that have already been reported are modeled after experimental designs used in electrophysiological research. As such they can be grouped into three types.

The first involves observation of fluctuations in spontaneous activity generated in specific brain regions that is associated with performance in cognitive tasks, in an attempt to identify whether and to what degree the region in question mediates the cognitive operations required by the task. The work of Kaufman et al.[2] is a fine example of the use of spontaneous magnetoencephalographic activity to address a cognitive issue. The issue they addressed was whether mental images of objects are akin to actual percepts—specifically, whether they involve activation of the visual system, as does the process of visual perception, or whether they are propositional in nature, consisting of nonsensory, abstract features. If the latter is the case, the visual system may not be engaged during their creation or manipulation.

Regional cerebral engagement during cognitive tasks has been assessed on the basis of blockage or relative suppression of the alpha rhythms in EEG recordings over the engaged region versus other, less engaged regions. Hemispheric differences during a variety of cognitive tasks have been assessed in this manner.[3-7] Inferences from relative alpha reduction or enhancement of higher EEG frequencies over a hemisphere or smaller cerebral region about the engagement of that hemisphere or region in the cognitive task can be hazardous because they entail the tacit assumption that activity recorded over a given region is activity generated predominantly in that region. This assumption can often be incorrect in view of the fact that activity recorded at any scalp site is due to volume-conducted currents that may originate in brain sites distal to the scalp recording site. The inference becomes even more problematic in cases where the source of a particular type of spontaneous activity is not independently known and where the brain area presumably engaged is quite restricted, as is indeed the case of the visual cortex.

The advantage of MEG in this connection is that the source of the spontaneous alpha activity can be estimated, and reduction of alpha produced at that specific source can be assessed during the specific cognitive task of interest. This advantage was exploited by Kaufman et al.[2] who presented their subjects with a sequence of random polygon shapes, instructing them to remember these shapes in order to compare them with a "probe" shape presented later. One second following the presentation of a series of three polygons a warning signal appeared, remained on the screen for two seconds, and was then substituted by the "probe" or test polygon. Subjects were instructed to either press a button as soon as the probe stimulus appeared independent of whether that stimulus was a member of the set previously shown (simple reaction time task), or to press one button if the probe was a member of the set and a different button if it was not (choice reaction time task). The former task does not require comparison of the probe stimulus with memory images of the previously presented polygons whereas the latter does.

The magnetic field over the occipital and parietal regions was sampled during the period preceding and following presentation of the "probe" stimulus. The fluctuation of alpha power content of the field over the entire epoch was calculated during the simple and choice reaction time tasks, and the locus of the alpha activity source was estimated to lie near the longitudinal fissure. Suppression of alpha power was observed following presentation of the probe stimulus, as compared to the pre-stimulus baseline during both tasks. However, during the choice reaction time task that calls for comparison of a percept to visual images, suppression of alpha was prolonged. It is important to note that the activity suppressed was demonstrably produced in the visual cortex, that is, the region mediating visual perception, rather than in other possible alpha sources. Thus the experiment constitutes a demonstration of the involvement of the visual cortex in the manipulation of visual images.

PROBE MAGNETIC EVOKED FIELDS

In a second type of MEG applications, indirect use has been made of magnetoencephalographic activity, in this case evoked rather than spontaneous, with the goal of establishing whether and to what degree particular brain areas are engaged in specific cognitive operations. This MEG application is also modeled after the electrophysiological EP probe procedure.[8-10] This procedure involves recording of EPs to sensory stimuli, over both hemispheres, during a control condition where the subjects are instructed to attend to those stimuli and during cognitive tasks where the subjects are instructed to ignore them and engage exclusively in the cognitive operations demanded by the task. The procedure is grounded on the premise that the information processing required by the cognitive task will compromise the efficiency of neuronal systems in processing the concurrent, task-irrelevant probe stimulus. In several experiments it has been demonstrated that the amplitude of the probe EPs is suppressed to a greater degree over the left hemisphere during linguistic tasks. Alternatively, during visuospatial and affective tasks, probe EP suppression is greater over the right hemisphere.[11-15] The degree of task-specific suppression of the probe stimulus in a hemisphere has been interpreted as an index of engagement of that hemisphere in the relevant cognitive task. This interpretation rests on the fundamental assumption that probe EPs recorded over a hemisphere are, in fact, generated in that hemisphere. Yet volume conduction and reference problems associated with EP recordings render that assumption questionable.[14] One MEG study[15] demonstrated the viability of that assumption by replicating previous probe EP results using probe magnetic evoked fields (MEFs), the source of which was confined to the temporal region of each hemisphere.

The experiment consisted of two parts. In the first part MEFs to a tone probe stimulus were recorded over both hemispheres, and the source location of the N1m and P2m components of the MEFs was estimated, on the basis of isofield maps, to fall in the vicinity of the auditory area of each hemisphere. In the second part, in addition to the tones, subjects were presented with a set of materials, tape-recorded in a language unfamiliar to them, which contained 30 target sounds, tokens of the phonological complex /na/. During a control condition the subjects were instructed to ignore the unintelligible verbal material and attend to the probe stimulus, whereas during the task condition they were to ignore the probe and try to detect and count the phonological target items embedded in the verbal material. MEFs to the probe stimulus were obtained from the previously established field maxima over both hemispheres. Subsequently the amplitude of the N1m and P2m in each hemisphere during the two conditions were compared. It was found that the N1m component amplitude was suppressed equally in both hemispheres during the phonological task, whereas the amplitude of the P2m component was significantly more suppressed in the left hemisphere. These results corroborate previous EP findings regarding task- and hemisphere-specific suppression of probe responses. Since the hemisphere-specific source of each probe response was not simply assumed (as in the case of EPs) but directly established, the explanation of their reduction in terms of degree of task-specific hemispheric engagement becomes more credible.

INFORMATION PROCESSING AND MEF COMPONENTS

A third type of MEG studies, modeled, once again, after electrophysiological paradigms, has also been conducted, with the intention to show direct cognitive, operation-specific changes of MEFs. These range from attempts to establish differences in MEFs and their source characteristics to speech versus non-speech stimuli, to attempts to investigate MEF changes to attended versus non-attended stimuli, and to attempts at recording establishing the source of late MEF components such as the P3m, which is the equivalent of the P3 component of EPs and is believed to reflect higher, cognitive processing of special stimuli.

Several preliminary attempts to investigate differences in brain responses to various speech versus non-speech sounds have been reported. For example, in one experiment[16] MEFs to the word /hei/ and to noise bursts were recorded from seven subjects. MEFs to the tone bursts were characterized by the N1m and P2m components with latencies of 100 and 200 msec, respectively. However, at the same latencies, the MEFs to the speech sound featured two components of the same polarity, namely, N1m and N2m. This peculiar MEF waveform to the word was interpreted by the authors as possibly indicative of a feature detection process specific to speech stimuli.

Yet such peculiar MEFs to speech sounds were not obtained in another study.[17] Rather, these authors obtained waveforms similar to those evoked by tonal stimuli featuring both the N1m and the P2m components. Nevertheless, the source location of the N1m component of MEFs varied for the different speech sounds used (i.e., /a/, /ka/, /ba/, and /pa/). According to the authors, this suggests that the different phonological features of the initial consonants activate different neural units in the auditory cortex.

The discrepancy of the raw MEF waveforms obtained in the two studies makes it difficult to decide whether different sources in the auditory cortex are responsible for the N1m component to non-speech and various speech stimuli, or simply, whether the locus of the N1m component source varies slightly as a function of the purely physical or acoustic features of the stimuli.

Variation in the N1m as well as in later MEF components as a function of attention to the evoking stimulus has also been reported.[18-21] In general, the N1m and/or the P2m to attended stimuli, whether visual or auditory, are higher in amplitude than those of non-attended stimuli. In that sense the MEG studies corroborate EP findings regarding enhancement of brain responses to "selected" versus "rejected" channels.[22]

A greater challenge faced by MEG investigators has been the identification of the source of the P3 component. This is a late positive component of EPs to rare or unpredictable stimuli with an approximate latency of 300 msec and constitutes a unique and striking feature of EPs to such special stimulus events. Unlike earlier components, common to both rare and frequent stimuli, the P3 changes less readily as a function of the physical parameters of the evoking stimuli, and it can be obtained in all sensory modalities. These attributes of the P3 have led to the notion that it represents higher, cognitive processing of unique stimulus events and to the correlated notion that its source must be outside the modality-specific sensory cortices, most likely in the hippocampi.

The P3 waveform can be recorded electrically from a variety of scalp locations; it is usually maximal in amplitude near the vertex and increases in latency at more posterior scalp locations. Depth recordings in neurosurgical patients have shown that a P3 response can be obtained from the vicinity of the hippocampus.[23-24] However, these intracranially recorded signals are not the same as those obtained from scalp recordings, making direct comparisons difficult.

Okada and associates[25] were the first to use magnetoencephalography in an attempt to localize the source of the P3 noninvasively. A visual oddball task was employed using sinusoidal gratings of 2 cycles/degree for the frequent stimulus (0.8 probability) and 1 or 1.7 cycles/degree for the rare stimulus (0.2 probability). Using a single-channel SQUID system, MEFs to these stimuli were recorded over the entire head surface in two subjects. EPs were also recorded simultaneously at the vertex and showed an N2 at about 300 msec and a P3 at about 450 msec. Such long latencies were thought to be caused by the difficulty in discriminating similar stimuli. The P3m component showed a reversal only on the right side of the head for both subjects. Contour maps, showing the extrema, were prepared from data filtered between 2-10 Hz and interpolated. Superimposition of fields from two dipoles in the occipital regions made interpretation of the data more difficult. Using a generic brain atlas, the authors estimated that the P3m source was located in the posterior portion of the hippocampal formation in both subjects.

Okada[26] also reported difficulties in an attempt to localize the source of the auditory P3m, chiefly due to the fact that the maximum extremum of the P3m could not be found, although the minimum was found above the temporal region of the scalp.

Another group of investigators, Gordon *et al.,*[27] were apparently more successful in localizing the source of the auditory P3m component. They used an oddball paradigm in which tone bursts of either 1.5 kHz (frequent) or 2 kHz (rare) were presented binaurally at 80 dB SPL and at 1-sec intervals. The frequent stimulus appeared with a probability of .85 and the rare with a probability of .15. Using a single-channel SQUID system, MEFs were recorded at 28 locations over the right hemisphere in two subjects. Simultaneously recorded electric signals from the vertex showed a P3 occurring near 300 msec. Magnetic signals were bandpassed 1-20 Hz and showed a P3m peak near 375 msec. Signals near the minima were of much greater amplitude than those near the maxima. The disparity in latency between the electric and magnetic P3 components was explained as the result of the magnetic signals being passed through an additional bandpass filter. However, such filtering would only be expected to alter the latency a few milliseconds at the most. For one subject, the P3m source was determined to be in the temporal lobe 2.7 cm deep and 2 mm posterior to area T4. Similar, but not specified, results were reportedly obtained from a second subject.

All three aforementioned studies suffer from the problem of generalizing on the basis of data obtained from extremely small numbers of subjects. However, the recent introduction of multiple-sensor SQUID systems has made it easier to study larger numbers of subjects. Taking advantage of this technological improvement, Lewine *et al.*[28] utilized a seven-channel system to record the P3m from both visual and auditory stimuli in 13 subjects. A complex protocol was used involving several manipulations designed to balance differences in responses to rare and frequent visual and auditory stimuli. In all subjects electric recordings were made at Fz, Cz, and Pz. In nine subjects magnetic field measurements were made at 56 locations over each hemisphere, and for four subjects in whom the electric or magnetic P3 was missing or was of poor quality, over the left hemisphere only. Auditory P3 peak latencies occurred at 280-330 msec for both the electric and magnetic responses. P3 peak latencies for the visual stimulus occurred later, at 380-450 msec. Reversal of the P3m component occurred in at least two subjects. Contour maps for these two subjects showed multiple extrema over each hemisphere. A high degree of interhemispheric and intersubject variability was observed in the position and amplitude of the response at the extema, and the authors caution that this may indicate that either multiple sources or a common extended structure is responsible for generating the P3m component. In any event, the authors concluded that the sources for the auditory and visual P3m are possibly located within the hippocampus.

Although none of the above studies used structural imaging (CT scans or MRIs) to localize precisely the P3m source in each individual, they all made attempts to describe its location in generic head models. Moreover, there is a discrepancy between the findings of Okada et al.[25] and Lewine et al.[28] on the one hand, and those of Gordon et al.[27] on the other. The former two point to the hippocampus as the likely P3m source for both visual and auditory responses, and the latter to the temporal cortex, at least in the case of the auditory response.

These inconsistencies prompted us to make yet another attempt to record clear MEF waveforms containing the P3m component and to identify subsequently its source in eight normal subjects. (The study was recently completed and is not yet published.) We employed the standard auditory oddball paradigm involving presentation of a frequent, 1-kHz tone and a rare, 2-kHz tone with probabilities of 0.8 and 0.2, respectively, at a rate of 1/sec. The stimuli were delivered through insert earphones to the left ear while continuous white noise was channeled to the right ear. EPs to both tones were recorded from Cz while MEFs were simultaneously recorded over the right hemisphere as well as in occipital, midline sites.

We obtained clear MEFs to the rare tone containing a pronounced P3m component in all eight subjects within the latency range in which the P3 component of the EPs appeared. Moreover, unlike the EPs to the frequent tone, which did not contain a P3 component, MEFs to the frequent tone featured a P3m response in six of the eight subjects. Isofield maps at successive time points ranging from 340 to 420 msec were suggestive of a series of sequentially active single dipolar sources for the P3m to both tones. Source localization attempted at these successive latencies revealed that a series of equivalent current dipoles extending in the medial to lateral direction, mostly on the floor of the Sylvian fissure, can account for the P3m to both tones.

The orientation of the dipoles to the frequent stimulus P3m was similar to that of the N1m component, whereas the orientation of the P3m dipole to the rare tone was almost at right angles to the N1m dipole and pointing towards Pz. This difference in dipole orientation may well account for the fact that EPs to frequent stimuli do not contain a P3 and that the P3m has the same "polarity" as the N1m rather than the P2m. When an equivalent dipole points towards the superior surface of the head, anywhere from Fz to Pz, the resulting EP peak will appear positive as is the case of the P2 to both tones and the P3 to the rare tones. When it points in the opposite direction, it results in negative EP peaks as is the case of the N1 to both tones and a negative peak appearing after the P2 at about 300 msec in the frequent tone EPs (that is, in the latency range where a P3 should appear). Thus the mistaken notion has emerged that frequent stimuli in the oddball paradigm do not result in late brain responses, but only rare stimuli do. The orientation of the P3m dipole also explains why in the MEF waveforms the polarity of the P3m is the same as that of the N1m, rather than the P2m.

In conclusion, this study resulted in two basic findings: (1) that the P3m occurs within the same latency range as the electrical P3, and for most of its duration can be accounted for, most readily, by a series of successively activated dipolar sources located approximately in the floor of the Sylvian fissure (where the sources of the earlier N1m and P2m components are also located) rather than in the hippocampus, and (2) that the P3m is not unique to rare stimuli. Rather, it is a feature of the brain's response to both frequent and rare stimuli. These findings may well precipitate new attempts to apply the MEG procedure to the study of cognitive processes.

Two other types of brain activity have received some attention on the part of MEG investigators, namely, the contigent negative variation (CNV) and the readiness potential that precedes voluntary movement, both of which have been obtained electro-encephalographically and have been interpreted as indices of the psychological states of orientation, arousal, anticipation, expectancy, and preparation to execute a deliberate motor act. The few preliminary MEG studies of CNV and the readiness potential were undertaken with the purpose of discovering the intracranial sources of these slow responses, a task for which electrophysiological procedures have proved to be less than sufficient. None of the MEG findings can be considered as definitive, yet all of them appear promising and intriguing. Weinberg and colleagues,[29] for example, succeeded in recording the MEF counterpart of CNV and attributed it to two intracranial sources corresponding to the early (or "orientation") and the late (or "response preparation") components of the CNV.

An MEF component corresponding to the readiness potential preceding finger movement was reported by Deecke *et al.*[30] Unlike the electrical readiness potential that can be recorded over both hemispheres, the magnetic field was restricted to the hemisphere contralateral to the moving finger, and its distribution was suggestive of a source close to the hand area in the central fissure. Deecke and associates[31] also estimated that the source of the magnetic response preceding toe movement is located in the mesial surface of the hemisphere contralateral to the moving toe. According to Deecke *et al.,*[32] complex finger-tapping movements are preceded by magnetic fields that can best be accounted for by two sources, one located in the primary motor and the other in the supplementary motor area.

CONCLUDING REMARKS

The dominant theme of most MEG applications surveyed is identification of the brain areas mediating particular cognitive operations. None of the other general issues outlined earlier in the INTRODUCTION has as yet received serious consideration.

Attempts to identify cerebral regions engaged in information processing have generally followed two basic methodological approaches, both borrowed from the electrophysiological literature. The one approach entails monitoring the spontaneous or evoked activity of a particular area, observing the changes in that activity precipitated by a concurrent cognitive task, and inferring, on the basis of such changes, the degree of engagement of that area in the cognitive task. The other approach consists in recording MEFs to stimuli presented under circumstances that induce the subject to process them in various ways, identifying those MEF components that vary with a particular type of processing, and localizing their sources in specific brain areas. Since the latter approach is more direct, it has been employed most frequently in MEG studies, though the former indirect approach may, in the long run, prove more efficient in addressing the variety of issues outlined earlier.

In view of the pragmatic constraints presently restricting the use of MEG in studies of cognition, the amount of work already accomplished leaves little doubt about the actual and potential contributions of this new, functional imaging technology to the study of neurophysiological correlates of cognitive operations.

REFERENCES

1. JAMES, W. 1980. The Principles of Psychology. Holt. New York, NY.
2. KAUFMAN, L., B. SCHWARTZ, C. SALUSTRI & S. J. WILLIAMSON. 1990. Modulation of spontaneous brain activity during mental imagery. J. Cogn. Neurosci. **2:** 124-132.
3. GLASS, A. 1964. Mental arithmetic and blocking of the occipital alpha rhythm. Electroencephalogr. Clin. Neurophysiol. **16:** 595-603.
4. BUTLER, S. R. & A. CLASS. 1974. Asymmetries in the electroencephalogram associated with cerebral dominance. Electroencephalogr. Clin. Neurophysiol. **36:** 481-491.
5. DOYLE, J. C., R. ORNSTEIN & D. GALIN. 1974. Lateral specialization of cognitive mode: EEG frequency analysis. Psychophysiology **11:** 567-578.
6. GALIN, D. & R. ORNSTEIN. 1972. Lateral specialization of cognitive mode: An EEG study. Psychophysiology **8:** 412-418.
7. PAPANICOLAOU, A. C., D. L. LORING, G. DEUTSCH & H. M. EISENBERG. 1986. Task-related EEG asymmetries: A comparison of alpha blocking and beta enhancement. Int. J. Neurosci. **30:** 81-85.
8. GALIN, D. & R. ELLIS. 1975. Asymmetry in evoked potentials as an index of lateralized cognitive processes: Relation to EEF and asymmetry. Neuropsychologia **13:** 45-50.
9. PAPANICOLAOU, A. C. 1980. Cerebral excitation profile in language processing: The photic probe paradigm. Brain Lang. **9:** 269-280.
10. PAPANICOLAOU, A. & J. JOHNSTONE. 1984. Probe evoked potentials: Theory, method and application. Int. J. Neurosci. **24:** 107-131.
11. PAPANICOLAOU, A. C., H. S. LEVIN, H. M. EISENBERG & B. D. MOORE. 1983. Evoked potential indices of selective hemispheric engagement in affective and phonetic tasks. Neuropsychologia **21:** 401-405.
12. PAPANICOLAOU, A. C., B. D. MOORE, G. DEUTSCH, H. S. LEVIN & H. M. EISENBERG. 1988. Evidence for right hemisphere involvement in recovery from aphasia. Arch. Neurol. **45:** 1025-1029.
13. PAPANICOLAOU, A. C., G. DEUTSCH, W. T. BOURBON, K. W. WILL, D. W. LORING & H. M. EISENBERG. 1987. Convergent evoked potential and cerebral blood flow evidence of task-specific hemispheric differences. Electroencephalogr. Clin. Neurophysiol. **66:** 515-520.
14. NUNEZ, P. 1981. Electrical Fields of the Brain. Oxford University Press. New York, NY.
15. PAPANICOLAOU, A. C., G. F. WILSON, C. BUSCH, P. DEREGO, C. ORR, I. DAVIS & H. M. EISENBERG. 1988. Hemispheric asymmetries in phonological processing assessed with probe evoked magnetic fields. Int. J. Neurosci. **39:** 275-281.
16. HARI, R., M. HAMALAINEN, E. KAUKORANTA, J. MAKELA, S. L. JOUTSINIEMI & J. TIIHONEN. 1989. Selective listening modifies activity of the human auditory cortex. Exp. Brain Res. **74:** 463-470.
17. KURIKI, S., M. MURASE & F. TAKEUCHI. Specificity of neuromagnetic responses in the human auditory cortex to consonants of monosyllable speech sounds. *In* Advances in Biomagnetism. L. Kaufman, S. Williamson & G. Stroink, Eds. Plenum Press. New York, NY. In press.
18. CURTIS, S., L. KAUFMAN & S. WILLIAMSON. 1987. Divided attention revisited: Selection

based on location or pitch. *In* Biomagnetism. K. Atsumi, M. Kotani, S. Veno, T. Katila & S. Williamson, Eds.: 138-141. Tokyo Denki University Press. Tokyo.

19. AINE, C., J. GEORGE & E. FLYNN. 1987. Latency differences and effects of selective attention to gratings in the central and right visual fields. *In* Biomagnetism. K. Atsumi, M. Kotani, S. Veno, T. Katila & S. Williamson, Eds.: 242-245. Tokyo Denki University Press. Tokyo.

20. ARTHUR, D., S. A. HILLYARD, E. FLYNN & A. SCHMIDT. 1989. Neural mechanisms of selective auditory attention. *In* Advances in Biomagnetism. S. J. Williamson, M. Hoke, G. Stroink & M. Kotani, Eds.: 113-116. Plenum Press. New York, NY.

21. LUBER, B., L. KAUFMAN & S. WILLIAMSON. 1989. Brain activity related to spatial analysis. *In* Advances in Biomagnetism. S. J. Williamson, M. Hoke, G. Stroink & M. Kotani, Eds.: 213-216. Plenum Press. New York, NY.

22. PICTON, T. W. & S. A. HILLYARD. 1988. Endogenous event-related potentials. *In* Human Event-Related Potentials. T. W. Picton, Ed.: 361-426. Elsevier. New York, NY.

23. McCARTHY, G., C. C. WOOD, P. D. WILLIAMSON & D. D. SPENCER. 1989. Task-dependent field potentials in human hippocampal formation. J. Neurosci. **9:** 4253-4268.

24. HALGREN, E., N. K. SQUIRES, C. S. WILSON, J. W. ROHRBAUGH, T. L. BABB & P. H. CRANDALL. 1980. Endogenous potential generated in the human hippocampal formation and amygdala by infrequent events. Science **210:** 803-805.

25. OKADA, Y. C., L. KAUFMAN & S. J. WILLIAMSON. 1983. The hippocampal formation as a source of the slow endogenous potentials. Electroencephalogr. Clin. Neurophysiol. **55:** 417-426.

26. OKADA, Y. C. 1983. Inferences concerning anatomy and physiology of the human brain based on its magnetic field. Nuovo Cimento **2(2):** 379-409.

27. GORDON, E., G. SLOGGETT, I. HARVEY, C. KRAIUHIN, C. PENNIE, C. YIANNIKAS & R. MEARES. 1987. Magnetoencephalography: Locating the source of P300 via magnetic field recording. Clin. Exp. Neurol. **23:** 101-110.

28. LEWINE, J. D., S. B. W. ROEDER, M. T. OAKEY, D. L. ARTHUR, C. J. AINE, J. S. GEORGE & E. R. FLYNN. A modality-specific in neuromagnetic P3. *In* Advances in Biomagnetism. L. Kaufman, S. Williamson & G. Stroink, Eds. Plenum Press. New York, NY. In press.

29. WEINBERG, H., P. BRICKETT, L. DEECKE & J. BOSCHERT. 1983. Slow magnetic fields of the brain preceding movements and speech. Nuovo Cimento **2:** 495-504.

30. DEECKE, L., H. WEINBERG & P. BRICKETT. 1982. Magnetic fields of the human brain accompanying voluntary movement: Bereitschaftsmagnetfeld. Exp. Brain Res. **48:** 144-148.

31. DEECKE, L., J. BOSCHERT, H. WEINBERG & P. BRICKETT. 1983. Magnetic fields of the human brain (Bereitschaftsmagnetfeld) preceding voluntary foot and toe movements. Exp. Brain Res. **52:** 81-86.

32. DEECKE, L., J. BOSCHERT, P. BRICKETT & H. WEINBERG. 1985. Magnetoencephalic evidence for possible supplementary motor area participation in human voluntary movement. *In* Biomagnetism: Application and Theory. H. Weinberg, G. Stroink & T. Katila, Eds.: 369-372. Pergamon Press. New York, NY.

Positron Emission Tomography: Basic Principles and Applications in Psychiatric Research[a]

NORA D. VOLKOW,[b,c] JONATHAN BRODIE,[d] AND
BERNARD BENDRIEM [e]

[b]*Medical Department*
Brookhaven National Laboratory
Upton, New York 11973

[c]*Department of Psychiatry*
State University of New York at Stony Brook
Stony Brook, New York 11794

[d]*Department of Psychiatry*
New York University School of Medicine
New York, New York 10016

[e]*Chemistry Department*
Brookhaven National Laboratory
Upton, New York 11973

INTRODUCTION

Positron emission tomography (PET) is a tracer technique that makes it possible to detect accurately and noninvasively *in vivo* concentrations of positron-labeled compounds.[1] Since various biological and pharmacological compounds can be labeled with positron-emitting nuclides, PET can be utilized to assess functional and biochemical regional characteristics of tissue in various organs.[2] In the brain, it provides a unique technique to quantify directly cerebral function and to monitor various biochemical pathways, receptors, and enzymes.[3] PET has already proven useful in detecting abnormalities heretofore unrecognized in patients with mental disorders.[4]

In this paper, we will first discuss the basic principles behind PET technology since this knowledge is needed in order to appreciate the potentials and limitations of PET, and then we will discuss the major applications of PET in psychiatric research.

[a]Supported by the U.S. Department of Energy under Contract No. DE-AC02-76CH000016.

BASIC PRINCIPLES OF PET

Imaging and quantitation with PET are feasible because of the unique characteristics of positron emitters. Positron emitters are unstable radionuclides that decay by positron emission. The positrons travel a short distance through tissue (mean-free path) before colliding with an electron to generate two annihilation photons (gamma rays), which are simultaneously emitted in almost opposite directions (180° angle) with an energy of 511 keV.[5] Thus, the presence of a positron is established by the simultaneous registration of these two annihilation photons by a series of radiation detectors placed in a circular fashion about the object. Photons will be registered by the PET camera only if they occur "in coincidence," that is, if they occur within the time window of the instrument (5-20 nsec) in two opposing detectors. Events that are emitted outside the volume delineated by the two coincident detectors will not be registered by the camera. This allows the location of the annihilation event within the volume delineated by the pair of coincident detectors.[6]

To optimize counting, each detector of the PET camera is operated in coincidence with several detectors. Usually these detectors are arranged around the object in multiple rings to obtain multiple images of the whole object at the same time. The radiation detectors are crystals, such as bismuth germanate, barium fluoride, cesium fluoride, sodium iodide, etc., that fluoresce when exposed to ionizing radiation. This fluorescence is converted into an electrical pulse by a photomultiplier tube that is attached to the crystal. The signals are then sent to a computer that stores the data and reconstructs it into an image.[7-9] The image represents the three-dimensional distribution of the radiocompound into the studied organ.

Isotopes and Radiopharmaceuticals

The positron emitters most commonly used for clinical PET are carbon-11, oxygen-15, fluorine-18, and nitrogen-13. These can be utilized to label almost any physiologic or radiopharmaceutical compound without altering its chemical properties. These radionuclides have short half-lives—20.4, 2.03, 110, and 9.96 min, respectively—which enable their utilization with minimal radiation exposure to a subject.[10] Another advantage of these four radionuclides is that the degradation of spatial resolution due to the distance the positron travels before colliding with an electron (mean free path) is minimal because the emitted positrons have relatively low beta energies. Since the source of the photons is localized a small distance from where the positrons are emitted, it introduces a nonreducible source of error in precise location of the order of one to two millimeters.[6]

A cyclotron is required to produce most of the radionuclides currently used in PET. Because of the short half-life of these radionuclides, the cyclotron needs to be in the vicinity of the PET camera. The radionuclides can be utilized as such as in the case of ^{15}O to measure oxygen metabolism or they can be used to label molecules as in the case of ^{18}F to label deoxyglucose. Radiotracer development is a fundamental aspect of PET methodology because biochemical assessments are based on the utilization of an appropriate tracer. The data on the distribution of the tracer within the tissue are then transformed into metabolic or biochemical information applying a mathematical model.

There are various possible tracers and various models that can be used to study a given biochemical parameter. A number of reviews address varied aspects of radiopharmaceuticals and mathematical models in PET technology.[10,11]

Positron emitters have been utilized to label various radiopharmaceutical compounds that enable measurement of metabolism, neurotransmitters, blood flow, and enzymes in the central nervous system. In the brain, major emphasis has been placed on studying regional brain metabolism, cerebral blood flow (CBF), and receptor location and concentration. Energy metabolism in the brain has been studied with glucose and oxygen as markers. The glucose analog deoxyglucose, labeled with fluorine-18 (FDG) or with carbon-11 (CDG),[12,13] has been used to identify abnormalities in glucose metabolism in patients with various neurological and psychiatric disorders.[14–18] Indeed, FDG has become the most widely used compound for PET studies. Assessment of oxygen metabolism has been done utilizing [15]O as a tracer.[19] Although it has not been used as widely as FDG, this tracer has been effective in assessing metabolism in brain tumors,[20] in ischemic tissue,[21] and in epilepsy.[22]

The techniques used to measure CBF with PET can be divided into those that utilize equilibrium models[23] versus those that utilize dynamic models.[24] Oxygen-15-labeled water has been one of the most widely utilized tracers to investigate CBF and has been administered to psychiatric and neurological patients as well as normal subjects to assess the effects of stimulation on regional activation in the brain.[25] Measurement of brain metabolism and CBF are particularly useful because these variables reflect functional activity of the nervous tissue.[26]

Assessment of neurotransmitter abnormalities is of interest in the investigation of psychiatric disorders because many of the hypotheses underlying the mechanism of these disorders implicate neurotransmitter derangement. To date, the most widely investigated neurotransmitter has been dopamine. Various compounds have been developed to study dopamine activity in the brain. The concentration of dopamine has been measured using FDG-labeled L-DOPA.[27] Dopamine receptor activity has been investigated using positron-labeled dopamine antagonists such as N-methylspiroperidol (NMSP), which has been labeled both with CDG and FDG.[28,29] Other derivatives of spiroperidol as well as haloperidol (haldol)[30] and other dopamine antagonists such as phenothiazines (chlorpromazine), benzamides (raclopride),[31,32] and clozapine[33] have been labeled with positron emitters to assess postsynaptic receptors. Nomifensine labeled with ^{11}C has been proposed to evaluate presynaptic dopamine receptors.[34] Examples of other receptors being investigated with PET include benzodiazepine,[35,36] GABA, opiates,[37] and acetylcholine.[38]

New efforts are also being developed to assess with PET other biochemical pathways in the brain, such as protein synthesis[39,40] and fatty acid metabolism.[41] Positron emitters have been synthesized to measure the concentration and turnover of individual enzymes such as the enzyme monoamine oxidase.[42]

Quantitation with PET

It is unfortunate that much of the clinical scientific literature that uses PET as a major investigative tool presents conclusions based on data acquisition and analysis in which the only critical tests applied are to the size of the sample, the magnitude of the reported effects, and the statistical significance of the conclusions. However, the validity of the tracer model, the precision and accuracy of the data acquisition, the propagation of errors in an experiment, and the assumptions used for image reconstruction and analysis are probably even more important if one is to evaluate critically the literature and reconcile the many disparate and confusing conclusions that have already been reported. In the sections that follow, we shall attempt to introduce the reader to some of these necessary concepts.

Accurate location and quantitation of positron emitters are not only limited by the mean-free path of the positrons but by certain characteristics inherent to gamma rays and the detection procedure used in PET. We will address the main variables that can influence the precision of the measurements with PET. One of them has to do with the coincidence time window of the instrument during which period of time two events are registered as coincidental; this leads to a non-null probability for two photons originating from different positrons to be detected simultaneously by accident. These detected events are "random coincidences" in contrast to "true coincidences" and represent a large portion of the total radiation detected by the detectors. Actually, the number of randoms is proportional to the square of the concentration of radioactivity as compared with the number of true counts, which is related linearly to the total concentration of radioactivity.[43] Randoms represent an important source of error in the PET image, because they decrease the contrast of the image by adding a background level of activity over the field of view. Randoms are of particular concern in the studies involving high count rates such as in studies with ^{15}O. Several mathematical corrections have been proposed to alleviate this problem.[44]

Another source of error in the quantitation of positron emitters is generated by the interactions of the photons as they travel through the tissue, which can alter the original direction of the photons as well as their energy. The most probable types of interactions of the photons are Compton scattering and attenuation.[45,46] Scattering occurs when a photon collides with a "free electron," losing part of its energy and changing its original direction. Scattering constitutes a source of error because it leads to mislocation of the positron source in the object due to assignment of incorrect lines of coincidence. The size of the error due to scattered events will depend on the concentration and distribution of radioactivity and on the characteristics of the tissue where the photons are emitted.[47] The diameter of the ring that holds the detectors (gantry) will also influence the amount of scatter. The smaller the diameter of the gantry the larger the problem with scatter.[7] Several mathematical corrections have been proposed for scatter correction.[47–49] In the brain where the morphology is characterized by an intricate pattern of areas with different tissue characteristics, scatter can introduce considerable error in regional quantitation. Failure to correct for scatter will result in blurring of boundaries among areas with degradation of contrast between regions with different amounts of radioactivity.

Another form of interaction of the photons is attenuation, which occurs when the photons interact with electrons leading to a decrease in their energy. When totally absorbed, no energy reaches the detector; thus, a reduced number of photons is registered. The degree of absorption or attenuation of the photons is dependent on the density of the tissue and can be corrected by performing a transmission scan. This is done by placing a source of positron emitters around the object and calculating the attenuation correction coefficient by obtaining the ratio of the measurement obtained from the positron source with or without the attenuation object.[7]

In evaluating images obtained with PET, it is important to consider the statistical quality of the image. Statistical variation of the radiation counts in the images is described by a Poisson distribution.[50] This distribution predicts that the noise due to the number of photons detected is related to the square root of the total number of photons. The ratio of true signal-to-noise is important because if this ratio is small, true differences in concentration of radioactivity among areas will not be detected as they will be hidden by the noise. The signal-to-noise ratio determines the number of counts that should be obtained in a given volume of tissue for an accurate quantitation. The number of counts can be increased by increasing the duration of the scanning, by delivering a higher dose of radioactivity, or by improving the sensitivity of the camera. When using compounds labeled with ^{18}F (110 min), it is feasible to increase the length of the scanning period. This translates into better quality images than the ones obtained with isotopes with shorter half-life. With ^{15}O-labeled compounds, the time of data collection is reduced by the fast decay of this isotope (121 sec), which requires the injection of higher doses of radioactivity to get a sufficient number of counts to overcome the statistical noise. The time of collection is also limited by the mathematical model employed, i.e., use of the intravenous bolus injection of H_2O for measurement of cerebral blood flow requires the scanning time be limited to 40-60 sec.[51]

Instrument Characteristics

The characteristics of the PET camera will also affect the quantitation of the positron emitters. Spatial resolution, temporal resolution, and sensitivity vary from instrument to instrument and are important in determining the precision of the measurement. Spatial resolution refers to the capacity of the camera to separate adjacent structures and resolve sharp detail. The term full-width half-maximum (FWHM) is used as a measurement of spatial resolution, and it refers to the distance separating two point sources where the number of counts is equal to half the maximum number of counts detected. Spatial resolution is important inasmuch as two sources separated by a distance equivalent to one FWHM will not be revealed as separate sources in the image. Currently, the radial resolution (in plane resolution) of PET systems used for clinical studies averages 5-6 mm. The axial resolution is the resolution obtained in the direction perpendicular to the plane of the image, and it defines the plane thickness for the image. Accurate measurement of activity in a region can only be attained if the size of the region is at least two times the resolution in all directions. Since in the brain, the regions of interest (ROI) are three-dimensional, randomly oriented, and usually smaller than two times the FWHM of the in-plane and the axial resolution[52] of current instruments, the delineation of small ROI will lead to misidentification of anatomical structures, blurring of boundaries between closely lying structures, and averaging of activities from surrounding areas outside the area of interest.

The spatial resolution of the camera is affected by the size, the number, and the arrangement of the detectors. In general, high spatial resolution can be achieved using small crystals closely packed in circular arrays. Bismuth germanate (BGO), a crystal with high density, is widely used to optimize detection efficiency and counteract the loss of sensitivity when using small crystals.[6] There is a great deal of effort under way to increase spatial resolution.

Temporal resolution refers to the speed of the camera which is determined by the number of counts it can collect without saturation of the system. This variable is very much dependent on the decay constant of the crystal. The decay constant refers to the amount of time required for a crystal to go from an excited state when it has absorbed a photon to a free state where it can again detect an event. The decay time constant of the crystal will also impose limitations on the coincidence resolving time of the instrument.[53] Time resolution becomes a pertinent variable when performing studies that involve administration of high doses of radioactivity as in the case of studies using dynamic models with ^{15}O-labeled compounds such as the intravenous bolus injection of $H_2^{15}O$ to assess CBF. An optimal dose of radioactivity needs to be delivered to obtain an adequate number of counts without saturation of the system because this would lead to underestimation of areas of high CBF.

The sensitivity of the camera refers to the ability of the system to detect as many of the true coincidences as possible for a given amount of radioactivity. The sensitivity of the camera is affected by the efficiency of the detector, which is dependent on the type and size of the crystal. The higher the atomic number of the crystal, the higher its ability to stop the photons once they hit the detector. Bismuth germanate, which has the highest density among the crystals used for PET, yields the highest detection efficiency. The larger the size of the crystal, the higher the probability of a photon interaction. On the other hand, the resolution is adversely affected by increased crystal size.

Although we have focused mainly on the crystals, there are other variables in the instrument that will affect its spatial resolution as well as its time resolution and sensitivity. For example, the electronic circuit can affect the sensitivity of the instrument because several signals have to be processed simultaneously. If there are not enough coincidence circuits in the camera, it can lead to periods where events are being registered by the detectors and not processed by the electronics. These periods of time where no events are registered are referred to as dead time and can be due to electronic circuits, the crystal, or the computers. They are important because they lead to diminished efficiency and can require the administration of higher doses of radioactivity to the patient to correct for these losses.

Image Reconstruction and Analyses

Finally, the reconstruction process and the analyses of the images will also affect the measurements obtained with PET. The computer reconstructs the image based on the measurements taken of the object at different angles by sorting the activity registered by pairs of coincident detectors for the different angles. Each measurement represents the sum of the activity in the volume of the space in between the pair of coincidence detectors. This method is similar to the one used for conventional X-ray and involves the use of the "convolution" or "filter back projection" reconstruction algorithms.[54,55] The filter utilized to reconstruct the image will affect the resolution and the noise in the image as well as its contrast and edge delineation.[56]

Once an image is obtained, the procedure to extract regional values will also affect the regional quantitation. The most common procedure is to delineate an anatomical area into the PET scan images and then obtain its average value. The size and geometry of the regions of interest will affect the quantitative values obtained. Size is important because in order to obtain adequate quantitation the dimension of the ROI should be at least twice the spatial resolution of the system. In brain studies attempting to quantify gray matter activity, this will introduce a source of error because the mean width of the cortex is 3 mm. Cortical regions will include activity from surrounding areas.[57] On the other hand, delineation of ROI with a size twice that of the spatial resolution of the instrument will lead to information from heterogeneously functional areas.[58] The shape of the region utilized to quantitate the image will also affect the values obtained. Because of the convoluted geometry of the brain, the use of squares or circles as opposed to irregular shapes increases the misidentification of structure due to averaging of activity in surrounding areas, which is known as the partial volume effect.[58]

When reviewing clinical studies with PET, it is important to realize that even similar studies differ not only in the size and shape of their ROI but also in their anatomical location within the image. Indeed, precise location of an anatomical area in a PET image is extremely difficult not only because of the lack of precise boundaries among brain areas but also because of the normal anatomical variability among individuals.[59] In general, the smaller the ROI the more imprecise its location, particularly as it approaches the resolution of the instrument.

CLINICAL APPLICATIONS IN PSYCHIATRIC RESEARCH

In the brain, PET provides a unique tool, for it allows direct evaluation of brain function and cerebral organization in a noninvasive way with far better spatial resolution and sensitivity than that obtained with other functional imaging techniques. In the case of psychiatric disorders, it is particularly useful because these disorders involve *functional* cerebral derangements that are not always detected with the available morphological imaging techniques such as CT or MRI. In fact, its utilization in psychiatric research has already proven to be of value in detecting functional and neurochemical derangements in psychiatric disorders which have heretofore gone unrecognized. Some of the initial research with PET focused on the investigation of metabolic abnormalities in schizophrenic patients. This area of investigation has now extended into the evaluation of other patient populations. Although it would be useful to reexamine previous work done with PET in psychiatric patients in light of the restrictions imposed by PET methodology, we do not have the data to be able to do so in an accurate fashion (e.g., size of the ROI, number of counts per region). Therefore, we will only describe the findings claimed in PET investigation in psychiatric patients.

Schizophrenia

PET research in the area of schizophrenia was an extension of the initial work begun by Kety *et al.*,[60] who investigated differences in global brain glucose utilization between normal and schizophrenic subjects. These studies did not report global differences in glucose metabolism in the brains of schizophrenics. Evaluation of regional differences in brain function was made feasible by the introduction of the cerebral blood flow techniques which allowed regional quantitation of CBF with use of ^{133}Xe as a tracer. Using these techniques, Ingvar and Franzen reported that chronic schizophrenics showed decreased CBF in the frontal cortex.[61] The utilization of the CBF technique with ^{133}Xe is limited by poor spatial resolution and by poor sensitivity to subcortical flow. These limitations were partially overcome with the introduction of PET which extended its application beyond measurement of CBF into direct regional assessment of glucose metabolism for the evaluation of brain function.[62] The initial studies with PET on chronic schizophrenics also revealed decreased glucose metabolism in the frontal cortex of these patients.[63,64] These findings have since been extended.[65,66] However, there have also been studies which have failed to show metabolic hypofrontality.[67,68] In general, the studies that have failed to show the hypofrontality differ from the ones that reported it in that the patients studied were less chronically ill and had a more florid symptom pattern or were not medicated.

The studies investigating glucose metabolic abnormalities in schizophrenic subjects have also reported increased metabolism in the basal ganglia.[69,70] Increased activity in the basal ganglia has been reported in schizophrenics with and without neuroleptic treatment. Furthermore, increased basal ganglia metabolism has also been found in schizophrenics who have never received neuroleptic treatment and who did not show hypofrontality.[71,72] These findings suggest that basal ganglia defects in schizophrenics may be independent of neuroleptic treatment and in some cases may precede the hypofrontality observed in these patients. The lack of hypofrontality in never-treated schizophrenics raises the question of the effect of neuroleptic treatment on the genesis of the metabolic hypofrontality. Indeed, studies evaluating chronic neuroleptic treatment on regional glucose metabolism have reported an accentuation of the hypofrontality after treatment.[67,72] Clinical correlations have shown that metabolic hypofrontality is related to the chronicity of the illness, to age, and hence to exposure of neuroleptic treatment. In one report, hypofrontality was accentuated in those schizophrenics who showed predominance of negative symptoms.[65]

Abnormalities on the temporal cortex[66,73] and on the parietal cortex,[74] as well as a predominance of defects of the left hemisphere,[70] have been described to occur in subgroups of schizophrenic patients. Metabolic studies with PET have also shown that schizophrenics have altered regional metabolic interactions as compared with normal subjects. Specifically, chronic schizophrenics showed a decreased relation between the anterior and the posterior areas as well as between the thalamic and the cortical areas.[75,76]

The metabolic studies in schizophrenic subjects can be summarized by the following results:

1. Chronic schizophrenics with a past history of neuroleptic exposure show decreased metabolic activity in the frontal cortex.
2. Schizophrenics both with and without neuroleptic medication show increased basal ganglia activity as compared to normal subjects.
3. A subgroup of schizophrenics also shows abnormalities in other cortical areas, i.e., the temporal and parietal cortex.
4. Metabolic defects in schizophrenics have not been traced to a single locus.
5. To date, the effects of neuroleptic treatments cannot be separated from the effects of the disease process.

Another major area in PET research has been the investigation of dopamine receptors in schizophrenic subjects. Preliminary studies used the labeled dopamine antagonist NMSP to measure the concentration of activity in the striatum and the concentration of the radioactivity in the cerebellum.[77] The ratio of striatal versus cerebellar radioactivity provides an index of the number of dopamine receptors because it reflects specific versus nonspecific binding of the label (the cerebellum lacks dopamine receptors). These preliminary studies revealed a decrease in dopamine receptors with aging[78] but were unable to show initially any difference in dopamine receptors between normal and schizophrenic subjects.[79]

Use of a similar strategy to assess dopamine receptors demonstrated a linear relation between the concentration of neuroleptic in the blood and the uptake of NMSP in the basal ganglia.[80] Furthermore, the uptake of NMSP was not different between schizophrenic patients who responded to neuroleptic treatment and those who did not.[81] This is of particular importance because failure to respond to neuroleptics is often equated with a lack of delivery of neuroleptic into the brain; medication is then often increased as a way of increasing the delivery of the drug into the brain. However, this preliminary study would suggest that this is not the case and provides an example of how PET strategies can be used to investigate significant clinical problems.

A new model to measure dopamine receptors that involves two PET scans (one done with NMSP alone and the other done after the injection of cold haloperidol) has been developed.[82] This method was developed because it was stated that failure to find differences between schizophrenics and normal subjects using the striatum/cerebellar ratio was because of the effects of CBF on this model. Using the double-scan strategy, it has been shown that naive schizophrenics showed increased uptake of radiotracer in comparison with normal subjects, which is indicative of an increased number of receptors.[82] Another group using the double-scan strategy with a different dopamine antagonist (raclopride) failed to show any increased number of dopamine receptors in naive schizophrenics.[83] The discrepancy in results could be a result of differences in the compounds utilized as well as to differences in patient population. Further studies need to be done to assess the validity of this methodology in determining the density of dopamine receptors *in vivo*.

Studies done with PET using radiolabeled haloperidol and clozapine to visualize postsynaptic dopamine receptors show a widespread uptake of the label throughout the brain.[30,33] This pattern of uptake in drugs that are powerful neuroleptics raises the question of other possible receptors being implicated in the antipsychotic properties of these compounds.

Affective Disorders

There have been several studies in which metabolic abnormalities have been found in patients with affective disorders. One study was done in a group of 11 patients, 10 with a DSM III diagnosis of bipolar disease and one with unipolar disease. These were compared with a group of 19 normal controls.[84] There were no differences in overall glucose metabolism among groups; however, the affective disorder patients showed decreased metabolic activity in the anterior/posterior gradient of the brain when compared with normal subjects. This decrease of activity in the anterior area was more marked in the superior areas of the brain. Since similar findings have been reported in schizophrenic subjects, it raises the question of the specificity of decreased anterior/posterior activity with respect to disease processes.[84]

Another study was done in a group of 24 patients, 11 with a DSM III diagnosis of unipolar disease, five with bipolar disease, five with mania, and three with a mixed disorder. These were compared with a group of nine normal controls.[85] Patients with a bipolar disorder showed decreased glucose metabolism when compared with normal subjects or with patients with unipolar depression. The decrease in glucose metabolism was significant for the frontal cortex, temporal, occipital, and parietal, as well as subcortical structures (caudate and thalamus). All of the subjects showed increased metabolic activity when they were rescanned during an euthymic phase or during a manic episode. A similar pattern has been reported using ^{133}Xe, in which the decreased cerebral blood flow observed in bipolar patients during a depression phase increased during the manic phase.[86] These findings suggest that the global hypometabolism seen in the depressed patient is associated with a state rather than with a trait characteristic of depression because glucose metabolism increases when the patient returns to an euthymic state or becomes manic. Indeed, differences in results obtained in the above PET studies could represent differences in the period of disease in which patients were scanned. Three of the patients in the latter study of Baxter *et al.*[85] also showed left frontal asymmetry characterized by decreased glucose metabolism on the left frontal cortex. Although this was seen in only three patients, similar findings have been reported using [133] Xe studies in which decreased blood flow in the left frontal cortex was seen in depressed patients.[86] Baxter *et al.* [86a] have recently replicated their previous findings in a larger group of patients and demonstrated a significant correlation between the intensity of depressive symptoms and the decreases in metabolic activity in the left frontal cortex.

A study was also done in a group of four unipolar depressed patients who were undergoing electroconvulsive treatment for depression.[87] The patients were tested before and after 24 h of a complete series of ECT treatments. The pre-ECT images for glucose metabolism and CBF showed decreased activity in the frontal cortex of three of the four patients; this defect was more accentuated in the left hemisphere. After ECT, three of the patients showed further reduction in CBF and glucose metabolism of the frontal cortex, which then showed a symmetric hypometabolic pattern. The regional decrease in CBF and glucose metabolism corresponded to the areas where the maximal electric activity is achieved with bilateral ECT.

The results obtained with PET in affective disorders are still preliminary, and more work needs to be done to replicate further previous findings. The studies, however, do suggest that there is a metabolic distinction between patients with unipolar and bipolar depression and that for a subgroup of depressed patients, left frontal hypoactivity may be related to the depressed state of the patients.

Obsessive Compulsive Disorders

A study done on 14 patients with a DSM III diagnosis of obsessive compulsive disorder showed that these patients had increased global metabolic rates throughout the brain when compared with 14 normal subjects or when compared with a group of 11 unipolar depressed patients.[88] Regional metabolic increase was significantly higher in the orbital gyri and was more marked in the left hemisphere than in the right. Patients with obsessive compulsive disorder also showed increased activity in the head of the caudate nuclei when compared both with normal subjects and with unipolar depressed patients. Treatment of these patients did not reveal any significant change in the hyperactivity of the caudate nuclei or of the orbital gyri. The relative value of the caudate versus the whole hemisphere revealed a difference between those patients who responded and those who did not. Patients who responded to treatment showed an increase in the ratio, whereas the nonresponders decreased the ratio both for the left and right hemispheres.

Alcoholism

Three preliminary reports have been done describing metabolic defects of chronic alcoholics. One of the studies was done on patients with Korsakoff's and Wernicke's encephalopathy[89] and showed decreased glucose metabolism on the parietal and temporal cortical areas of these patients. The other two PET studies investigated chronic alcoholics with no evidence of neurological impairment. One study showed decreased glucose metabolism on the prefrontal cortex of these subjects[90] and the other study showed a widespread decrease in glucose metabolism in the brain of chronic alcoholics.[91] The defects in metabolism were larger in the right hemisphere and were more accentuated in the older patients.

The effects of acute alcohol intoxication on cerebral blood flow have also been investigated with PET and ^{15}O-labeled water.[92] This study showed a heterogeneous response from the various brain areas to the effects of alcohol. The cerebellum appeared to be particularly sensitive to alcohol, which lowered the CBF, whereas the prefrontal cortex showed increased CBF after alcohol. Decreased CBF in cerebellum was associated with poor muscle coordination.

Cocaine Abuse

Cerebral blood flow was investigated in a group of 20 chronic cocaine abusers.[93] These patients showed widespread defects of flow, suggestive of cerebrovascular pathology. These findings were explained by the vasoactive properties of cocaine. Indeed, cocaine administration has been shown to induce vasculitis, stroke, and hemorrhages on cerebral vessels.[94] The defects on CBF were predominantly localized in anterior areas of the brain and in the left hemisphere. Repeated scans done after 10 days of cocaine detoxification continued to show the cerebral blood flow defects.

The effects of chronic cocaine consumption on dopamine brain activity have recently been investigated using PET and NMSP. This study revealed decreased dopamine-receptor availability in recently detoxified cocaine abusers.[95]

Miscellaneous Disorders

Studies done on patients with a history of panic attacks have been investigated after lactate infusion with PET to assess cerebral blood flow. Patients who experienced panic attacks secondary to lactate infusion showed decreased left versus right blood flow in the parahippocampal gyrus.[96] This effect was not seen either in normal subjects or in patients who did not experience panic attacks with the lactate infusion. A preliminary report on two patients with a history of panic attacks showed evidence of temporal lobe dysfunction as assessed with CBF, glucose metabolism, and EEG.[97]

Brain function in patients with a history of repetitive, purposeless violent behavior has been evaluated both for glucose metabolism and CBF.[98] This preliminary study showed defects in brain function, which could not be recognized with CT scan or EEG. These defects were widespread and were different in the various patients. All subjects, however, showed evidence of abnormalities of the temporal lobes, which occurred with more frequency in the left hemisphere.

CONCLUSION

Because of the complexity of the technology and the difficulty in comparing experimental conditions among laboratories, it is not surprising to find discrepancies among investigators. Furthermore, the complexity of the technique has limited its use to research studies done in relatively small numbers of subjects. In studies done with PET on psychiatric patients, the heterogeneity of the populations investigated adds further to the difficulty in the interpretation of the data obtained with PET.

Much work needs to be done before conclusive statements can be obtained from research work done with PET in psychiatric patients. This work will not only require careful evaluation and selection of the patients to be investigated but also standardization procedures for data acquisition and image analyses so that comparisons can be made among investigators. PET is a powerful tool for investigating brain function, organization, and neurochemistry in normal and pathological conditions. Its correct utilization in the investigation of psychiatric illnesses will require that we understand its potentials and its limitations.

ACKNOWLEDGMENTS

The authors are appreciative of Dr. A. Wolf for his review of the manuscript.

REFERENCES

1. TER POGOSSIAN, M. M., M. E. PHELPS, E. J. HOFFMAN & N. A. MULLANI. 1975. A positron-emission transaxial tomograph for nuclear imaging (PETT). Radiology **14:** 89-98.
2. WOLF, A. P. 1981. Special characteristics and potential for radiopharmaceuticals for positron emission tomography. Sem. Nucl. Med. **11:** 2-12.
3. PHELPS, M. E. & J. C. MAZZIOTTA. 1985. Positron emission tomography: Human brain function and biochemistry. Science **228:** 799-809.
4. VOLKOW, N. D. & L. R. TANCREDI. 1986. Positron emission tomography: A technology assessment. Int. J. Technol. Assessment Health Care **2:** 577-594.
5. FRIEDLANDER, G., J. KENNEDY, E. MACIAS & M. MILLER. 1981. Nuclear and Radiochemistry. John Wiley. New York, NY.
6. VOLKOW, N. D., N. A. MULLANI & B. BENDRIEM. 1988. PET instrumentation and clinical research. Am. J. Physiol. Imaging. **3:** 142-153.
7. HOFFMAN, E. & M. PHELPS. 1986. Positron emission tomography: Principles and quantitation. *In* Positron Emission Tomography and Autoradiography Principles and Application for the Brain and Heart. M. Phelps & J. Mazziotta, Eds.: 237-286. Raven Press. New York, NY.
8. BUDINGER, T. F., G. T. GOLLBERG & R. H. HUESMAN. 1979. Emission computed tomography. *In* Topics in Applied Physics. Vol. 32. Image Reconstruction from Projections, Implementation and Applications. G. T. Herman, Ed.: 147-246. Springer-Verlag. Berlin.
9. TER POGOSSIAN, M. M. 1977. Basic principles of computed axial tomography. Sem. Nucl. Med. **7:** 109-127.
10. FOWLER, J. S. & A. P. WOLF. 1986. Positron emitter-labeled compounds: Priorities and problems. *In* Positron Emission Tomography and Autoradiography: Principles and Application for the Brain and Heart. M. Phelps, J. Mazziotta & H. Schelbert, Eds.: 391-450. Raven Press. New York, NY.
11. HUANG, S. & M. PHELPS. 1986. Principles of tracer kinetic modeling in positron emission tomography and autoradiography. *In* Positron Emission Tomography and Autoradiography: Principles and Application for the Brain and Heart. M. Phelps, J. Mazziotta & H. Schelbert, Eds.: 287-346. Raven Press. New York, NY.

12. REIVICH, M., A. ALAVI, A. P. WOLF, J. H. GREENBERG, J. FOWLER, D. CHRISTMAN, R. MACGREGOR, S. C. JONES, J. LONDON, C. SHIVE & Y. YONEKURA. 1981. Use of 2-deoxy-D-^{11}C glucose for the determination of local cerebral glucose metabolism in humans: Variations within and between subjects. J. Cereb. Blood Flow Metab. **2**: 307-317.

13. REIVICH, M., D. KUHL, A. P. WOLF, J. GREENBERG, M. PHELPS, T. IDO, V. CASELLA, E. HOFFMAN, A. ALAVI & L. SOKOLOFF. 1979. The [^{18}F] fluorodeoxyglucose method for the measurement of local cerebral glucose utilization in man. Circ. Res. **44**: 127-137.

14. PATRONAS, N. J., G. DICHIRO, C. KUFTA, D. BAKAMIAN, P. L. KORNBLITH, R. SIMON & S. M. LARSON. 1985. Prediction of survival of glioma patients by means of positron emission tomography. J. Neurosurgery. **62**: 816-822.

15. ENGEL, J., JR. 1984. The use of PET scanning in epilepsy. Ann. Nuerol. 15(Suppl.): S180-S191.

16. FOSTER, N. L., T. N. CHASE, P. FEDIO, N. J. PATRONAS, R. BROOKE & G. D. CHIRO. 1983. Alzheimer's disease: Focal cortical changes shown by positron emission tomography. Neurology **33**: 961-965.

17. VOLKOW, N. D., J. D. BRODIE & F. GOMEZ-MONT. 1985. Applications of PET to psychiatry. In Positron Emission Tomography. M. Reivich & A. Alavi, Eds.: 311-327. Alan R. Liss. New York, NY.

18. MAZZIOTTA, J. C. & M. E. PHELPS. 1986. Positron emission tomography studies of the brain. In Positron Emission Tomography and Autoradiography. M. E. Phelps, J. Mazziotta & H. Schelbert, Eds.: 493-579. Raven Press. New York, NY.

19. JONES, T., D. A. CHOSLER & M. M. TER POGOSSIAN. 1976. The continuous inhalation of oxygen-15 for assessing regional oxygen extraction in the brain of man. Br. J. Radiol. **49**: 339-343.

20. RHODES, C. G., R. J. WISE, J. M. GIBBS, R. S. FRACKOWIAK, J. HATAZAWA, A. J. PALMER, D. G. THOMAS & T. JONES. 1983. In vivo disturbance of the oxidative metabolism of glucose in human cerebral gliomas. Ann. Neurol. **14**: 614-626.

21. LENZI, G. L., R. S. FRACKOWIAK & T. JONES. 1982. Cerebral oxygen metabolism and blood flow in human cerebral ischemic infarction. J. Cereb. Blood Flow Metab. **2**: 321-335.

22. BERNARDI, S., M. R. TRIMBLE, R. S. FRACKOWIAK, G. L. LENZI & T. JONES. 1983. An interictal study of partial epilepsy using positron emission tomography and the oxygen-15 inhalation technique. J. Neurol. Neurosurg. Psychiatry **46**: 473-477.

23. JONES, T., D. A. CHESLER & M. M. TER POGOSSIAN. 1976. The continuous inhalation of oxygen-15 for assessing regional oxygen extraction in the brain of man. Br. J. Radiol. **49**: 339-343.

24. RAICHLE, M. E., P. HERSCOVITCH, M. A. MINTUN & W. R. W. MARTIN. 1985. Dynamic measurement of local blood flow and metabolism in man with positron emission tomography. In The Metabolism of the Human Brain Studied with Positron Emission Tomography. T. Greitz, Ed.: 159-164. Raven Press. New York, NY.

25. MAZZIOTTA, J. C., S.-C. HUANG, M. E. PHELPS, R. E. CARSON, N. S. MACDONALD & K. MAHONEY. 1985. A noninvasive positron computed tomography technique using oxygen-15 labeled water for the evaluation of neurobehavioral task batteries. J. Cereb. Blood Flow Metab. **5**: 70-78.

26. SIESJO, B. K. 1978. Brain energy metabolism. John Wiley. New York, NY.

27. FIRNAU, G., E. S. GARNETT, R. CHIRAKAL, S. SOUD, C. NAHMIAS & G. SCHROBLIGER. 1986. [^{18}F] fluoro-L-Dopa for the in vivo study of intracerebral dopamine. J. Appl. Radiat. Isot. **37**: 669-675.

28. WAGNER, H. N. 1986. Quantitative imaging of neuroreceptors in the living human brain. Sem. Nucl. Med. **16**: 51-62.

29. ARNETT, C. D., A. P. WOLF, C. Y. SHIUE, J. S. FOWLER, R. R. MACGREGOR, D. R. CHRISTMAN & M. SMITH. 1986. Improved delineation of human dopamine receptor using ^{18}F-N-methylspiroperidol and PET. J. Nucl. Med. **27**: 1878-1882.

30. KOOK, C. S., M. F. REED & G. A. DIGENIS. 1975. Preparation of [^{18}F] haloperidol. J. Med. Chem. **18**: 533-535.

31. MAZIERE, M., J. L. SAINT LAUDY, M. CROUZEL & D. COMAR. 1975. Synthesis and distribution kinetics of ^{11}C-chloropromazine in animals. In Radiopharmaceutical.

G. Subramanian, B. Rhodes, J. Cooper & V. Sodd, Eds.: 189-195. New York Society of Nuclear Medicine. New York, NY.

32. FARDE, L., E. EHRIN, L. ERIKSSON, T. Y. GREITZ, H. HALL, C. G. HEDSTROM, J. E. LITTON & G. SEDVALL. 1985. Substituted benzamides as ligands for visualization of dopamine receptor binding in the human brain by positron emission tomography. Proc. Natl. Acad. Sci. **82**: 3863-3867.

33. HARTVIG, P., S. A. EKERNAS, L. LIONDSTRON, B. EKBLOM, U. BONDESSON, H. LUNDQVIST, C. HALLDIN, K. NAGREN & B. LANGSTROM. 1986. Receptor binding of N-(methyl-^{11}C) clozapine in the brain of Rhesus monkey studied by positron emission tomography (PET). Psychopharmacology **89**: 248-252.

34. AQUILONIUS, S. M., K. BERGSTROM, S. A. ECKERNAS, P. HARTVIG, K. L. LEENDERS, H. LUNDQVIST, G. ANTONI, A. GEE, A. RIMLAND, J. UHLIN, B. LANGSTROM. 1987. *In vivo* evaluation of striated dopamine reuptake sites using ^{11}C-nomifensin and positron emission tomography. Acta Neurol. Scand. **76**: 283-287.

35. COMAR, D., M. MAZIERE, J. M. GODOT, J. M. CEPEDA, C. MENINI & R. NAQUET. 1979. Visualization of ^{11}C-flunitrazepam displacement in the brain of the live baboon. Nature **280**: 329-331.

36. PERSSON, A., E. EHRIN, L. ERIKSSON, L. FARDE, C.-G. HEDSTROM, J. E. LITTON, P. MINDUS & G. SEDVALL. 1985. Imaging of ^{11}C-labelled RO 15-1788 binding to benzodiazepine receptors in the human brain by positron emission tomography. J. Psychiatr. Res. **19**: 609-622.

37. FROST, J. J., H. N. WAGNER, R. F. DANNALS, H. HAVERT, J. M. LINKS, A. A. WILSON, H. D. BURNS, D. F. WONG, R. W. McPHERSON, A. E. ROSENBAUM, M. J. KUHAR & S. H. SNYDER. 1985. Imaging opiate receptors in the human brain by positron emission tomography. J. Comput. Assist. Tomogr. **9**: 231-236.

38. VORA, M. M., R. D. FINN, T. E. BROOTHE, D. R. LISKOWSKY & L. T. POTTER. 1983. [N-methyl-^{11}C]scopolamine: Synthesis and distribution in rat brain. J. Lab Comp. Radiopharmaceut. **20**: 1229-1236.

39. BARRIO, J. R., M. E. PHELPS, S. C. HUANG, R. E. KEEN & N. S. MacDONALD. 1982. 1-[^{11}C]-L-leucine and the principles of metabolic trapping for the tomographic measurement of cerebral protein synthesis in man. J. Labelled Compd. Radiopharm. **19**: 1271-1272.

40. BUSTANY, P., T. SARGENT, J. M. SANDUBRAY, J. F. HENRY, E. CABANNIS, F. SOUSSALINE, M. CROUZEL & D. COMAR. 1981. Regional human brain uptake and proteins incorporation of ^{11}C-L-methionine studied *in vivo* with PET. J. Cereb. Blood Flow Metab. **1** (Suppl 1): S17-S18.

41. WELCH, M. J., C. S. DENCE, D. R. MARSHALL & M. R. KILBOURN. 1983. Remote system for production of carbon-11 labeled palmitic acid. J. Labelled Compd. Radiopharm. **20**: 1087-1095.

42. FOWLER, J. S., R. R. MacGREGOR, A. D. WOLF, C. D. ARNETT, S. L. DEWEY, D. SCHLYER, D. CHRISTMAN, J. LOGAN, M. SMITH, H. SACHS, S. M. AQUILONIUS, P. BJURLING, C. HALLDIN, P. HARTVIG, K. L. LEENDERS, H. LUNDQUIST, L. ORELAND, C. G. STALNACKE & B. LANGSTROM. 1987. Mapping human brain monoamine oxidase A and B with ^{11}C-suicide inactivators and positron emission tomography. Science **235**: 481-485.

43. TER POGOSSIAN, M. 1985. Positron emission tomography instrumentation. *In* Positron Emission Tomography. M. Reivich & A. Alavi, Eds. Alan R. Liss. New York, NY.

44. GRAHAM, M. C. & R. E. BIGLER. 1983. Principles of positron emission tomography. *In* Physics of Nuclear Medicine. D. V. Rao, R. Chandra & M. C. Graham, Eds. American Institute of Physics. New York, NY.

45. CHANDRA, R. 1976. Interactions of high energy radiation with matter. *In* Introductory Physics of Nuclear Medicine.: 57-70. Lea and Febiger. Philadelphia, PA.

46. COMPTON, A. H. 1961. The scattering of x-rays as particles. Am. J. Phys. 817.

47. BENDRIEM, B., F. SOUSSALINE, R. CAMPAGNOLO, B. VERREY, P. WAGNBERG & A. SYROTA. 1986. A technique for the correction of scattered radiation in a PET system using time of flight information. J. Comput. Assist. Tomogr. **10**: 287-297.

48. BERGSTROM, M., L. ERIKSSON, C. BOHM, G. BLOMQUIST & J. LITTON. 1983. Correction
     for scattered radiation in a ring detector positron camera by integral transformation of
     the projections. J. Comput. Assist. Tomogr. 7: 42-50.
49. ENDO, M. & T. ILINUMA. 1984. Software correction of scatter coincidence in positron CT.
     Eur. J. Nucl. Med. 9: 391-396.
50. FEINBERG, B. N. 1986. Engineering aspects of radiation. In Applied Clinical Engineering.:
     345-375. Prentice-Hall. Englewood, NJ.
51. HOWARD, B. E., M. D. GINSBERG, W. R. HASSEL, A. H. LOCKWOOD & P. FREED. 1983.
     On the uniqueness of cerebral blood flow measured by the in vivo autoradiographic strategy
     and positron emission tomography. J. Cereb. Blood Flow Metab. 3: 432-441.
52. MAZZIOTTA, J. C., M. E. PHELPS, D. PLUMMER, et al. 1981. Quantitation in positron
     emission computed tomography: Five physical-anatomical effects. J. Comput. Assist.
     Tomogr. 5: 734-743.
53. BROWNELL, G. L., C. A. BURNHAM, S. WILENSKY, S. ARONOW, H. KAZEMI & D.
     STRIEDER. 1968. New developments in positron scintigraphy and the application of
     cyclotron-produced positron emitters. In Proceedings of the Symposium on Medical
     Radioisotope Scintigraphy.:163-176. IAEA. Salzburg, Vienna.
54. BROOKS, R. A. & G. DICHIRO. 1976. Principles of computer-assisted tomography (CAT)
     in radiographic and radioisotopic imaging: Review article. Phys. Med. Biol. 21: 689-732.
55. RAMACHANDRAN, G. N. & A. V. LAKSHMINARAYANAN. 1971. Three-dimensional recon-
     struction from radiographs and electron micrographs: Application of convolution instead
     of Fourier transforms. Proc. Natl. Acad. Sci. USA 68: 2236.
56. BUDINGER, T. F., G. T. GULLBERG & R. H. HUESMAN. 1979. Emission computed tomogra-
     phy. In Topics in Applied Physics. Vol. 32. Image Reconstruction from Projections:
     Implementation and Applications. G. T. Herman, Ed.: 147-246. Springer-Verlag. Berlin.
57. HOFFMAN, E. J., S. C. HUANG & M. E. PHELPS. 1979. Quantitation in positron emission
     computed tomography: I. Effect of Object Size. J. Comput. Assist. Tomogr. 3: 299-308.
58. JAGUST, J. W., T. F. BUDINGER, R. H. HUESMAN, R. P. FRIEDLAND, B. M. MAZOYER, B. L.
     KNITTEL. 1986. Methodological factors affecting PET measurements of cerebral glucose
     metabolism. J. Nucl. Med. 27: 1358-1367.
59. BLINKOV, S. M. & I. I. GLEZER. 1968. The human brain in figures and tables. A quantitative
     handbook. Plenum Press. New York, NY.
60. KETY, S. S. & C. E. SCHMIDT. 1948. The nitrous oxide method for the quantitative determi-
     nation of cerebral blood flow in man: Theory, procedure and normal values. J. Clin.
     Invest. 27: 476-483.
61. INGVAR, D. H. & G. FRANZEN. 1974. Distribution of cerebral activity in chronic schizo-
     phrenics. Lancet 2: 1484-1486.
62. BRODIE, J. D., N. D. VOLKOW & J. ROTROSEN. 1983. Principles and applications of positron
     emission tomography in neurosciences. In Handbook of Neurochemistry. A. Lajtha, Ed.:
     331-347. Plenum. New York, NY.
63. BUCHSBAUM, M. S., D. H. INGVAR, & R. KESSLER. 1982. Cerebral glucography with
     positron tomography: Use in normal subjects and in patients with schizophrenia. Arch.
     Gen. Psychiatry 39: 251-259.
64. FARKAS, T., A. P. WOLF & J. JAEGER. 1984. Regional brain glucose metabolism in chronic
     schizophrenia. Arch. Gen. Psychiatry 41: 293-300.
65. VOLKOW, N., P. VAN GELDER, A. P. WOLF, J. D. BRODIE, J. E. OVERALL, R. CANCRO
     & F. GOMEZ-MONT. 1987. Phenomenological correlates of metabolic activity is chronic
     schizophrenics. Am. J. Psychiatry 144: 151-158.
66. WOLKIN, A., J. JAEGER, J. D. BRODIE, A. P. WOLF, J. FOWLER, J. ROTROSEN, F. GOMEZ-
     MONT & R. CANCRO. 1985. Persistence of cerebral metabolic abnormalities in chronic
     schizophrenia as determined by positron emission tomography. Am. J. Psychiatry 142:
     564-571.
67. SHEPPARD, G., J. GRUZELIER, R. MANCHANDA, S. R. HIRSH, R. WISE, R. FRACKOWIAK
     & T. JONES. 1983. ^{15}O positron emission tomography scanning in predominantly never-
     treated acute schizophrenic patients. Lancet 2: 1448-1452.
68. WIDEN, L., G. BLOMQUIST, T. GREITZ, J. E. LITTON, M. BERGSTROM, E. EHRIM, S.

ELANDER, K. ERICSON, L. ERIKSSON, D. H. INGVAR, L. JOHANSSON, J. L. G. NILSSON, S. STONE-ELANDER, G. SEDVALL, F. WIESEL & G. WIIK. 1983. PET studies of glucose metabolism in patients with schizophrenia. Am. J. Neuroradiol. **4:** 550-552.

69. VOLKOW, N. D., J. D. BRODIE, A. P. WOLF, F. GOMEZ-MONT, R. CANCRO, P. VAN GELDER, J. A. G. RUSSELL & J. OVERALL. 1986. Brain organization of schizophrenics. J. Cereb. Blood Flow Metab. **6:** 441-446.

70. GUR, R. E., S. M. RESNICK, A. ALAVI, R. C. GUR, S. CAROFF, R. DANN, F. L. SILVER, A. J. SAYKIN, J. B. CHAWLUK, M. KUSHNER & M. REIVICH. 1987. Regional brain function in schizophrenia: A positron emission tomography study. Arch. Gen. Psychiatry **44:** 119-125.

71. VOLKOW, N. D., J. D. BRODIE, A. P. WOLF, B. ANGRIST, J. RUSSELL & R. CANCRO. 1986. Brain metabolism in schizophrenics before and after acute neuroleptic administration. J. Neurol. Neurosurg. Psychiatry **49:** 1199-1202.

72. EARLY, T. S., E. M. REIMAN, M. E. RAICHLE & E. SPITZNAGEL. 1987. Left globus pallidus abnormality in never-medicated patients with schizophrenia. Proc. Natl. Acad. Sci. **84:** 561-563.

73. DeLISI, L. E., H. H. HOLCOMB, R. M. COHEN, D. PICKAR, W. CARPENTER, J. M. MORIHISA, A. C. KING, R. KESSLER & M. S. BUCHSBAUM. 1985. Positron emission tomography in schizophrenic patients with and without neuroleptic medication. J. Cereb. Blood Flow Metab. **5:** 201-206.

74. KISHIMOTO, H., H. KUWAHARA, S. OHNO, O. TAKAZU, H. NAKANO, K. SAKURA, T. ISHII & S. YOKOY. 1987. Decreases in association areas found in chronic schizophrenics using ^{11}C-glucose PET in cerebral dynamics laterality and psychopathology. R. Takahashi, P. Flor-Henry, J. Gruzelier & S. Niwa, Eds.: 555-560. Elsevier. New York, NY.

75. CLARK, C. M., R. KESSLER, M. S. BUCHSBAUM, R. S. BARGOLIN & H. H. HOLCOMB. 1984. Correlational methods for determining regional coupling of cerebral glucose metabolism. Biol. Psychiatry **19:** 663-678.

76. VOLKOW, N. D., A. P. WOLF, J. D. BRODIE, R. CANCRO, J. E. OVERALL, H. RHOADES & P. VAN GELDER. 1988. Brain interactions in chronic schizophrenics under resting and activation conditions. Schizophrenia Res. **1:** 47-54.

77. WAGNER, H. N., D. BURNS, R. F. DANNALS, D. F. WONG, B. LANGSTROM, T. DUEHLER, J. J. FROST, H. T. RAVERT, J. M. LINKS, S. B. ROSENBLUM, S. E. LUKAS, A. V. KRAMER & M. J. KUHAR. 1984. Imaging dopamine receptors in the human brain by positron tomography. Science **221:** 1264-1266.

78. WONG, D. F., H. N. WAGNER, R. F. DANNALS, J. M. LINKS, J. J. FROST, H. T. RAVERT, A. A. WILSON, A. E. ROSENBAUM, A. GJEDDE, K. H. DOUGLAS, J. D. PETRONIS, M. F. FOLSTEIN, J. K. T. TOUNG, H. D. BURNS & M. J. KUHAR. 1984. Effects of age on dopamine and serotonin receptors measured by positron tomography in the living human brain. Science **226:** 1393-1396.

79. WONG, D. F., H. N. WAGNER, G. D. PEARLSON, L. JUNE & H. WAGNER. 1985. Dopamine receptor binding of C-11-3-N-methylspiroperidol in the caudate in schizophrenia: A preliminary report. Psychopharmacol. Bull. **21:** 595-598.

80. SMITH, M., A. P. WOLF, J. D. BRODIE, C. D. ARNETT, F. BAROUCHE, C. Y. SHIUE, J. S. FOWLER, J. A. G. RUSSELL, R. R. MacGREGOR, A. WOLKIN, B. ANGRIST, J. ROTROSEN & E. PESELOW. Serial [^{18}F] N-methylspiroperidol PET studies to measure changes in antipsychotic drug D-2 receptor occupancy in schizophrenic patients. Biol. Psychol. In press.

81. WOLKIN, A., F. BAROUCHE, A. P. WOLF, *et al.* 1987. Dopamine blockade and clinical response: Evidence for two biological subgroups of schizophrenia (abstract). 26th Annual Meeting of American College of Neuropsychopharmacology. December.

82. WONG, D. F., H. N. WAGNER, L. E. TUNE, R. F. DANNALS, G. D. PEARLSON, J. M. LINKS, C. A. TAMMINGA, E. P. BROUSOLLE, H. T. RAVERT, A. A. WILSON, J. K. T. TOUNG, J. MALAT, J. A. WILLIAMS, L. A. O'TUAMA, S. H. SNYDER, M. H. KUHAR & A. GJEDDE. 1986. Positron emission tomography reveals elevated D$_2$ dopamine receptors in drug-naive schizophrenics. Science **234:** 1558-1563.

83. FARDE, L., F. A. WEISEL, S. STONE-ELANDER, C. HALLDIN, A. L. NORDSTROM, H. HALL

& G. SEDVALL. 1990. D$_2$ dopamine receptors in neuroleptic naive schizophrenic patients: A positron emission tomography study with ^{11}C raclopride. Arch. Gen. Psychiatry **47:** 213-216.

84. BUCHSBAUM, M. S., L. DELISI, H. HOLCOMB, CAPPELLETTI, A. KING, J. JOHNSON, E. HAZLETT, S. DOWLING-ZIMMERMAN, R. POST, J. MORIHISA, W. CARPENTER, R. COHEN, D. PICKAR, D. WEINBERGER, R. MARGOLIN & R. KESSLER. 1984. Anteroposterior gradients in cerebral glucose use in schizophrenia and affective disorder. Arch. Gen. Psychiatry **41:** 1159-1166.

85. BAXTER, L. R., M. E. PHELPS, J. MAZZIOTTA, J. M. SCHWARTZ, R. H. GERNER, C. E. SELIN & R. M. SUMIDA. 1985. Cerebral metabolic rates for glucose in mood disorders. Arch. Gen. Psychiatry **42:** 441-447.

86. MATTHEW, R. J., J. S. MEYER, D. J. FRANCES, K. M. SEMCHUK, K. MORTEL & J. L. CLAGHORN. 1980. Cerebral blood flow in depression. Am. J. Psychiatry **137:** 1449-1450.

86a. BAXTER, L. R., J. M. SCHWARTZ, M. E. PHELPS, J. C. MAZZIOTTA, B. H. GUZE, C. E. SELIN, R. H. GERNER & R. M. SUMIDA. 1989. Reduction of prefrontal cortex glucose metabolism common to three types of depression. Arch. Gen. Psychiatry **46:** 243-250.

87. VOLKOW, N. D., S. BELLAR, N. MULLANI & L. GOULD. 1988. Effects of electroshock on brain glucose metabolism: A preliminary study. Convulsive Ther. **4:** 199-205.

88. BAXTER, L. R., M. E. PHELPS, J. MAZZIOTTA, B. H. GUZE, J. M. SCHWARTZ & C. E. SELIN. 1987. Local cerebral glucose metabolic rates in obsessive-compulsive disorders. Arch. Gen. Psychiatry **44:** 211-218.

89. KESSLER, R. M., E. S. PARKER, C. M. CLARK, P. R. MARTIN, D. T. GEORGE, H. WEINGARTNER, L. SOKOLOFF, M. H. EBERT & M. MISHING. 1984. Regional cerebral glucose metabolism in patients with alcoholic Korsakoff's syndrome (abstract). **10:** 541. Society of Neuroscience. Washington, D.C.

90. SAMSON, Y., J. C. BARON, A. FELINE, J. BARIES & C. H. CRAUZEL. 1986. Local cerebral glucose utilization in chronic alcoholics: A positron tomographic study. J. Neurol. Neurosurg. Psychiatry **49:** 1165.

91. SACHS, H., J. A. G. RUSSELL, D. R. CHRISTMAN & B. COOK. 1987. Alteration of regional cerebral glucose metabolic rate in non-Korsakoff chronic alcoholism. Arch. Neurol. **44:** 1242-1251.

92. VOLKOW, N. D. 1987. Effects of alcohol and cocaine on cerebral blood flow as measured with positron emission tomography. In Cerebral Dynamics, Laterality and Psychopathology. R. Takahashi, P. Flor Henry, J. Gruzelier & S. Niwa, Eds. 463-475. Elsevier. Amsterdam.

93. VOLKOW, N. D., N. MULLANI, L. K. GOULD, S. ADLER & K. KRAJEWSKI. 1988. Cerebral blood flow in chronic cocaine users: A study with positron emission tomography. Br. J. Psychiatry **152:** 641-648.

94. LANGSTON, W. J. & E. B. LANGSTON. 1986. Neurological consequences of drug abuse. In Diseases of the Nervous System. A. K. Asburg, G. M. McKhann, W. I. McDonald, Eds: 1333-1340. W. B. Saunders. Philadelphia, PA.

95. VOLKOW, N. D., J. S. FOWLER & A. P. WOLF. 1990. Effects of chronic cocaine abuse on postsynaptic dopamine receptors. Am. J. Psychiatry **147:** 719-724.

96. REIMAN, E. M., M. E. RAICHLE, F. K. BUTLER, P. HERSCOVITCH & E. ROBINS. 1984. A focal brain abnormality in panic disorder: A severe form of anxiety. Nature **310:** 683.

97. VOLKOW, N. D., A. HARPER & A. C. SWANN. 1986. Temporal lobe abnormalities and panic attacks. Am. J. Psychiatry **143:** 1484-1485.

98. VOLKOW, N. D. & L. TANCREDI. 1987. Neural substrates of violent behavior: A preliminary study. Br. J. Psychiatry **151:** 668-673.

Probing the Human Brain with a Simple Positron Detection System[a]

ALDEN N. BICE

Department of Radiology
University of Washington
Seattle, Washington 98195

INTRODUCTION

Noninvasive, quantitative *in vivo* measurements of human brain chemistry were limited until the development of the transaxial imaging process known as positron emission tomography (PET).[1-3] This imaging technique is based on the detection of annihilation radiation (photons) resulting from positron emission, and it provides a method of accurately quantifying radiotracer concentrations within the body. Since positron-emitting radioisotopes exist for several elements of biological interest (e.g., ^{11}C, ^{13}N, ^{15}O, and ^{18}F, a hydrogen substitute), the potential number of biomedical applications of PET is large. Recent applications of PET to the study of the human brain include the noninvasive measurement of neuroreceptors and the measurement of regional cerebral function.[4-12]

As an imaging modality PET is an invaluable research and clinical tool,[13-15] and the prevalence of PET machines continues to increase. Nevertheless, there are practical considerations that presently limit the location and use of PET devices to larger hospitals or clinics. One consideration is the high cost of PET technology. Another is the level of administered radioactivity necessary to produce the transaxial images with adequate resolution and signal-to-noise ratio. Typically, 5-80 mCi quantities of the short-lived (2-109 min half-life) radiotracers are administered in a PET study. A suitable accelerator (usually a cyclotron) must be located in close proximity to the PET device to insure that sufficient quantities of the radiotracer are available when needed.

Results from selective PET studies of brain chemistry and radiotracer kinetics suggested that, in certain instances, a high spatial resolution image of the distribution of the positron-emitting radionuclide was not needed to obtain valuable data. If the time course of an injected positron-emitting radiotracer in a relatively large region of the brain, such as the frontal lobe, constituted adequate information, then a simple nonimaging device, which requires far lower levels of administered radioactivity, could be used.

This paper describes the simplest of positron detection systems—a two-detector coincidence-counting system developed for the study of the pharmacokinetics of positron-labeled drugs in the living human brain. This inexpensive, relatively high-efficiency coincidence-counting system requires that only a few hundred microcuries of labeled drug be administered to the subject, thereby allowing for multiple studies

[a]Supported, in part, by NIH grants CA42593 and CA42045.

145

without an excessive radiation dose. Measurement of the binding of [¹¹C]carfentanil, a high affinity synthetic opiate, to opiate receptors in the presence and in the absence of a competitive opiate antagonist exemplifies the use of this system for estimating different degrees of receptor binding of drugs in the brain. The instrument has also been used for measuring the transport of other positron-emitting radiotracers into the brain. We illustrate how such a simple system might be used to study brain biochemistry and function.

MATERIALS AND METHODS

The principles of positron detection for imaging applications have been discussed in detail by others.[16-18] Basically, all detection techniques capitalize on the unique property of positron radiation—two identical photons (each 511 keV in energy) are emitted colinearly from the point of positron annihilation. The photons are easily detected by a pair of scintillation detectors. FIGURE 1 illustrates the arrangement of the scintillation detectors in the prototype high-efficiency annihilation detection system (HEADS)[19] used in this work. Two standard 3″ × 3″ sodium iodide (NaI) crystals, positioned in cylindrical lead collimators, were used for the coincident detection of the photon pairs. The requirement of coincident detection of the annihilation photons limited the field of view for positron activity to the volume between the scintillation detectors. Therefore, subjects were positioned so that the volume of the brain to be monitored was located between the two crystal faces. An adjustable headrest mounted between the detectors facilitated subject positioning. The headrest and detectors were mounted on the upper table of a portable elevating stand that could be adjusted in height to match most patient stretchers.

Unlike PET, which provides detailed spatial information about the radiotracer accumulation in a transaxial anatomical slice, a HEADS instrument measures, as a function of time, a weighted average of the radioactivity (i.e., tracer) in the volume between the two crystals. Improvements in spatial resolution of the simple HEADS system are possible,[20] but in general this type of detector is best suited for measuring positron-emitting radiotracers that distribute themselves widely in the brain and show marked differences in brain accumulation under different physiological conditions.

Human studies were performed with a HEADS system and several suitable positron-emitting tracers. Described here are studies with two tracers, [¹¹C]carfentanil and L-[¹¹C]methionine. Details of these studies are discussed extensively elsewhere[19,21,22] and are summarized below.

Twenty-eight normal volunteers were studied (with consent) using [¹¹C]carfentanil,[7] a derivative of the opiate fentanyl, with a high affinity for mu-type opiate receptors. All studies were performed with the subject's head positioned in the HEADS system such that the thalamus and corpus striatum were located near the center of the field of view. Time activity curves of ¹¹C activity (FIG. 2) were obtained for at least 60 min postinjection. The administered dose of [¹¹C]carfentanil ranged between 200 and 400 μCi (0.1-0.6 μg).

Four types of patient studies were performed. Each subject performed a baseline study where only [¹¹C]carfentanil was injected intravenously (i.v.). In a second study, subjects were administered 1 mg/kg naloxone (i.v.) 5 min prior to a [¹¹C]carfentanil injection. In the third type of study, subjects were administered naloxone intravenously (either 1, 0.1, or 0.01 mg/kg of body weight) 15 min after the [¹¹C]carfentanil. Subjects in the fourth study group received injections of [¹¹C]carfentanil at predefined times (1,

48, 72, 120, and 168 h) after oral administration of 50 mg of naltrexone (an opiate receptor antagonist used in the treatment of opioid dependence).

The transport into the brain of the positron-labeled large neutral amino acid L-[¹¹C]-methionine was investigated in four subjects. Each subject received intravenously 360-410 μCi of L-[¹¹C]methionine, and the accumulation of radioactivity in the mid-temporal regions of the brain was monitored for 40-60 min post-tracer injection. Three hours later a second methionine uptake measurement was performed after an oral dose of 100 mg/kg of L-phenylalanine.

RESULTS

Curve 1 in FIGURE 2 represents a typical time activity curve for a study in which [¹¹C]carfentanil was given alone. The lower curve (Curve 3) is an example of the activity

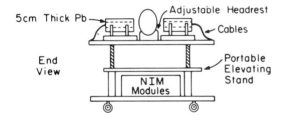

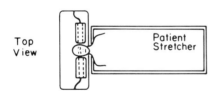

FIGURE 1. HEADS hardware: the arrangement of the two collimated sodium iodide crystals used for detecting coincident 511-keV annihilation photons from positron-emitting radiotracers in the human head. Detectors and electronics (NIM modules) are mounted on a portable elevating stand that can be adjusted in height to match patient stretchers. From Bice *et al.*,[19] with permission.

in the same subject when pretreated with 1 mg/kg (i.v.) of naloxone, a competitive antagonist, which inhibits the specific binding of carfentanil to mu-type opiate receptors in the brain. Curve 2 represents a competitive displacement study in the same subject in which 0.1 mg/kg of naloxone was administered (i.v.) 15 min after the [¹¹C]carfentanil. All curves are scaled to the same injected activity.

Curve 1 of FIGURE 2 represents the time course of the total binding of the radiolabeled ligand. Curve 3 represents the time course of the nonspecific binding. The difference between Curves 1 and 3 represents the specific binding kinetics of carfentanil. Curve 2 represents the total binding kinetics of carfentanil when a competitive mu-type opiate receptor-binding ligand is present in the brain and indicates that the simple HEADS instrument is capable of measuring a quantity related to receptor binding.[19]

FIGURE 3 depicts [¹¹C]carfentanil kinetic data in subjects who also received naltrexone. The six normalized time-activity curves (averaged over subjects) from the control

FIGURE 2. Three time-activity curves obtained with the same subject using the HEADS instrument and an opiate receptor-binding radiopharmaceutical. For each measurement the subject was positioned such that the corpus striatum and thalamus were centrally located in the field of view. Curve 1 represents the normal uptake of [^{11}C]carfentanil. Curve 3 represents the uptake of [^{11}C]carfentanil after intravenous pretreatment with 1 mg/kg of naloxone. Curve 2 represents the time course of carfentanil in the brain when 0.1 mg/kg of naloxone is administered intravenously 15 min after the carfentanil (indicated by the vertical arrow). The curves are normalized for differences in injected activity, which ranged from 200 to 290 μCi. The statistical errors (± 1 σ) are less than the size of the data points. There was no change measured in the absolute sensitivity of the HEADS instrument between studies. PI, post-carfentanil injection. Adapted from Bice *et al.*,[19] with permission.

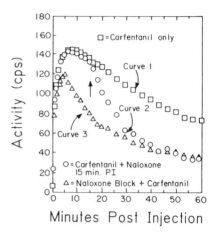

studies and the five different times after oral naltrexone are shown in the figure. The early portions of the curves are similar, reflecting delivery of the tracer to the brain. The [^{11}C]carfentanil accumulation curves obtained in studies 1 h after oral naltrexone are not significantly different from similar curves obtained after intravenous injection of naloxone (cf. FIG. 2). From these data it is possible to formulate an empirical index representing the percentage blockade of mu-type opiate receptors by naltrexone.[21]

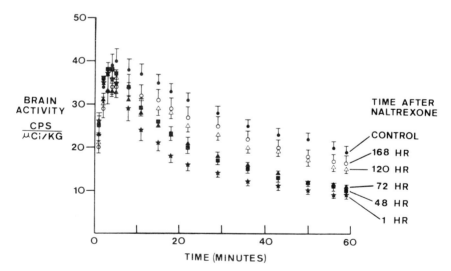

FIGURE 3. The normalized time-activity curves in control studies and 1, 48, 72, 120, and 168 h after oral administration of 50 mg of naltrexone (an opiate receptor antagonist). Each point shows mean + 1 S.E.M. The activity was normalized to the injected dose and subject's body weight. From Lee *et al.*,[21] with permission.

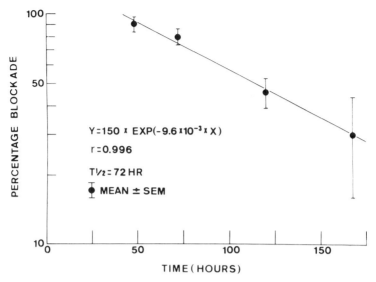

FIGURE 4. Semilogarithmic plot of the percentage of blockade of opiate receptors by naltrexone as a function of time (48, 72, 120, and 168 h) after oral administration of the antagonist. Each point shows mean + 1 S.E.M. With regression analysis, naltrexone bound to opiate receptors was eliminated monoexponentially with a correlation coefficient of 0.996 and an average half-time of 72 h. From Lee *et al.,*[21] with permission.

FIGURE 4 depicts the percentage blockade at various times after naltrexone administration and indicates the prolonged "action" of this antagonist and its metabolites.

FIGURE 5 illustrates the accumulation over time of the methionine tracer in the brain with and without the presence of L-phenylalanine. This graph, which represents a mathematical transformation of the original time-activity data,[23,24] indicates that a simple positron detection system is capable of monitoring differences in blood-brain

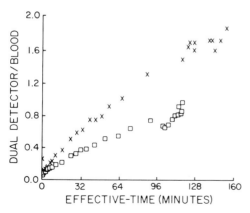

FIGURE 5. Representative integral plots for the brain accumulation of L-[¹¹C]-methionine in a normal volunteer in the presence and absence of a saturating dose of L-phenylalanine. The curves were derived (*see* text) by transforming the time-activity data measured with the **HEADS** instrument. The upper curve reflects the rate of tracer transport into the brain under baseline (fasting) conditions. The lower curve reflects the rate of tracer transport into the brain 60 min after the subject ingested 100 mg/kg of L-phenylalanine. Abscissa: normalized, integrated blood tracer concentration; ordinate: ratio of tissue tracer concentration to blood concentration. From O'Tuama *et al.,*[22] with permission.

barrier transport rates.[22] The initial slope of each curve is proportional to the rate of transport of L-[11C]methionine into the brain. The lower curve reflects the L-methionine transport rate under saturation conditions. The slope of the latter portion of each kinetic curve is related to the trapping of L-[11C]methionine in the brain and presumably its incorporation into proteins. FIGURE 5 also demonstrates the high temporal resolution (seconds) achievable with a dual-detector system.

DISCUSSION

The monitoring of opiate receptor occupancy by different drugs or the transport and accumulation of large neutral amino acids in the brain are but two examples of the potential uses for a portable, nonimaging device. The dual-detector system (HEADS) used in the studies described here cost less than $20,000 to construct and was simple to operate. The present results suggest that some biomedical problems can be addressed without a PET machine.

The sensitivity of a HEADS-type system is an important feature because it allows for many studies of the same subject, something that is less easily justified on a routine basis with PET because of the much higher radiation dose to the subject. The possibility of multiple studies on the same individual implies that, when appropriate, each subject could act as his own control, as was illustrated in FIGURES 2, 3, and 5. The smaller amounts of activity needed in HEADS-type studies suggests that community clinics or hospitals, without PET, could receive deliveries of positron-emitting drugs from a nearby medical accelerator and thereby benefit from the growing availability of selective positron-labeled tracers.

It is important to recognize that the major limitation of the simplified coincidence system is the lack of imaging capability. Only integrated tracer kinetics in a large tissue volume are measured. Therefore, a HEADS-type system often will be an adjunctive device to a PET scanner, especially when detailed spatial information about the tracer distribution is required.

Under favorable conditions PET can detect changes in regional tracer accumulation of a few percent. Because of its sensitivity a HEADS instrument is capable of detecting differences of tracer accumulation in the field of view of a few percent or less. The amount of radioactivity between the coincident detectors defines the statistical accuracy of each measurement. It also affects the ability of a dual-detector system to discern changes in count rate due to changes in tracer accumulation in localized volumes within the field of view. Any alterations in local tissue tracer kinetics (relative to a control study) must be of sufficient magnitude so that the weighted sum of all events from the field of view is measurably different from the corresponding sum in the control measurement.

Following this reasoning, it is clear that without additional information a dual-detector system cannot unambiguously attribute observed count rate differences (between control and other studies) to changes in tracer kinetics in specific areas within the field of view. However, Jeffries et al.[25] of the Maryland Psychiatric Research Center have demonstrated that a dual-detector system can provide estimates of tracer accumulation in specific brain regions if multiple studies are performed with a well-characterized tracer and subject neuroanatomical data are available. Using a receptor-binding ligand and anatomical data from magnetic resonance imaging, Jeffries et al.

were able to assess the occupancy of caudate D2-dopamine receptors by neuroleptic drugs and confirm these estimates with PET.

One tracer which we have only briefly investigated and which may prove amenable to studies with a dual-detector system is 2-deoxy-2-[^{18}F]fluoro-D-glucose (FDG). FDG, a glucose analog, has been used heavily in PET to measure cerebral glucose utilization under normal and abnormal brain pathology and physiology.[11] For example, Metz, Cooper and coworkers recently assessed the effects of ethanol on regional cerebral metabolic rate.[26,27] Subjects received two PET studies, one after the consumption of a beverage containing 0.5 g/kg ethanol. Mood changes in the subjects were accompanied with metabolic changes in the parietal and temporal lobes. Subjects with the largest elevations in measures of positive moods after ethanol were found to have decreased temporal lobe glucose metabolism and increased parietal lobe glucose metabolism. Subjects with feelings of anxiety, depression, and anger after ethanol had just the opposite changes in glucose metabolism. Such changes in regional metabolic behavior with changes in mood might be monitorable with a simple positron detection system. If so, multiple studies beyond the two normally allowed with PET might prove valuable.

The development of positron detection technology and highly specific positron-emitting radiotracers has provided another tool with which to examine the human body. Widespread application of these technological advances might hasten our understanding of the relationship between brain function and chemistry.

REFERENCES

1. TER POGOSSIAN, M. M., M. E. PHELPS, E. J. HOFFMAN, et al. 1975. A positron emission transaxial tomograph for nuclear medicine imaging. Radiology 114: 89-98.
2. PHELPS, M. E., E. J. HOFFMAN, N. A. MULLANI, et al. 1975. Applications of annihilation coincidence detection to transaxial reconstruction tomography. J. Nucl. Med. 16: 210-233.
3. PHELPS, M. E., E. J. HOFFMAN, N. A. MULLANI, et al. 1976. Design considerations for a positron emission transaxial tomograph (PET III). IEEE Trans. Biomed. Eng. 23: 516-522.
4. WAGNER, H. N., JR., H. D. BURNS, R. F. DANNALS, et al. 1983. Imaging dopamine receptors in the human brain by positron tomography. Science 221: 1264-1266.
5. WAGNER, H. N., JR., H. D. BURNS, R. F. DANNALS, et al., 1984. Assessment of dopamine receptor densities in the human brain with carbon-11-labeled N-methylspiperone. Ann. Neurol. 15(Suppl): 579-584.
6. FROST, J. J., H. S. MAYBERG, R. S. FISHER, et al. 1988. Mu-opiate receptors measured by positron emission tomography are increased in temporal lobe epilepsy. Ann. Neurol. 23: 231-237.
7. FROST, J. J., H. N. WAGNER, JR., R. F. DANNALS, et al. 1985. Imaging opiate receptors in the human brain by positron tomography. J. Comput. Assisted Tomogr. 9(2): 231-235.
8. FARDE, L., H. HALL, E. EHRIN, et al. 1986. Quantitative analysis of D2 dopamine receptor binding in the living human brain by PET. Science 231: 258-261.
9. PHELPS, M. E., J. C. MAZZIOTTA & S. C. HUANG. 1982. Study of cerebral function with positron computed tomography. J. Cereb. Blood Flow Metab. 2: 113-162.
10. FOX, P. T., M. A. MINTUN, M. E. RAICHLE et al. 1984. A noninvasive approach to quantitative functional brain mapping with $H_2{}^{15}O$ and positron emission tomography. J. Cereb. Blood Flow Metab. 4: 329-333.
11. PHELPS, M. E. & J. C. MAZZIOTTA. 1985. Positron emission tomography: Human brain function and biochemistry. Science 228: 799-809.
12. PHELPS, M. E., J. R. BARRIO, S. C. HUANG, et al. 1984. Criteria for the tracer kinetic measurement of cerebral protein synthesis in humans with positron emission tomography. Ann. Neurol. 15(Suppl): S192-S202.

13. AMA COUNCIL ON SCIENTIFIC AFFAIRS. 1988. Positron emission tomography in oncology. JAMA **259(14):** 2126-2131.
14. AMA COUNCIL ON SCIENTIFIC AFFAIRS. 1988. Application of positron emission tomography in the heart. JAMA **259(16):** 2438-2445.
15. AMA COUNCIL ON SCIENTIFIC AFFAIRS. 1988. Positron emission tomography—A new approach to brain chemistry. JAMA **260(18):** 2704-2710.
16. AMA COUNCIL ON SCIENTIFIC AFFAIRS. 1988. Instrumentation in positron emission tomography. JAMA **259(10):** 1531-1536.
17. BROWNELL, G. L. 1960. Localization of intracranial lesions using coincidence counting radiation detection equipment. *In* Medical Physics. Vol. III: 332-338. Year Book Medical Publishers. Chicago, IL.
18. BROWNELL, G. L., J. A. CORREAI & R. G. ZAMENHOF. 1978. Positron instrumentation. *In* Recent Advances in Nuclear Medicine. Vol. 5: 1-49. Grune and Stratton, New York, NY.
19. BICE, A. N., H. N. WAGNER, JR., J. J. FROST, *et al.* 1986. A simplified detection system for neuroreceptor studies in the human brain. J. Nucl. Med. **27(2):** 184-191.
20. LINKS, J. M., M. ANDREACO, J. YOUNG, *et al.* 1988. A new probe system with multiple region of interest capabilities for *in vivo* monitoring of positron-emitting tracers. J. Nucl. Med. **29:** 832.
21. LEE, M. C., H. N. WAGNER, JR., S. TANADA, *et al.* 1988. Duration of occupancy of opiate receptors by naltrexone. J. Nucl. Med. **29(7):** 1207-1211.
22. O'TUAMA, L. A., T. R. GUILARTE, K. H. DOUGLASS, *et al.* 1988. Assessment of [11C]-L-methionine transport into the human brain. J. Cereb. Blood Flow Metab. **8(3):** 341-345.
23. GJEDDE, A. 1982. Calculation of cerebral glucose phosphorylation from brain uptake of glucose analogs *in vivo:* A re-examination. Brain Res. Rev. **4:** 237-274.
24. PATLAK, C. S., R. G. BLASBERG & J. D. FENSTERMACHER. 1983. Graphical evaluation of blood-to-brain transfer constants from multiple-time uptake data.
25. JEFFRIES, K. J., C. A. TAMINGA, H. L. LOATS, *et al.* Private communication.
26. METZ, J., H. DE WIT, J. B. BRUNNER & M. D. COOPER. 1988. Effects of alcohol on regional cerebral metabolic rate in normal subjects. J. Nucl. Med. **29(5):** 840.
27. WAGNER, H. N., JR. 1988. Scientific highlights 1988: The future is now. J. Nucl. Med. **29(8):** 1329-1377.

Brain-Behavior Relationships in Aphasia Studied by Positron Emission Tomography[a]

E. JEFFREY METTER

Gerontology Research Center
National Institute on Aging
4940 Eastern Avenue
Baltimore, Maryland 21224

Language is uniquely human, so information regarding brain control of this function has resulted from human pathologic states or normal controls. Focal brain lesions that have caused aphasia have long been studied to understand the relationship between brain structure and language function. One major assumption was that the structural lesion was primarily responsible for the observed behavioral deficits in aphasic patients.

The most widely utilized anatomically based model and classification of aphasia[1,2] argues that the left hemisphere in most right-handed individuals is centrally involved with language processing. In particular, damage to left perisylvian structures results in aphasia. Specifically, damage to Broca's region (the posterior part of the third inferior frontal gyrus) results in nonfluent (Broca's) aphasia; damage to the posterior superior temporal lobe (Wernicke' region) results in fluent (Wernicke's) aphasia; damage to connections between the two structures (the arcuate fasciculus) leads to conduction aphasia; damage to regions around these principal sites (association cortex) results in transcortical and anomic aphasias. This anatomical model emphasizes specific cortical centers and cortical-to-cortical connections. Recently, the model has been expanded to include subcortical structures including the thalamus[3–6] and basal ganglia.[7,8]

Difficulties exist with the model. Although some aphasic syndromes suggest a lesion site with better-than-chance accuracy, the presence of a specific lesion does not necessarily imply the type of aphasia that is present.[1,9] These findings suggest that the model is limited in explaining the neuropathology of language behavior.

Positron emission tomography (PET) allows us to explore the physiologic effects of a structural lesion. Studies from PET and blood flow techniques have made it clear that anatomical information alone is not sufficient to understand the brain's role in either abnormal or normal language function. A focal lesion may cause diffuse, widespread functional changes in the brain, produce focal physiologic changes in specific distant regions, or varying combinations of these effects.[10] Changes in distant areas may result in altered behavioral function. The combining of both structural and functional considerations may provide a more complete picture of brain-behavior relationships.

In this review, I will focus on our studies of aphasic patients using positron emission tomography using (F-18)-fluorodeoxyglucose as a measure of glucose metabolism.

[a]Funded, in part, by Department of Energy Contract No. DE-AM03-76-SS00012, U.S. Public Health Service Research Grants R01-GM-24839 and P01-NS-15654, and the Veterans Administration Medical Research.

Glucose is the natural energy source used by the brain. It has been shown that neurons increase their utilization of glucose in direct proportion to their activity.[11-14] Therefore, we can assume that changes in glucose utilization reflect changes in tissue function, where function refers to those behavioral tasks that a region may carry out or perform.

POSITRON EMISSION TOMOGRAPHY

General Considerations

PET developed parallel to X-ray computed tomography (CT) and uses many of the same principles to create a brain image. Instead of using an external energy source (X-ray), it uses an internal energy source that is injected into the subject.

PET uses positron-emitting radioisotopes. When positrons (positive electrons) combine with normal negative electrons, both are annihilated and form two photons which travel 180° apart. Two detectors linked in coincidence can measure both photons and can determine the line of origin. Using multiple pairs of detectors allows for constructing a brain image of positron distribution. PET technology has shown dramatic improvement in resolution over the past decade and currently has a resolution of about 5 mm. A number of positron-emitting isotopes exist including oxygen-15, nitrogen-13, carbon-11, krypton-77, and fluorine-18. All have half-lives varying from 2 min to 110 min, which require the presence of a cyclotron for isotope production.

Quantitative Models

Understanding the distributional features of a positron-labeled molecule is necessary for a meaningful study. PET is currently used primarily to study glucose and oxygen metabolism, and cerebral blood flow (CBF). Other isotopes allow for determination of cerebral blood volume, protein synthesis, dopamine-receptor-ligand binding, and drug distribution. Thus a variety of physiologic processes can be studied.

Several models now exist for the measurement of regional cerebral blood flow using (O-15)-water or (O-15)-carbon dioxide.[15-20] In most cases, oxygen extraction (the amount of oxygen taken up by the brain) is measured using (O-15)-oxygen. Oxygen metabolism can then be calculated from the CBF and oxygen extraction scans. Their advantages include simplicity and short scanning times. The major disadvantage is poor resolution.

The other commonly used marker is (F-18)-fluorodeoxyglucose (FDG) which measures glucose metabolism. Quantitative models are based on the deoxyglucose method[21] adapted to man with (F-18)-fluorodeoxyglucose (FDG).[22,23] 2-deoxyglucose (DG) is a competitive substrate for glucose, that is, it is transported and metabolized as though it were glucose. Once transported into a cell, DG is phosphorylated but not metabolized further; it is trapped within the cell. The amount of DG accumulated is proportional to the amount of glucose utilized. Regional glucose utilization can be calculated in two ways.

1. Repeated scanning is done following injection to measure constants that are needed to calculate a metabolic rate. This approach is accurate but labor intensive and limited in the number of tomographic planes.
2. FDG is injected intravenously, and arterialized venous blood samples (i.e., the hand is warmed to cause venous blood to approximate arterial blood) are drawn to create an FDG and glucose blood curve. Scanning is started after 40 min when FDG has reached a steady state in the brain. Local cerebral metabolic rates of glucose (LCMRGlc) are then calculated using standardized constants usually derived from young control subjects. This is simple to do and is the commonly used approach.

The accuracy of the second approach is dependent on the stability of the constants in the equation. Recent studies have shown relative stability in several pathologic states and with aging.[24–27] The major advantage of the FDG method is that multiple, high-resolution images can be obtained after a single injection.

Scanning Approaches

PET can be used to study subjects in two types of states: "resting" and with controlled stimulation. Each approach has advantages and disadvantages. The state under which a patient is scanned is important as PET reflects the functional activity of the brain during the procedure. Most subjects are studied in a resting state, but such states vary between laboratories. Mazziotta, Phelps, Carson, and Kuhl[28] examined glucose metabolism in different resting states by studying subjects with ears plugged or unplugged and eyes covered or uncovered. With eyes and ears open cerebral glucose metabolism was found to be symmetric in the left and right hemispheres (i.e., a region in each hemisphere has the same metabolic rate). Changing the resting state by plugging both ears and covering the eyes resulted in significant right-left hemisphere asymmetry and a decline in global glucose metabolism. This study demonstrates that all resting states are not equivalent and shows the importance of knowing the state of the subjects in any study.

Performance of tasks during PET studies (activation studies) may show regional changes in LCMRGlc as compared to resting states. Auditory tasks cause different metabolic patterns determined by the stimulus and the perceptual or cognitive strategy employed in doing the task.[29] Verbal stimuli produced diffuse left hemisphere increases, plus focal bilateral superior and posterior temporal increases in glucose metabolism. Nonverbal stimuli (chords) resulted in diffuse right temporal and bilateral inferior parietal activation. Tone sequences produced variable responses dependent on the subject's strategy in analyzing the data. The interpretation was that subjects who used highly analytic strategies had greater left posterior temporal activations, while those using non-analytic strategies had greater right-sided activations.

All PET studies—whether while resting or doing a specific task—are activation studies because the brain continues to work even during the nonspecific stimulation during resting. The advantage of specific tasks is that all subjects are doing similar cognitive processing, so that some variables associated with brain function are controlled. Activation studies have some limitations. First, to measure activation two scans (resting and activation) need to be done. Second, it must be assumed that all individuals use similar cognitive processes during the task. This is not always the case, as Mazziotta *et al.*[29] demonstrated. In pathologic states such as aphasia, activation studies may be difficult to interpret. A pattern different from normal may imply transfer of the specific function under study to another brain region or involvement of other cognitive processes not generally or significantly involved during normal activity. Likewise, task difficulty and complexity may affect the degree and regions that are changed. As an example consider the right hemisphere response to a language task (e.g., naming or repetition) that has three levels of difficulty and assume that in normal subjects (1) for the simplest task there is a 20% increase in global, right hemisphere glucose metabolism (GMRGlc), (2) for the moderate task, a 40% increase, and (3) for the hardest task, a 60% increase. In an aphasic individual, assume the simplest task causes a 40% increase in right hemisphere GMRGlc. We could conclude that the right hemisphere compensates for left hemisphere damage and has increased its right hemisphere activity in a functional way to do the simple task. Alternatively, we could argue that the difficulty in doing the simple task by the aphasic patient was equivalent to the moderate task for the normal subject so that the right hemisphere change was a "normal" response based on difficulty. Finally, we could argue that the simple task was very difficult for the aphasic subject and that the 40% increase was less than the 60% increase that should have occurred as it did for the most difficult level of the task in normal subjects. As can be seen, all three interpretations are plausible, making a final judgment difficult.

PET IN THE STUDY OF APHASIA

General Considerations

Our studies of aphasic stroke patients with resting FDG PET (eyes open and ears unoccluded) have demonstrated that cerebral metabolic abnormalities consistently extend beyond the zone of infarction determined by CT (remote effects)[30,31] or at autopsy.[32] In our experience, metabolic abnormalities always exceed the limits of symptomatic structural lesions in aphasic patients. Such metabolic changes are observed chronically following a stroke (up to 15 yr),[31] though the metabolic pattern may change with time.

Explanations for remote metabolic effects were sought in a recent autopsy.[32] The patient was found to have lacunes in the basal ganglia region of both hemispheres. On the left, a lacune destroyed the anterior limb of the internal capsule and was associated with decreased glucose metabolism in the overlying frontal cortex. The destroyed anterior limb of the internal capsule contained both afferent and efferent tracts to the metabolically depressed frontal cortex, and disconnected the frontal region from other brain structures. Histologic evaluation of the frontal cortex showed no statistically significant loss of neuronal elements to account for the metabolic decline. Lacunes in the right basal ganglia spared the internal capsule and were associated with preserved frontal glucose metabolism. The slight difference in location of the left and right lesions resulted in a distinctly different frontal metabolic effect. Thus, the utility of resting FDG PET can be seen in understanding the brain-behavior relationship in clinical syndromes.

Metabolic Patterns

In our studies of approximately 65 stroke patients (the vast majority of them being aphasic patients with left hemisphere lesions), five patterns of metabolic abnormalities were found associated with the structural lesions.[10,33] Kushner et al.,[34] using a slightly different approach, noted similar patterns.

The first pattern found metabolic abnormalities restricted to the area of structural damage. These lesions were consistently found to be asymptomatic[35]—that is, to have no history of associated signs or symptoms. This pattern argues that for a structural lesion to be associated with a persistent clinical deficit, it must affect other brain regions. This finding emphasizes a new concept in studying brain-behavior relationships, namely, the focus must not be on the damaged region alone, but on the influence of the damage on other areas (remote effects).

The second and third patterns were those most commonly seen in aphasia. The second pattern showed measurable metabolic abnormalities in either temporoparietal or frontoparietal regions but not both (Kushner et al.[34] called these patients "lobar"). Structural lesions that caused this pattern tended to spare the lenticular nuclei and internal capsule. The third pattern showed measurable metabolic abnormalities in both temporoparietal and frontoparietal regions. The structural lesions tended to be larger than with the second pattern and to extend deeper into the lenticular and internal capsule. Small subcortical structural lesions produced either of these two patterns.

The fourth pattern was found with small thalamic lesions producing mild metabolic changes throughout the ipsilateral hemisphere. This pattern has been seen in several subjects including patient NA.[36,37] We believe that the cortical changes are independent of specific behavior, but rather may result from general thalamic influence on cortex. This pattern differs from the third pattern in the mildness and evenness of the metabolic asymmetry.

The fifth pattern was found on repeated studies of aphasic patients. Generalized metabolic changes that occur acutely following stroke tend to improve, that is, all regions show a relatively uniform increase in glucose metabolism. This pattern has been well described in the cerebral blood flow literature. In our experience, global glucose metabolic rates change by 20-40% form the first to seventh months post-stroke. This change involves all brain regions. It represents a generalized response to stroke and does not appear to be related directly to behavior, but rather to physiologic phenomena or to factors within the FDG model.

The patterns demonstrate that left hemisphere glucose metabolic changes occur that are not random and may differ between subjects. The patterns, in general, ignore the severity of the hypometabolism in each region, or how metabolic or structural changes in one region affect another. Such relational changes will be important to explore.

Consequences of Remote Effects

The implications of reduced metabolism in structurally non-damaged brain regions can be understood by considering what factors contribute to regional metabolism. Contributions to regional metabolism include the metabolic activity of neurons, glia, and dendritic innervation. The dendrites are derived from cell-cell interactions within a region, short-distance connections from adjacent brain regions, and long fibers arising from more distant regions. Metabolic activity depends on the summation of these individual contributions. A reduction in regional metabolism can occur from damage to one or more of these components or to changes in the firing patterns of neurons within the region. Firing changes would result from increases or decreases in either excitatory or inhibitory inputs to the region. Structural damage in one region can result in metabolic changes in a distant region based on damage to the message sent from the first to the second region (i.e., dendritic activity). Thus the distant effect can be indirect (decreased dendritic activity) or direct (loss of neuronal firing). The degree of contribution from each of these factors is difficult or impossible to determine. Likewise, lesions to white matter tracts resulting in a disconnection (as described above) would be associated with metabolic changes at sites that were connected by the white matter tracts. In the disconnection both proximal and distal regions presumably would function normally; what is destroyed in the communication between the two.

The contribution that a remote metabolic change may have on behavior may be distinctly different from that caused by direct structural and local metabolic damage. When damage is severe and tissue is destroyed, no regional function is possible although lesser degrees of structural damage may allow for partial function. Remote metabolic changes caused by a lesion may either cause functional loss similar to that which would be observed in the case of direct damage; or, alternatively, the functional integrity of the remote region may not be lost, but rather only modified in its ability to carry out its goals—that is, the distant region operates in a normal way but without, or with modified, information normally received from the structurally damaged area. Thus a 50% loss of metabolic activity at a structural lesion site may behaviorally manifest differently than a 50% metabolic reduction at a remote site with no structural damage. In this way, new concepts are needed to understand how remote metabolic effects are similar to and different from direct local effects of structural damage.

Behavioral Considerations

To examine the behavioral consequences of brain metabolic patterns, we have studied the traditional anatomic aphasic syndromes: Wernicke's, Broca's, and conduction aphasias.[38,39] The three aphasic syndromes differed in the depth of the structural lesions. Broca's aphasic patients showed slightly more anterior lesions, with deep extension into the lenticular nuclei and internal capsules. A specific difference between Broca's and non-Broca's patients with similar structural lesions was the extent of structural damage to the posterior internal capsule.[40] Conduction aphasia patients showed no involvement of the lenticular nuclei and basal ganglia, but involved the insula in some patients. Wernicke's aphasia patients occupied a middle ground in extent and depth of the structural lesion. Wernicke and conduction aphasic patients had lesions extending farther posteriorly into posterior temporal and lateral occipital lobes than did those with Broca's aphasia.

The glucose metabolic patterns were different between the three syndromes. All three had similar metabolic asymmetry in the temporoparietal regions. The three syndromes differed in the frontal lobe. Conduction aphasia showed mild, Broca's region metabolic asymmetry and none in prefrontal regions. Wernicke's aphasia showed mild-to-moderate glucose metabolic asymmetry in both Broca's and prefrontal regions. Broca's aphasia had severe glucose metabolic asymmetry in both areas.

The prefrontal metabolic differences are of striking interest because they distinguished the three syndromes and were not associated with structural damage, and because prefrontal areas have not been discussed as important in distinguishing these syndromes. A key question becomes: What effect do the prefrontal changes have in the behavioral differences between the three syndromes? In Broca's aphasia, the left prefrontal hypometabolism was frequently as severe as regions showing moderate-to-severe structural damage. This suggests that the frontal regions are behaving as though structurally damaged and that normal, frontal lobe function has been disrupted. This may explain some aspects of behavior in Broca's aphasia including slow, difficult motoric features and some of the difficulties in sequencing materials in speech. In Wernicke's and conduction aphasia, the left prefrontal hypometabolism is less apparent, suggesting less modification of the normal response in those regions when compared to Broca's aphasia. Since the prefrontal changes in Wernicke's aphasia are present but not marked, we can argue that frontal function is preserved but altered by loss of input information from temporoparietal regions and loss of the ability to send specific, integrated information to other brain regions. Thus prefrontal cortex has lost some influence on cerebral function. In Wernicke's aphasia, this may cause jargon output, where the patient talks excessively with little self-control or awareness of his own speech. In these individuals the frontal lobes may function with little assistance or monitoring by the left temporoparietal language regions.

Another observation we have made is a strong association of the head of the caudate and thalamus to frontal, parietal, and cerebellar metabolism.[41] Recent pathoanatomic studies have demonstrated the presence of aphasic syndromes with subcortical lesions in the region of lenticular nuclei and thalamus.[7,8] We have shown that such lesions are associated with temporoparietal hypometabolism,[31,36] particularly with posterior internal capsule and posterior lenticular nuclei lesions.[36,42] On close scrutiny,[36,43] the thalamus was more involved with the memory aspects of language, while the head of the caudate was more associated with frontal metabolism and was associated with more basic functions underlying but probably not specific to language. Mazziotta, Phelps, and Wapenski[44] had normal volunteers either write their name repeatedly while blindfolded or do a novel, finger-sequence task following the injection of FDG. They showed prominent increases in striatal metabolism as well as contralateral sensory-motor cortex with name writing, while showing only cortical activation with the novel sequence task. Huntington's disease (HD) subjects showed no striatal activation during the name-writing task but had cortical activation similar to the controls during the novel sequence task. The authors argue that with loss of striatal function, HD patients lose the semiautomated processes controlled by the basal ganglia and need to use motor system functions usually reserved for novel acts. These observations and the strong caudate correlation to frontal metabolism suggest a strong cortical-subcortical interrelationship in the executions of specific behaviors. Likewise in progressive supranuclear palsy, a disease with basal ganglia pathology, FDG PET studies have shown prominent metabolic reduction in the frontal lobes, showing important relationships between these structures.[45] Such patients show a "subcortical dementia" characterized by slowness of thought and response, with slow, delayed recall, apathy, but no aphasia or apraxia.[46]

These observations argue that basal ganglia-cortical integration is involved with speech.[47] Most aphasia models discuss speech in regard to content rather than execution, that is, the motor sequencing and patterning to create speech. Much of speech is based on overlearned, well-planned sequences of movements. What is unique in any connected speech output is the sequencing of well-learned phonemes and larger units (morphemes, words). Speech production depends on movements controlled at one level by the basal ganglia and at another by cortical regions and cortical-cortical communication. The control can be at the level of output planning or in programming the execution of a planned output. This is consistent with the observations of Friedman, Alexander, and Naeser[48] on transcortical motor aphasia. Damage to either cortical or subcortical structures or connections will result in disordered communication though not necessarily "aphasia."

Another observation in comparing the three aphasic syndromes worthy of discussion was the presence of a similar degree of temporoparietal metabolic asymmetry in all three. As demonstrated in the second pattern, we had found two subjects who had frontoparietal hypometabolism without clear temporal hypometabolism. Thus the parietal changes may be the most consistent region of metabolic abnormality. At present, however, we have not found any aphasic patients without metabolic changes in the left temporoparietal region.

A major debate over the past hundred years has been whether aphasia is a unitary phenomena or whether multiple types of aphasia exist. Differences in the two points of view depend on whether the focus is on features common to all aphasic patients (regardless of severity) or on features that differ between patients. From the PET data, there is evidence supporting both viewpoints. Common changes in temporoparietal glucose metabolic asymmetry are consistent with unitary language abnormalities occurring in all aphasia. Language functions were found to correlate with involvement of the posterior temporal and inferior parietal regions.[49] Different patterns of glucose asymmetry were found in prefrontal regions and each were associated with different aphasic syndromes. It is difficult at present to be certain whether frontal changes are directly associated with language or other functions that modify language behavior. Thus both sides of the traditional debate can be supported, and the advantages of each might profitably be integrated to create a more realistic model of brain-behavior relationships.

CONCLUSION

PET studies demonstrate that current anatomical models of aphasia need to be expanded. Such changes are occurring as seen by the efforts of Crossen.[6] The most popular current model of aphasia has been based on left hemisphere dominance for language and on cortical-cortical connections between centers.[1] This model is linear in nature: Sound is received, processed in superior temporal lobe, reprocessed in temporoparietal areas, and then transferred to posterior inferior frontal cortex for a response. However, recent evidence has shown that deep lesions can cause aphasia or aphasia-like syndromes. These observations have shown that not only cortical-cortical but cortical-subcortical connections are critical for language performance. PET observations are consistent with these ideas, leading us to acknowledge new dimensions in brain function: specifically, remote metabolic effects and their relationship to behavioral dysfunction.

Such observations lead to the hypothesis that language abnormalities in aphasia are associated with temporoparietal changes no matter where the structural lesion is located, while features that distinguish syndromes are associated with the extent and nature of changes occurring in other brain regions, including subcortical structures and prefrontal regions. We need to expand existing models to account for the multiple interactions that are needed for even simple tasks. In this way PET will improve our understanding of brain-behavior relationships.

SUMMARY

Positron emission tomography allows for the study of human brain physiology and chemistry including cerebral blood flow, oxygen or glucose metabolism. We applied PET to study glucose metabolism using aphasia as a model of neurobehavior. The most striking observation was that the extent of cerebral glucose metabolic changes in aphasic patients consistently involve brain regions that are not structurally damaged. The remote metabolic effects can be predicted depending on the location and extent of structural damage. Two observations were made: (1) In our experience, all right-handed aphasic patients with left hemisphere structural lesions have metabolic abnormalities in the left temporoparietal region, and (2) metabolic abnormalities are variably found in undamaged, left prefrontal lobe, basal ganglia, and thalamus. Variations in clinical aphasic syndromes were found to relate to these frontal metabolic changes, suggesting that aspects of the aphasia result from differences in prefrontal function rather than directly from structural damage to perisylvian or deep structures.

ACKNOWLEDGMENTS

I would like to thank Drs. Wayne Hanson and Diana Van Lancker for review of the manuscript.

REFERENCES

1. BENSON, D. F. 1979. Aphasia, Alexia, Agraphia. Churchill/Livingston. New York, NY.
2. BENSON, D. F. & N. GESCHWIND. 1985. The aphasias and related disturbances. *In* Clinical Neurology. A. B. Baker & R. J. Joynt, Eds. Harper & Row. Philadelphia, PA.
3. BROWN, J. W. 1975. On the neural organization of language: Thalamic and cortical relationships. Brain Lang. **2:** 18-30.
4. MOHR, J. P., W. C. WATTERS & G. W. DUNCAN. 1975. Thalamic hemorrhage and aphasia. Brain Lang. **2:** 3-17.
5. VAN BUREN, J. M. 1975. The question of thalamic participation in speech mechanisms. Brain Lang. **2:** 31-44.
6. CROSSON, B. 1984. Role of the dominant thalamus in language: A review. Psychol. Bull. **9:** 491-517.

7. NAESER, M. A., M. P. ALEXANDER, N. HELM-ESTABROOKS, H. L. LEVINE, S. A. LAUGH-
    LIN & N. GERSCHWIND. 1982. Aphasia with predominantly subcortical lesion sites. Arch.
    Neurol. **39:** 2-14.
8. DAMASIO, A. R., H. DAMASIO, M. RIZZO, N. VARNEY & F. GERSCH. 1982. Aphasia with
    nonhemorrhagic lesions in the basal ganglia and internal capsule. Arch. Neurol. **39:** 15-20.
9. BASSO, A., A. R. LECOURS, S. MORASCHINI & M. VANIER. 1985. Anatomoclinical correla-
    tions of the aphasias as determined through computerized tomography: Exceptions. Brain
    Lang. **26:** 201-229.
10. METTER, E. J., W. R. HANSON, W. H. REIGE, C. JACKSON, J. MAZZIOTTA, M. E. PHELPS
    & D. E. KUHL. 1985. Remote metabolic effects in aphasia stroke patients. *In* Clinical
    Aphasiology 1985. R. H. Brookshire, Ed.: 126-135. BRK Press. Minneapolis, MN.
11. FREYGANG, W. H. & L. SOKOLOFF. 1958. Quantitative measurement of regional circulation
    in the central nervous system by use of radioactive inert gas. Adv. Biol. Med. Physiol. **6:**
    263-279.
12. SÁLFORD, L. G., T. E. DUFFY & F. PLUM. 1973. Altered cerebral metabolism and blood
    flow in response to physiological stimulation. Stroke **4:** 351-362.
13. DESROSIERS, M. H., C. KENNEDY, C. S. POTLAK, K. D. PETTIGREW, L. SOKOLOFF & M.
    REIVICH. 1974. Relationship between local cerebral blood flow and glucose utilization in
    the rat. Neurology **24:** 389.
14. YAROWSKY, P., M. KADEKARO & L. SAKOLOFF. 1983. Frequency-dependent activation of
    glucose utilization in the superior cervical ganglion by electrical stimulation of cervical
    sympathetic trunk. Proc. Natl. Acad. Sci. **80:** 4179-4183.
15. HUANG, S. C., R. E. CARSON & M. E. PHELPS. 1982. Measurement of local blood flow and
    distribution volume with short-lived isotopes: A general input technique. J. Cereb. Blood
    Flow Metab. **2:** 99-108.
16. JONES, T., D. A. CHESLER & M. M. TER-POGOSSIAN. 1976. The continuous inhalation of
    oxygen-15 for assessing regional oxygen extraction in the brain of man. Br. J. Radiol. **49:**
    339-343.
17. ALPERT, M. M., R. H. ACKERMAN, J. A. CORREIA, J. C. BARON, G. L. BROWNELL &
    J. M. TAVERAS. 1977. Measurement of rCBF and $rCMRO_2$ by continuous inhalation of
    150-labelled CO_2 and O_2. Acta Neurol. Scand. **56** (Suppl. 72): 186-187.
18. BARON, J. C., D. COMAR, F. SOUSSALINE, A. TODD-POKROPEK, M. G. BOUSER, P. CAS-
    TAIGNE & C. KELLERSHOHN. 1979. Continuous 150 inhalation technique: An attempt to
    quantify CBF, EO_2 and $CMRO_2$. Acta Neurol. Scand. **60** (Suppl. 72): 194-195.
19. FRACKOWIAK, R. S. J., G. L. LENZI, T. JONES & J. D. HEATHER. 1980. Quantitative
    measurement of regional cerebral blood flow and oxygen metabolism in man using 150
    and positron emission tomography: Theory, procedure and normal values. J. Comput.
    Tomogr. **4:** 727-736.
20. LAMMERTSMA, A. A., T. JONES, R. S. J. FRACKOWIAK & G. L. LENZI. 1981. A theoretical
    study of the steady-state model for measuring regional cerebral blood flow and oxygen
    utilization using oxygen-15. J. Comput. Assist. Tomogr. **5:** 544-550.
21. SOKOLOFF, L., M. REIVICH, C. KENNEDY, M. H. DESROSIERS, C. S. PATLAK, K. D.
    PETTIGREW, O. SAKURADA & H. SHINOHARA. 1977. The (C-14)deoxyglucose method
    for the measurement of local cerebral glucose utilization: Theory, procedure and normal
    values in the conscious and anesthetized albino rat. J. Neurochem. **28:** 897-916.
22. REIVICH, M., D. KUHL, A. WOLF, J. GREENBERG, M. PHELPS, T. IDO, V. CASELLA, J.
    FOWLER, E. HOFFMAN, A. ALAVI, P. SOM & L. SOKOLOFF. 1979. The (F18)-
    fluorodeoxyglucose method for the measurement of local cerebral glucose utilization in
    man. Circ. Res. **44:** 127-137.
23. PHELPS, M. E., S. C. HUANG, E. J. HOFFMAN, C. S. SELIN, L. SOKOLOFF & D. E. KUHL.
    1979. Tomographic measurement of local cerebral metabolic rate in humans with (F-189
    2-fluoro-2-deoxyglucose: Validation of method. Ann. Neurol. **6:** 371-388.
24. REIVICH, M., A. ALAVI, A. WOLF, J. FOWLER, J. RUSSEL, C. ARNETT, R. R. MACGREGOR,
    C. Y. SHIUE, H. ATKINS, A. ANAND, R. DANN & J. H. GREENBERG. 1985. Glucose
    metabolic rate kinetic model parameter determination in humans: The lumped constants
    and rate constants for (18F)fluorodeoxyglucose and (11C)deoxyglucose. J. Cereb. Blood
    Flow Metab. **5:** 179-192.

25. HAWKINS, R. A., J. C. MAZZIOTTA, M. E. PHELPS, S. C. HUANG, D. E. KUHL, R. E. CARSON, E. J. METTER & W. H. REIGE. 1983. Cerebral glucose metabolism as a function of age in man: Influence of the rate constants in the flurodeoxyglucose method. J. Cereb. Blood Flow Metab. **3:** 250-253.

26. HAWKINS, R. A., M. E. PHELPS, S. C. HUANG & D. E. KUHL. 1981. Effect of ischemia on quantification of local cerebral glucose metabolic rate in man. J. Cereb. Blood Flow Metab. **1:** 37-51.

27. FRIEDLAND, R. P., T. F. BUDINGER, Y. YANO, R. H. HUESMAN, B. KNITTEL, S. E. DERENZO, B. KOSS & B. A. OBER. 1983. Regional cerebral metabolic alterations in Alzheimer-type dementia: Kinetic studies with 18-fluorodeoxyglucose. J. Cereb. Blood Flow Metab. **3**(Suppl. 1): S510-S511.

28. MAZZIOTTA, J. C., M. E. PHELPS, R. E. CARSON & D. E. KUHL. 1982. Tomographic mapping of human cerebral metabolism: Sensory deprivation. Ann. Neurol. **12:** 435-444.

29. MAZZIOTTA, J. C., M. E. PHELPS, R. E. CARSON & D. E. KUHL. 1982. Tomographic mapping of human cerebral metabolism: Auditory stimulation. Neurology **32:** 921-937.

30. KUHL, D. E., M. E. PHELPS, A. P. KOWELL, E. J. METTER, C. SELIN & J. WINTER. 1980. Effect of stroke on local cerebral metabolism and perfusion: Mapping by emission computed tomography of 18FDG and 13NH3. Ann. Neurol. **8:** 47-60.

31. METTER, E. J., C. G. WASTERLAIN, D. E. KUHL, W. R. HANSON & M. E. PHELPS. 1981. 18FDG positron emission computed tomography in a study of aphasia. Ann. Neurol. **10:** 173-183.

32. METTER, E. J., J. C. MAZZIOTTA, H. H. ITABASHI, N. J. MANKOVICH, M. E. PHELPS & D. E. KUHL. 1985. Comparison of x-ray CT, glucose metabolism and post-mortem data in a patient with multiple infarctions. Neurology **35:** 1695-1701.

33. METTER, E. J., C. A. JACKSON, D. KEMPLER, W. R. HANSON, J. C. MAZZIOTTA & M. E. PHELPS. 1986. Remote glucose metabolic patterns in chronic stroke lesions. Neurology **36**(Suppl. 1): 349.

34. KUSCHNER, M., M. REIVICH, C. FRESCHI, F. SILVER, J. CHAWLUK, M. ROSEN, J. GREENBERG, A. BURKE & A. ALAVI. 1987. Metabolic and clinical correlates of acute ischemic infarction. Neurology **37:** 1103-1110.

35. METTER, E. J., D. KEMPLER, C. A. JACKSON, W. H. RIEGE, W. R. HANSON, J. C. MAZZIOTTA & M. E. PHELPS. 1987. Are remote glucose metabolic effects clinically important? J. Cereb. Blood Flow Metab. **7**(Suppl. 1): 5196.

36. METTER, E. J., W. H. RIEGE, W. R. HANSON, D. E. KUHL, M. E. PHELPS, L. R. SQUIRE, C. G. WASTERLAIN & D. F. BENSON. 1983. Comparisons of metabolic rates, language and memory in subcortical aphasia. Brain Lang. **19:** 33-47.

37. BARON, J. C., R. D'ANTONA, P. PANTANO, M. SERDARU, Y. SAMSON & M. G. BOUSSER. 1986. Effects of thalamic stroke on energy metabolism. Brain **109:** 1243-1259.

38. METTER, E. J., D. KEMPLER, C. JACKSON, W. R. HANSON, J. C. MAZZIOTTA & M. E. PHELPS. 1986. Cerebral glucose metabolism: Differences in Wernicke's, Broca's and conduction aphasias. *In* Clinical Aphasiology 1986. R. H. Brookshire, Ed.: 97-104. BRK Publishers. Minneapolis, MN.

39. METTER, E. J., D. KEMPLER, C. A. JACKSON, W. R. HANSON, J. C. MAZZIOTTA & M. E. PHELPS. 1989. Cerebral glucose metabolism in Wernicke's, Broca's and conduction aphasias. Arch. Neurol. **46:** 27-34.

40. METTER, E. J., D. KEMPLER, C. A. JACKSON, W. R. HANSON, J. C. MAZZIOTTA & M. E. PHELPS. 1987. A study of Broca's aphasia by 18F-fluorodeoxyglucose positron emission tomography. Ann. Neurol. **22:** 134.

41. METTER, E. J., D. KEMPLER, C. A. JACKSON, W. R. HANSON, W. H. RIEGE, L. CAMRAS, J. C. MAZZIOTTA & M. E. PHELPS. 1987. Cerebellar glucose metabolism in chronic aphasia. Neurology **37:** 1599-1606.

42. METTER, E. J., C. JACKSON, D. KEMPLER, W. H. RIEGE, W. R. HANSON, J. C. MAZZIOTTA & M. E. PHELPS. 1986. Left hemisphere intracerebral hemmorrhages studies by (F-18)-fluorodeoxyglucose positron emission tomography. Neurology **36:** 1155-1162.

43. METTER, E. J., W. H. RIEGE, W. R. HANSON, M. E. PHELPS & D. E. KUHL. 1988. Evidence for a caudate role in aphasia from FDG positron computed tomography. Aphasiology **2:** 33-43.

44. MAZZIOTTA, J. C., M. E. PHELPS & J. WAPENSKI. 1985. Metabolic differences of motor system responses found between normal subjects and patients with basal ganglia disease. Neurology 35(Suppl. 1): 110.

45. D'ANTONA, R., J. C. BARON, Y. SAMSON, M. SERDARU, F. VIADER, Y. AGID & J. CAMBIER. 1985. Subcortical dementia: Frontal cortex hypometabolism detected by positron tomography in patients with progressive supranuclear palsy. Brain 108: 785-799.

46. ALBERT, M. L., R. G. FELDMAN & A. L. WILLIS. 1974. The "subcortical dementia" of progressive supranuclear palsy. J. Neurol. Neurosurg. Psychiatry 37: 121-130.

47. GORDON, W. P. 1985. Neuropsychologic assessment of aphasia. In Speech and Language Evaluation in Neurology: Adult Disorders. J. K. Darby, Ed. Grune & Stratton. Orlando, FL.

48. FRIEDMAN, M., M. P. ALEXANDER & M. A. NAESER. 1984. Anatomic basis of transcortical motor aphasia. Neurology 34: 409-417.

49. METTER, E. J., W. H. RIEGE, W. HANSON, L. CAMRAS, D. E. KUHL & M. E. PHELPS. 1984. Correlations of cerebral glucose metabolism and structural damage to language function in aphasias. Brain Lang. 19: 33-47.

Imaging Dementia with SPECT

B. LEONARD HOLMAN,[a,b,e] J. STEVAN NAGEL,[a,e]
KEITH A. JOHNSON,[d] AND THOMAS C. HILL[c,e]

Department of Radiology,
[a]*Brigham and Women's Hospital and*
[c]*New England Deaconess Hospital;*
[d]*Department of Neurology,*
Massachusetts General Hospital; and
[e]*Harvard Medical School,*
Boston, Massachusetts 02113

Lewis Thomas has called Alzheimer's disease the disease of the century.[1] The increasing interest has come about as awareness of its malignancy and prevalence has heightened.[2] Alzheimer's disease is the primary cause of the severe dementia affecting at least 5% of Americans over the age of 65 and 20% over the age of 80.[3] The disastrous impact of the disease on the lives of its patients and their families is compounded by its enormous financial cost to society. Currently, half of the nursing care in the United States, worth over 20 billion dollars, goes to the treatment of the other dementias. Over 50 million dollars is spent annually for research on the dementias in the U.S. alone.[4] Perhaps most important, millions of dollars are spent annually on psychometric and clinical testing in only a marginally successful attempt to diagnose and stage Alzheimer's disease.

The signs and symptoms of Alzheimer's disease are nonspecific: (1) dementia without prominent focal neurologic defects and (2) a steadily progressive course. Neurofibrillary tangles and senile plaques are present but may be seen in other conditions including trauma and normal aging. While it is possible to diagnose Alzheimer's disease in some patients with 90% certainty based on a constellation of clinical and laboratory observations, approximately half the patients with Alzheimer's disease cannot be accurately categorized at the time of their initial visit. In these patients, it may require years of follow-up study before these patients can be correctly diagnosed.

Radiotracer methods have been used to measure blood flow and metabolism in patients with Alzheimer's disease for several decades. Initially, investigators using the inert gas washout method observed that blood flow was reduced globally in Alzheimer's disease. More recently, studies carried out at a number of positron emission tomography (PET) facilities have suggested that the abnormalities in flow and metabolism are focal and most extensive in the posterior temporoparietal area.

Those techniques that have been developed to study regional brain perfusion and metabolism in Alzheimer's disease have used either positron-emitting tracers or radioactive gases. Both methodologies require special-purpose instrumentation and are technically difficult to perform with precision and accuracy. PET is an exceedingly costly

[b]Address correspondence to B. Leonard Holman, M.D., Chairman, Department of Radiology, Brigham and Women's Hospital, 75 Francis Street, Boston, MA 02115.

technology and is inappropriate for patient screening. PET should be restricted to helping us better understand the physiology of the disease process and to developing potential applications that will lead to the development of appropriate commercially available single-photon radiotracers.

A family of amines has been developed which accumulates in the brain proportional to cerebral blood flow. I-123 IMP (isopropyl iodoamphetamine) and its related radio-compounds have an initial distribution related to regional cerebral blood flow. The tracers remain within the brain without significant clearance for sufficiently long intervals so that tomography can be performed either using special-purpose instrumentation or the more generally available rotating gamma camera. With I-123 IMP or the more recently introduced Tc-99m-labeled cerebral perfusion agents, we can begin to explore the potential clinical role of cerebral profusion imaging in the dementias.

IMAGING TECHNIQUES

Cerebral perfusion SPECT (single photon emission computed tomography) imaging is the process by which cerebral blood flow is demonstrated with tomographic single-photon scintigraphic techniques. The radiopharmaceuticals that have been used most extensively for this purpose are I-123 N-isopropyl-p-iodoamphetamine (IMP or iofeta-mine) and Tc-99m HMPAO. IMP was developed by Winchell et al.[5] and has been studied extensively to measure cerebral perfusion. The typical intravenous dose of IMP is 3 to 5 mCi (111-185 MBq). Because of its lipophilicity, IMP localizes in the brain in approximate proportionality to the regional cerebral blood flow and thus behaves similarly to a "chemical microsphere."[6] The complex kinetics of I-123 IMP, including significant lung uptake, affects brain uptake which varies from 6% to 9% of the injected dose. IMP uptake in various regions of the brain can be compared to determine relative blood flow.

The macrocyclic amine, propyleneamine oxine (PnAO), has been labeled with technetium-99m.[7] This lipophilic compound crosses the blood-brain barrier, but it has a very rapid clearance from the brain, precluding tomographic imaging. However, significant improvements in brain residence time has been observed with newer PnAO derivatives. One such derivative, Tc-99m HMPAO, has a moderately high first-pass extraction through the cerebral circulation.[7,8]

The brain uptake of Tc-99m HMPAO is also proportional to cerebral blood flow, but unlike I-123 IMP, Tc-99m HMPAO does not undergo cerebral redistribution, remaining fixed in the brain for at least 6 h after intravenous injections. Because the dosimetry of Tc-99m is more favorable than I-123, higher doses can be administered with marked improvement in image quality, especially with special-purpose brain imaging systems. Because Tc-99m HMPAO is labeled from kit preparations on-site, it is available for both routine and emergency studies. Blood clearance of Tc-99m HMPAO is slower than I-123 IMP clearance. As a result, image contrast is not as good as with I-123 IMP.[9] Also the radiocompound is unstable and must be used soon after preparation. Other Tc-99m-labeled compounds with superior biologic characteristics are currently undergoing clinical trials and will further improve the quality and simplicity of SPECT perfusion imaging of the brain.

INSTRUMENTATION

Single photon emission computed tomography of the brain can be performed using either special purpose or rotating gamma camera systems. Each imaging system has its advantages; the choice of equipment depends on the level of utilization and on the purposes to which the technique will be applied.

The high collection coefficiency of the special purpose systems makes rapid scanning (5-7.5 min) of an entire slice possible. The primary advantage of this system is its high sensitivity, resulting in high spatial resolution and rapid imaging. As a result, SPECT perfusion images of the brain can be obtained with a spatial resolution of 8 mm (full width at half-maximum) in the plane of the slice. The special purpose systems would, therefore, be the preferred instruments for the studies requiring high spatial resolution, regional quantification, or rapid sequential imaging.

The rotating gamma camera approach is preferable for routine clinical imaging, because of its availability and because it can be used for other types of tomographic and non-tomographic imaging. The major constraint on rotating gamma camera tomography is sensitivity. The low sensitivity for each tomographic slice is compensated by the fact that the gamma camera collects volumetric information as opposed to the single-slice information obtained with the multidetector system. Improvements in collimator design (the slant-hole, long-bore, and fan-beam collimators, for example) and in reconstruction algorithms have substantially improved the quality of SPECT perfusion images using the Anger-type gamma camera. Satisfactory tomographic imaging has been achieved with the rotating gamma camera using all of the perfusion agents described above. Multiheaded systems have been introduced recently, with corresponding improvement in sensitivity and resolution.

IMAGE ACQUISITION

Careful quality control is essential with SPECT. The relatively low photon flux from the target organ and the scattered radiation from the high energy gamma rays of I-123 stretch the imaging process to its limits.

Between 3-5 mCi I-123 IMP is injected intravenously (or, alternatively, 10-20 mCi of Tc-99m HMPAO). Imaging begins 10-20 min after injection with the patient supine and the head centered in the field of view. The patient's head should be placed in a holder to ensure that it does not move during the 30-40 min of data acquisition. The patient should be placed on a comfortable couch so that movement is reduced to a minimum during data acquisition.

For the rotating gamma camera, a 64-frame, 360° study is acquired with the detector as close to the head as possible using a collimator optimized to the energies of the radionuclide. The total image requires 20-30 min.

Reconstruction is performed using a ramp filter. A three-dimensional Butterworth filter is then applied to the reconstructed images to reduce the noise introduced from the out-of-slice planes as well as from the plane of the image. Image reconstruction from the 3D-data set may be performed along any plane of interest, depending on the clinical situation. Typically, reconstructions are performed along the plane parallel to the orbitomeatal line and in the coronal and sagittal planes.

NORMAL PATTERNS

Patients without central nervous system disease and with a normal X-ray CT examination demonstrate bilaterally symmetrical activity on the SPECT perfusion images (FIG. 1). Activity is greatest along the convexity of the frontal, temporal, parietal, and occipital lobes corresponding anatomically to cortical gray matter. Activity is also high in the regions corresponding to the basal ganglia and thalamus. The regions between the basal ganglia and the convexity corresponding anatomically to cortical white matter and the ventricles have less activity.

Attention must be paid to achieving a reproducible baseline state. We inject the tracer with the patient's eyes open, with the room dimly lit, and with white noise in the background. This state of activation is maintained during the 10-20 min before image acquisition. Strong arguments have been made for covering the patient's eyes and ears in order to reduce outside stimulants which might increase blood flow and metabolism. The injection protocol will depend on the information that is being sought, but once the protocol is established, it must be followed diligently.

SPECT IN THE DEMENTIAS

More than 15 years ago, investigators using the inert gas washout method observed that blood flow was reduced in Alzheimer's disease.[10,11] Studies carried out at various PET facilities suggested that these abnormalities in flow and metabolism were focal and most extensive in the parietal area. (A number of groups have suggested that the changes in metabolism seen with PET could be repeated with the single-photon tracer I-123 IMP.)[12–14]

The first use of the single-photon-emitting radiopharmaceutical I-123 IMP for the scintigraphic diagnosis of Alzheimer's disease and multi-infarct dementia (MID) patients in comparison to normal control subjects was made by Cohen et al.[12] They described studies initially performed using a portable gamma camera equipped with a rotating slant-hole collimator; subsequently a rotating single-headed gamma camera and conventional SPECT technique were used. The IMP SPECT scans of Alzheimer's patients were noted to have extensive, symmetric cortical deficits in IMP uptake while multi-infarct dementia patients had multiple, discrete asymmetric cortical defects. Recent work by several observers have corroborated Cohen's initial findings and demonstrated that parietal IMP deficits are the most reliable pattern for diagnosing Alzheimer's disease (FIG. 2).[13,14]

Semiquantitative analysis of I-123 IMP uptake in the cortex has been performed by several observers. Johnson and associates defined cortex-to-cerebellum I-123 IMP ratios using 2- by 4-pixel rectangular regions of interest placed in the parietal, frontal, temporal, and occipital lobes as well as the cerebellum on transaxial cross sections.[13] Alzheimer's patients averaged 27% less relative I-123 IMP uptake in the parietal lobe than control subjects. Similar but less striking temporal and frontal lobe I-123 IMP deficits were seen in patients with Alzheimer's disease; occipital lobe and cerebellar uptake of I-123 IMP was normal. The severity of the parietal lobe deficits was demonstrated with IMP. Using a cutoff value of 0.66, below which the parietal cortex:cerebellum ratio was abnormal, this quantitative method was 76% sensitive and 78% specific when applied to a group of 37 mild to severely symptomatic Alzheimer's patients and

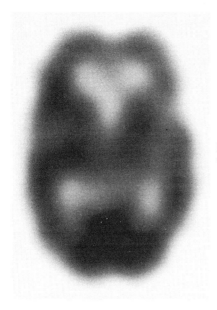

FIGURE 1. Transaxial perfusion SPECT in a normal subject.

FIGURE 2. Transaxial perfusion SPECT in a patient with Alzheimer's disease. Note decreased uptake bilaterally in the association cortex of the parietal, frontal, and posterior temporal lobes.

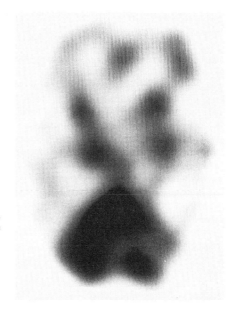

nine control subjects.[15] These data showed that parietal deficits are the most reliable markers for Alzheimer's, but they are also seen in some normal subjects.

Several other groups have also reported accurate detection of Alzheimer's disease. Hellman *et al.* have reported a method of quantitating cortical uptake on transaxial cross sections with an elliptical, 2-cm thick, ring-shaped cortical region of interest that is divided into 12 equal annular segments.[16] Comparison also was made to total hemispheric and cerebellar counts by summing cross sections. Using a cutoff value for parietal:cerebellar ratio of 0.60, Alzheimer's patients were correctly distinguished from normal controls with a high degree of accuracy. Jagust and coworkers[17] have reported a quantitative method for measuring I-123 IMP uptake based on the ratio of the mean of the cortical uptake seen in left and right temporoparietal (TP) regions compared to the uptake in the whole tomographic slice (WTS) chosen at the midventricular level. A TP:WTS ratio of ≤ 1.0 separated nine of nine Alzheimer's patients from normal controls and MID patients.

The diagnostic dilemma is not the detection of Alzheimer's disease when its clinical manifestations are obvious, but rather, diagnosis early in its clinical course when symptoms are mild. We have found that subjective interpretation of the SPECT whole-brain image set is more accurate than interpretation from quantitative indices—with subjective assessment, sensitivity is 88% and specificity is 87% (compared to 76% and 78% with quantitative indices). Furthermore, sensitivity is 80% in mild Alzheimer's disease (Blessed Dementia Scale ≤ 10).

Parietal deficits are present on perfusion SPECT in the majority of clinically diagnosed Alzheimer's patients and appear to be the most constant scintigraphic finding for Alzheimer's disease on I-123 IMP SPECT (FIG. 2). However, recent experience has shown that considerable asymmetry may be present; rarely the parietal defect may be unilateral. Further parietal defects can extend contiguously into the temporal lobe in a fashion that produces a "hockey stick"-shaped temporoparietal defect on the parasagittal images. Although parietal deficits are the characteristic finding in Alzheimer's, discrete frontal and temporal lobe deficits also are common and can be unilateral. Basal ganglia deficits are variable, occurring occasionally in association with prominent ipsilateral cortical defects. In severely demented patients, cortical I-123 IMP uptake may be globally decreased.

PET studies have shown that focal and asymmetric metabolic deficits in the dominant frontal, temporal, and parietal lobes are associated with memory and language dysfunction. Similarly, perfusion SPECT has shown focal defects inferiorly in the left temporal lobes of individual patients who have aphasia. Visual-spatial cognitive dysfunction has been seen in Alzheimer's disease patients with focal occipital lobe IMP defects. An important characteristic of IMP SPECT in Alzheimer's disease is that it involves the association areas of the cerebral cortex, including the sensorimotor strip, the primary auditory cortex in the temporal lobe, and the primary visual cortex of the occipital lobe. Lesions that involve only the primary cortex are not typical of Alzheimer's disease and point to other diagnoses. Preservation of the sensory-motor cortex in Alzheimer's disease is seen most easily on the parasagittal views.

Johnson *et al.*[15] found a significant association between reduced iofetamine I-123 uptake and dementia severity in the parietal region but not in the temporal, frontal, or occipital regions. Their data suggest that among cortical regions, decreased cerebral perfusion in the parietal lobes is most strongly associated with functional disability and cognitive impairment in Alzheimer's disease, and this is consistent with observations from neuropathologic studies.[18] Several PET studies have assessed the relationship between cerebral functional activity and illness severity in Alzheimer's disease. Frackowiak *et al.*[19] reported decrements in regional brain oxygen metabolism in a group of 13 patients with degenerative dementia; the greatest decrease was in posterior temporal and parietal regions bilaterally. Image abnormalities in all brain regions were greater in severely demented patients with Alzheimer's disease than in patients with less severe Alzheimer's disease, and decreases in frontal and parietal regions were greatest in the severely demented. Similar results were reported by DeLeon *et al*.[20] In contrast to these reports, Foster *et al*.[21] did not find an association between parietal hypometabolism and dementia severity. They studied 20 patients with Alzheimer's disease with PET and 18-fluorodeoxyglucose and reported that comparisons of metabolic rates in mildly and severely demented patients failed to yield statistically significant differences. These conflicting data may result from differences in estimating dementia severity or from differences in image analysis.

SPECT SCANNING IN MULTI-INFARCT DEMENTIA

Multi-infarct dementia is characterized by one or more scattered perfusion defects that can be either unilateral or bilateral, are generally asymmetric in distribution, can involve any part of the cortex including the primary cortex, and do not have a predilection for the parietal lobes. When large, the perfusion defects of multi-infarct dementia can conform to vascular anatomy, such as the territory supplied by the middle cerebral artery in the temporal, posterior frontal, and parietal lobes. Twenty percent of all MCA infarct patients suffer from dementia. Vascular dementia also can follow bilateral anterior cerebral artery infarcts or a unilateral anterior cerebral artery infarction of the dominant hemisphere. Basal ganglia deficits can be seen as a remote effect of large cortical infarcts, but many occur as isolated lesions. Diminished uptake in the cerebellar hemisphere contralateral to a cortical infarct is called cerebellar diaschisis and can be seen in multi-infarct dementia or in asymmetric Alzheimer's disease; isolated cerebellar infarction also may occur.

Not all patients are distinguishable as having Alzheimer's disease, multi-infarct dementia, or other disorders based on the pattern of SPECT uptake. For example, normal images may be seen in mildly symptomatic patients. In some cases, an asymmetric presentation of Alzheimer's disease may be indistinguishable from the pattern of a cerebral infarction seen in another patient. The presence of a parietal deficit may favor the diagnosis of Alzheimer's disease and involvement of the motor cortex may favor multi-infarct dementia; however, some patients may have a mixture of both diseases. Even if a stroke has occurred, it is not certain that a patient's dementia is due to that event. Thus, evidence of multi-infarct dementia does not rule out Alzheimer's disease. Similarly, patients with bilateral parietal defects, which are presumably due to Alzheimer's disease, may have other perfusion defects due to stroke.

IMAGING OTHER DEMENTIAS

Many other diseases produce dementia but are somewhat less common than Alzheimer's disease and multi-infarct dementia. These include Parkinson's disease, Huntington's disease, progressive supranuclear palsy, as well as cognitive deficits associated with Jakob-Creutzfeldt disease, Korsakoff's psychosis, and systemic lupus erythematosus. The characteristic parietal and temporoparietal lobe defects seen in Alzheimer's disease are probably not unique to that disease. A characteristic finding in Huntington's disease is bilaterally decreased basal ganglia IMP uptake, particularly in the area of the caudate nuclei.[22] In the later stages of Huntington's disease, the cortical uptake can be decreased globally.

To date, only small numbers of patients with Parkinson's disease have been studied. Some mild to moderately symptomatic patients had normal scans, and some severely diseased subjects had Alzheimer's-like parietal deficits but were clinically distinguishable by their motor symptoms.

Progressive supranuclear palsy is characterized clinically by dementia, parkinsonism, and a gaze disorder. Preliminary imaging results in progressive supranuclear palsy suggest asymmetric basal ganglia and predominantly frontal lobe cortical deficits. Bilateral parietal deficits are not a characteristic finding in Korsakoff's psychosis or in encephalopathies such as Jakob-Creutzfeldt disease where tracer uptake can be globally decreased. With systemic lupus erythematosus, the cerebral tracer uptake may be normal or diffusely heterogeneous, reflecting widespread small vessel disease. In severe cases of systemic lupus erythematosus, Alzheimer's-like parietal lobe defects can be seen along with defects in other lobes as the multiple small perfusion defects coalesce into larger geographic defects. However, distinguishing between systemic lupus erythematosus and Alzheimer's disease at this point is usually not a difficult clinical problem. Large focal cortical deficits also may be present in systemic lupus erythematosus, representing areas of infarction.

Depression can mimic dementia. In one study of patients admitted for evaluation of dementia, 10% were found to have depression. These psychiatric patients may be distinguished from Alzheimer's disease on perfusion SPECT by the absence of parietal deficits. Phelps et al.[23] have shown frontal lobe metabolic deficits in some depressed patients on PET scans. Preliminary work by van Royen et al.[24] suggests similar findings using SPECT and the cerebral perfusion tracer T1-201 DDC (dithiocarbamate). Finally, Van Heertum et al.[25] report variable cortical deficits, including frontal lobe IMP deficits, in depression.

What is the value of a screening test in Alzheimer's disease? There is no cure and in fact no effective management for the disease. Clinical criteria can be useful in the diagnosis, and many other life-threatening diseases can be excluded by CT or MR. The vast majority of the patients are elderly, well beyond their financially productive years. But patients and their families have a right to know whether or not they have a disease and what that disease is. In only half of the patients with Alzheimer's disease can a diagnosis be established with an 80% to 90% certainty at the time of the initial workup. To deprive patients in whom the diagnosis cannot be established clinically of an accurate test because the disease itself cannot be treated condemns them to years of financial and emotional vulnerability and uncertainty. Furthermore, the underlying disease may not be Alzheimer's after all; it may be a benign process or a treatable disease, such as depression and vascular dementia. In either case, it is essential for the patient, his clinician, and his family to have the information necessary to prepare for the future. To offer less is to submit to a dehumanizing process lacking in compassion and foresight.

The experience that we are gaining in applying SPECT to the evaluation of the dementias will be of immeasurable value as we begin to evaluate therapeutic maneuvers and pharmacologic interventions objectively. At this point, our assessment of the progress of the disease has been limited to measurements during the baseline state. As we begin to evaluate patients during the active stage of the disease and with pharmacologic interventions and as we refine our quantitative measures of tracer uptake and kinetics, SPECT will become increasingly useful as an objective measure of disease process and the effects of pharmacologic therapy.

REFERENCES

1. THOMAS, L. 1981. On the problem of dementia. Discover **2**: 34-36.
2. KATZMAN, R. 1976. The prevalence and malignancy of Alzheimer's disease. Arch. Neurol. **33**: 217-218.
3. BRUST, J. C. M. 1983. Dementia and cerebrovascular disease. *In* The Dementias. R. Mayeux & W. G. Rosen, Eds.: 131-147. Raven Press. New York, NY.
4. FINCH, C. E. 1985. Alzheimer's disease: A biologist's prospective. Science **230**: 1111.
5. WINCHELL, H. S., W. D. HORST, L. BRAUN, W. H. OLDENDORF, R. HATTNER & H. PARKER. 1980. *N*-isopropyl-[I-123]*p*-iodamphetamine: Single-pass brain uptake and washout; binding to brain synaptosomes; and localization in dog and monkey brain. J. Nucl. Med. **21**: 947-952.
6. HOLMAN, B. L., R. G. L. LEE, T. C. HILL, R. D. LOVETT & J. LISTER-JAMES. 1984. A comparison of two cerebral perfusion tracers, *N*-isopropyl I-123 *p*-iodamphetamine and I-123 HIPDM in the human. J. Nucl. Med. **25**: 25-30.
7. HOLMES, R. A., S. B. CHAPLIN, K. G. ROYSTON, T. J. HOFFMAN, W. A. VOLKERT, D. P. NOWONTNIK, L. R. CANNING, S. A. CUMMING, R. C. HARRISON, B. HIGLEY, G. NECHVATAL, R. D. PICKETT, I. M. PEPER & R. D. NEIRINCKX. 1985. Cerebral uptake and retention of Tc-99m-hexamethyl-propyleneamine oxime (Tc-99m-HM-PAO). Nucl. Med. Commun. **6**: 443-447.
8. ELL, P. J., J. M. L. HOCKNELL, P. H. JARRITT, I. CULLUM, D. LUI, D. CAMPOS-COSTA, D. P. NOWONTNIK, R. D. PICKETT, L. R. CANNING & R. D. NEIRINCKX. 1985. A Tc-99m-labelled radiotracer for the investigation of cerebral vascular disease. Nucl. Med. **6**: 437-441.
9. SHINICHI, N., K. KAZUO, J. SEISHI, H. HIROAKI & W. KATSUSHI. 1989. Comparative study of regional cerebral blood flow images by SPECT using xenon-133, iodine-123 IMP, and technetium-99m HM-PAO. J. Nucl. Med. **2(30)**: 157-164.
10. OBRIST, W. D., E. CHIVIAN, S. CRONQUIST & D. H. INGVAR. 1970. Regional cerebral blood flow in senile and presenile dementia. Neurology **20**: 315-322.
11. SIMARD, D., J. OLESEN, O. B. PAULSON, N. A. LASSEN & E. SKINHOJ. 1971. Regional cerebral blood flow and its regulation in dementia. Brain **94**: 273-288.
12. COHEN, M. B., L. S. GRAHAM, R. LAKE, E. J. METTER, J. FITTEN, M. K. KULKARNI, R. SEVRIN, L. YAMADA, C. C. CHANG, N. WOODRUFF & A. S. KLING. 1986. Diagnosis of Alzheimer's disease and multiple infarct dementia by tomographic imaging of I-123 IMP. J. Nucl. Med. **26(6)**: 769-774.
13. JOHNSON, K. A., S. T. MUELLER, T. M. WALSHE, R. J. ENGLISH & B. L. HOLMAN. 1985. Cerebral perfusion imaging in Alzheimer's disease with SPECT and I-123 IMP. Neurology **35**(Suppl. 1): 235.
14. SHARP, P., H. GEMMELL, G. CHERRYMAN, J. BESSON, J. CRAWFORD & F. SMITH. 1986. The application of I-123 labelled isopropylamphetamine to the study of brain dementia. J. Nucl. Med. **26**: 761-768.
15. JOHNSON, K. A., B. L. HOLMAN, S. P. MUELLER, T. J. ROSEN, R. ENGLISH, J. S. NAGEL & J. H. GROWDON. 1988. Single photon emission computed tomography in Alzheimer's disease: Abnormal iofetamine I-123 uptake reflects dementia severity. Arch. Neurol. **45**: 392-396.
16. HELLMAN, R. S., R. S. TIKOFSKY, B. D. COLLIER, *et al.* 1987. Quantitative differences between healthy subjects and patients with Alzheimer's disease in brain imaging with I-123 iodoamphetamine. Radiology **165**: 245.
17. JAGUST, W. J., T. F. BUDINGER & B. R. REED. 1987. The diagnosis of dementia with single photon emission tomography. Arch. Neurol. **44**: 258-262.
18. BRUN, A. & E. ENGLUND. 1981. Regional pattern of degeneration in Alzheimer's disease: Neuronal loss and histopathological grading. Histopathology **5**: 549-564.
19. FRACKOWIAK, R. S. J., C. POZZILLI, N. J. LEGG, G. H. DuBOULAY, J. MARSHALL, G. I. LENZI & T. JONES. 1981. Regional cerebral oxygen supply and utilization in dementia. A clinical and physiological study with oxygen-15 and positron tomography. Brain **104**: 753-778.

20. DeLeon, M. J., S. H. Ferris, A. E. George, et al. 1983. Computed tomography and positron emission transaxial tomography evaluations of normal aging and Alzheimer's disease. J. Cereb. Blood Flow Metab. **3:** 391-394.
21. Foster, N. L., T. N. Chase, P. Fedio, N. J. Patronas, R. A. Brooks & G. DiChiro. 1983. Alzheimer's disease: Focal changes shown by positron emission tomography. Neurology **33:** 961-965.
22. Nagel, J. S., K. A. Johnson, M. Ichise, R. J. English, T. M. Walshe, J. H. Morris & B. L. Holman. 1988. Decreased iodine-123 IMP caudate nucleus uptake in patients with Huntington's disease. Clin. Nucl. Med. **13:** 486-490.
23. Phelps, M. E., J. C. C. Mazziotta, L. Baxter, et al. 1984. Positron emission tomographic study of the affective disorders: Problems and strategies. Ann. Neurol. **15:** S149-S156.
24. van Royen, E. A., J. F. deBruine, T. C. Hill, et al. 1987. Cerebral blood flow imaging with thallium-201 diethyldithiocarbamate SPECT. J. Nucl. Med. **28:** 178-183.
25. Van Heertum, R. L. & R. A. O'Connell. 1988. The evaluation of psychiatric disease with IMP cerebral SPECT imaging. Adv. Functional Neuroimaging **1:** 4-11.

For Some Times, Less is More: Part III Overview, with Further Examples and Strategies

F. FRANK LeFEVER

Neuropsychology Laboratory
Helen Hayes Hospital
West Haverstraw, New York 10993

I've roughed up the smooth cliché to emphasize the times for which less may be more: these important times are the Brief, the Long, the Many, and the Right. Techniques described in the remaining papers, as well as some additional ones that I'll describe (for example, rheoencephalography, transcranial Doppler sonography, 40-Hz local EEG), tend to be simpler and cheaper than the elaborate imaging and mapping techniques described in Parts I and II, and may have advantages they lack. For example, those lacking the spatial *integration* of some mapping or imaging techniques may offer superior temporal integration. They may lack spatial *resolution,* but have very fine temporal resolution. They are thus not rivals but complementary techniques; that is, ones that may not just *supplement,* but complement in a dialectic in which each adds to and improves the other's effort.

There may be cases where one technique may be substituted for the other, and cases where one is clearly superior to the other, but I will try especially to show how an investigator might go back and forth between them as each refines targets for the other's special aim.

Less may be "more" for some *places* as well. Although varying in degree of simplicity, economy, and distribution, these simpler techniques tend to offer the possibility of large increments of time and talent invested in neuropsychological research, particularly in the many clinical settings that afford a wealth of patient types and clinical phenomena, and a wealth of clinical experience and insight, but limited technological resources.

For some kinds of questions, some simpler techniques offer enough freedom of exploration in time to compensate for their limitations in comprehensive surveillance of the brain, or to make them useful to those fine-tuning their more comprehensive surveillance. Some will offer greater freedom in choice of individuals or populations to study or in the choice of experimental conditions—settings, tasks, etc.

Most will offer a subtler but perhaps more important freedom: the freedom to explore questions that are not "important" or theoretically "sound" enough to justify the purchase and operation of, or even allocating time with, "super machines"—and yet may in some cases be used to test hypotheses derived from them or develop new ones for them to test.

Let me also say a word in favor of redundancy or apparent redundancy. I have so often seen patients with, for example, clearly identified right-hemisphere lesions do well on one visual/perceptual "right hemisphere" test and poorly on another that I am thankful I do not have to choose one "representative" test. Hypothetical constructs are best defined by relationships among several independent variables and dependent variables, each chosen from a population of possible manipulations and measures; however, it is easier and more common to restrict one's operational definition to one conventional procedure.

Much effort has gone into defining "brain activity" in terms of specific cognitive, sensory, or motor tasks and manipulations that can be related to, for example, cerebral electrophysiological changes. Demonstrations that this activity involved metabolic changes and that changes in local blood flow were tightly coupled to metabolic changes have had and continue to have a profound impact on the way we study the brain (viz., Part II of this volume). We are still expanding the list of subjects and conditions for which we can look at blood flow as if we were looking at brain activity.

Discordant findings from different laboratories are continually under examination, and attempts are made to determine which differences in subjects, tasks, or ways of indexing metabolic activity are relevant. From these attempts, a consensus may be reached, common standards may be adopted, and if one paradigm or measure does not emerge as sole arbiter, one may at least learn what adjustments to make for the special biases or limits of each. However, what potential is there in these comparisons and adjustments for identifying possible cases of failure in the normal parallels?

My sense of cellular physiology is too weak for me to guess whether it is meaningful to try to separate brain activity from brain metabolism even conceptually, but the separation between brain metabolism and brain nutrition/oxygenation is clear enough to make identification of the mechanisms by which they are coupled a provocative and important problem. Earlier discussions emphasized neurogenic control (e.g., noradrenergic), while much recent attention has been focused on adenosine. Different aspects of regional and fine local regulation may involve more than one mechanism; but whether one mechanism or several are involved, acting independently or interactively, wherever a mechanism exists there is a possibility of a broken mechanism.

Are there cases in which blood flow does *not* precisely match metabolic need? We now believe that this is not grossly the case in Alzheimer's dementia, and there is little enthusiasm now for treatments aimed at pumping more blood to tissues now thought too inactive to need it; but can we rule this out universally? More provocative to a neuropsychologist is the possibility of subtler weaknesses or lags in autoregulation on a scale relevant to the fine shifts in activity we seek to identify in our specific functional activation paradigms. The consequence of gross inadequacy of blood flow during high activity may be irreversible damage; but what of a slightly less than optimal blood flow response to the increment of activity appropriate to a specific task? Would the outcome be diminished efficiency or rate of processing, perhaps shown in slower or less accurate performance? Or would it be a shift of activity to another region, perhaps shown in an altered strategy (e.g., a "verbal" approach to a task normally done "nonverbally"), or in a shift of attention to things other than task?

What is the problem with "attention" in Attention Deficit Disorder? Is it "weak"? Is it directed to the wrong things just generally? Does it shift too soon? Only simultaneous measures of neural activity and blood flow, each with a temporal resolution in seconds, could tell us whether blood flow was minimal because "attention" (activity) shifted, or "attention" (activity) shifted because blood flow was minimal or increased too slowly.

IMPORTANT TIMES: THE BRIEF, THE LONG, THE MANY, THE RIGHT

Brief times of neuropsychological interest may range from less than a second to several minutes. The ability to maintain attention or maintain a given type of cognitive activity (e.g., grammatical judgments or mental spatial rotations) over a sufficient length of time for PET or rCBF localizations may be achieved in optimal settings with well-trained volunteers, but what can we devise subsequently to monitor localized activity in patients unable to maintain one or the other? Are there ways in which we can distinguish between "poor" attention or "weak" lateralization and attention or lateralized activity that varies from moment to moment?

Granted that various kinds of Continuous Performance Task (CPT)[1] can detect lapses of attention—*perhaps* as a general trait, more confidently as a state during a CPT, and most confidently as part of the response to that particular CPT—what can we say about lapses or shifts of attention during naturalistically more valid tasks (e.g., reading) or shifts of cognitive strategy/lateralized activity during neuropsychological tests allowing alternative strategies (e.g., right- and left-brain approaches to block design)? How finely can we cut it? Can we monitor responses to single words in a stream of words?

Long times of neuropsychological interest begin where the brief times end, and may be hours, days, months, etc. Split-screen EEG/video 24-hour monitoring to evaluate subtle or infrequent seizure phenomena has already set a new standard or at least introduced a broader concept of adequate observation time, as has Holter monitoring for even longer periods.

Ultradian rhythms in either general or lateralized brain activity, reportedly with periods of about 90 min[2,3] can be evaluated only with monitoring over at least most of a day, and circadian rhythms obviously require more than one or two days to detect. Beyond replicating and extending prior findings with normal subjects, what can we learn about possible alterations of ultradian or circadian rhythms in, for example, head-injured patients and patients with post-concussion or whiplash syndromes?

If we can validate monitoring procedures using normal volunteers to whom we are free to administer demanding multiple-form specialized tests many times a day for several days, could we then monitor neurological patients less stressfully (using one or more of the physiological indices to be described in this and other papers in this section), with only an occasional probe in the form of brief cognitive tests during periods of predicted good, poor, or hemispherically biased performance?

When "long" goes beyond a few hours or a few days, continuous monitoring even with unobtrusive techniques may not be practical—nor even desirable, given the excessive amounts of data we would accumulate. However, repeated measures on the same patient over many weeks or months may be desirable, if, for example, we are trying to evaluate changes from acute to later recovery and chronic periods; for this approach, the convenience, economy, and safety of repeated measures become important considerations.

The "right" time may emerge from studies of longer times: within a designated part of an ultradian cycle, a few minutes may be of special interest. When monitoring reading, the right time may not be the 1-3 sec after every word or after every sentence, but only after those which are misread or which require special attention later inferred to have been lacking. The right time might be the brief period of an absence attack. In other words, the right time might be identified in retrospect on the basis of behavioral data, or might be unexpectedly announced on the basis of an immediately detected physiological event or behavioral lapse. It will almost certainly be missed or obscured by averaging over many trials of, for example, presenting the same type of stimulus.

AUTONOMIC MEASURES

Venables (Part III, this volume) provides a valuable summary of both the limits and the advantages of autonomic measures in the study of brain function, and an authoritative review of technical requirements that must be met rigorously even with these "simple" procedures if results are to be replicable and useful. Beyond this, he provides heuristically valuable examples of applications to neuropsychological issues, including one which combines autonomic measures with dichotic techniques (see papers by Bruder and by Katz and Smith).

As a complement to Venable's critical review of concepts of how phasic heart rate changes are controlled, Levine and Gueramy (also in Part III) describe studies of cardiac deceleration and other aspects of the orienting reflex in head injury and other neurological conditions, as well as more general autonomic functioning which may be altered in special patient groups.

CARDIAC DECELERATION RESPONSE: POSSIBLE USES IN COMA, PERSISTENT VEGETATIVE STATE, AND LESS EXTREME CONDITIONS

Family members often insist that patients in a vegetative state understand what is said to them. As a cautious first step, I tried to determine whether the patients (or at least the two I studied) could discriminate one word from another, using the cardiac deceleration response.[4] Although studies cited by Levine and Gueramy and by Venables have averaged responses over many trials and/or many subjects, and Venables describes mathematical approaches to control for cyclic influences (e.g, due to respiration), I was limited to just a few trials with each subject.

When successive beat-to-beat durations were plotted graphically, cyclic "peaks" (long intervals) and "valleys" (short intervals) were obvious, and I adopted the simple-minded approach of comparing the peak just before a stimulus transition to the one just following it, and the valley just before the transition to the valley just following it. I believe this controls not only for the obvious cyclic influences of respiratory sinus arrhythmia, but also for slower drifts in heart rate or "local" perturbations of a few seconds around the time of the stimulus transition, and is therefore likely to be more sensitive than comparison of post-transition durations to average durations no matter how derived or adjusted. It leads naturally to yes/no decisions about the results of each presentation; in any one case, the decision may be wrong as regards its general implications, but any strong and reliable effect should be evident in a series of such decisions.

When 20 repetitions of one word (ca. 1 per sec) were followed by twenty of another, one patient's heart rate slowed briefly after 7 of 8 such transitions (p = 0.02, one-tailed); the other patient's trend in the same direction was not statistically reliable (4 rate decreases, 2 increases, 1 no change). In contrast, similar transitions between pure tones and silences (one patient) or between tones of different frequencies (the other patient) were followed by decreases or increases about equally. For the two patients combined, word transitions were followed by 13 decreased, 3 increased, and 1 unchanged rate, but tone transitions by 5 decreased, 6 increased, and 3 unchanged rates (word/tone difference, p = 0.03, two-tailed test).

If "no change" cases are ignored, the tendency for nonword transitions to produce more rate increases than word transitions is also statistically reliable (p = 0.025, two-tailed), which raises an important possibility: The patients may simply have failed to discriminate tone transitions or, alternatively, they may have discriminated them but sometimes found the transition to be startling or aversive. In contrast to other indices (autonomic or EEG) that require supplementary information, or comparison of recordings at more than one site (e.g., digital vs. cephalic changes), the cardiac response has the potential of differentiating between an "orienting" reflex (deceleration) and a "defensive" reflex (acceleration) in one measure at one site.

When EEG is the index, use of stimuli that are sufficiently intense or startling to produce gross "alerting" might be questioned on humanitarian grounds, as well as on grounds of the insensitivity and inflexibility of this strategy for evaluating subtler sensory discriminations. Moreover, this use of EEG seems to depend on well-defined alpha or theta rhythms as a background against which changes can be seen, and many patients who are alert and responsive may not meet this criterion.[5]

Few studies reporting use of EEG with comatose or persistently vegetative patients attempt phasic measures: Most focus on tonic patterns that correlate well with alertness or sleep in normal subjects but not in these patients. In only 5 of 20 cases reviewed by Chase et al.[5] was the question of phasic responses addressed. Of three "alert" patients, one who was "inattentive" but able to follow simple commands gave no EEG response to noise or light; a "cooperative" patient showed a shift from theta to alpha after "an aural arousal stimulus" on one occasion, and the third patient showed a "minimal" response of questionable relevance to awareness: photic driving. Of two "unresponsive" patients, one tended to show replacement of slow wave activity by better organized alpha rhythms after auditory or tactile stimulation.

Hawkes and Bryan-Smith[6] recommended EEG as a "rapid and simple way" to distinguish between the locked-in state and akinetic mutism or other "coma" conditions, and emphasized the importance of evaluating not just tonic EEG composition but reactivity of the EEG to "alerting stimuli." Noise, pain, and eye opening elicited EEG changes in most of their patients, but of two described as "rousable" and "locked-in," only one responded to noise and neither responded to pain or eye opening so far as the EEG could indicate.

Cardiac deceleration might prove to be a useful tool not just for initial evaluations of patients but for monitoring and evaluating rehabilitation procedures, such as the still controversial "coma stimulation" programs. For example, EEG changes following sensorimotor therapy with comatose patients have been claimed on the basis of brief samples (ten, each lasting 16 sec) before and after each therapy session.[7] If cardiac responses had been monitored during therapy sessions, they might have identified which interventions elicited responses on a moment-to-moment basis, categorized responses as "orienting" or "defensive," and provided a basis for identifying their relationship to possible long-term changes.

My attempt to separate word discrimination based simply on acoustic changes from discrimination based on meaning (a series of different words in a single category, spoken once, interrupted sporadically by a word from another category) was encouraging but inconclusive, because exploration using standard EKG had to be limited. Further explorations and routine clinical use of the cardiac deceleration response will require automatic, direct, and rapid recording of inter-beat time—not the "momentary" averages in commercially available instruments, but time between each successive beat. I offer the following recipe, surely not the most technologically advanced, strictly for its heuristic value.

1. A peak detector,[8] rather than a level detector or Schmitt trigger, because it is relatively independent of absolute current levels and thus does not require continued recalibration to compensate for "drift" in skin/electrode resistance; it is also relatively resistant to movement artifact (triggering by limb movement or respiration). Electrodes would not have to be placed on the chest wall, patients unable to restrict movements could be included, and clinical use would not presuppose the time and technical skill to monitor and recalibrate the instrument, allowing full attention to stimulus presentation and behavioral observation.

2. A digital beat-to-beat timer[9] would use pulses from the peak detector to initiate timing with one R wave and to conclude timing, record the value, reset and begin again with the next R wave. Rather than average or interpolated values, this yields the exact duration of each R-R interval, immediately upon its completion.

3. The digital value obtained by the beat-to-beat timer could be printed immediately and silently on thermal-sensitive paper, perhaps by the printer of a pocket-sized calculator. With even minimal programming capability, it might also do some automatic analysis of data as it is collected, allowing the user to detect responses at a glance. One calculator key could signal stimulus presentation, allowing more precise timing than, for example, manual marking of an EKG tape.

Other Applications

Although the cardiac deceleration response has been used mainly in laboratory studies to answer theoretical questions or to evaluate perceptual capacities of representative samples of normal human or animal groups, its potential for clinical evaluation of individuals has already been noted.[10] Its potential value when brain damage precludes comprehension of audiological testing instructions or reliable compliance with them is obvious. Moreover, aphasic patients who do comprehend sometimes confuse yes/no responses on a sporadic basis, and follow-up cardiac response verification or contradiction of hearing loss would be valuable. It is imperative that the rehabilitation and management of brain-injured patients not be complicated by inaccurate or incomplete assessments of basic sensory functions.

Attentional deficits manifested as smaller decelerations at critical points in attention-demanding tasks have been reported for patients with right-hemisphere lesions[11] and for hyperactive boys.[12]

AUTONOMIC ADDENDA

Although I have emphasized phasic responses, this section would be incomplete without reference to monitoring over long enough periods to assess overall variability of beat-to-beat values. Decreased respiratory sinus arrhythmia (i.e., reduction in the normal inhibition of heart activity by respiration, mediated by the vagus nerve) has been included in measures of peripheral autonomic neuropathy, as in diabetes, and also to assess central nervous system integrity, perhaps cholinergic function specifically.[13,14] It is known that geriatric patients are susceptible to cognitively significant anticholinergic effects of rather small amounts of many commonly prescribed medications, and correlations have been reported between serum or cerebral spinal fluid anticholinergic activity and some cognitive tests.[15] In contrast, it has been suggested that there is a *positive* relationship between cholinergic *hyperactivity* and "negative" schizophrenic symptoms.[16] Similarly, although we normally assume that anticholinergic "side effects" are detrimental to head-injured patients, it has been suggested that there is a subgroup among whom coma is maintained by an active cholinergic process.[17] If this is true, and if the process includes enhanced vagal outflow, measures of heart rate variability might help identify patients in this subgroup and monitor attempted interventions.

It would be advantageous to monitor cholinergic status and correlate it to behavioral or cognitive status, particularly during any changes due to treatment or disease progression, without subjecting the patient to repeated blood drawing or spinal tapping; monitoring of sinus arrhythmia is one candidate.

In contrast to parasympathetic measures, sympathetic measures have been emphasized by others to assess arousal level. In addition to those listed in the paper by Levine and Gueramy, there are other studies of, for example, head injury,[18] third ventricle enlargement in schizophrenia,[19] and developmental hyperactivity.[20] Of particular interest is the possibility that such monitoring can be used to determine *optimal* levels of arousal and perhaps predict drug response or be used to titrate drug dosage.[18,20]

Finally, mention must be made of a development in electrodermal measurement[21] too recent for evaluation and comment by Venables in his paper. Based on an alternating-current technique in which unbalancing of a self-balancing circuit is caused by impedance changes induced by sudomotor activity, it is said to avoid electrode polarization, electrochemical tissue attack, and sensitivity to noise and drift errors typical of the usual direct current procedures. In addition to what is claimed to be greater stability and reliability in amplitude measurements, greater precision of the latency measure, based on its independence from other factors, has been exploited to assess autonomic conduction velocities by comparing palmar and plantar latencies. Perhaps it will find a use in long-term monitoring and left/right comparisons, to detect tonic and phasic autonomic expressions of lateralized cerebral activation. As Venables points out, pending replication of Rippon's 1987 study, we cannot yet use electrodermal responses to track shifts in hemispheric activity because we are not yet sure whether such activity enhances or inhibits contralateral skin responses!

"BEDSIDE" CEREBRAL BLOOD FLOW MONITORING (MOMENT-TO-MOMENT)

Swift and Perlman[22] assumed increased brain activity would result in increased temperature measured at the tympanic membrane, and were disconcerted to obtain "inconsistent" results with verbal verses nonverbal tasks. In fact, their female subjects gave results similar to the predominantly female group of Meiners and Dabbs,[23] who had reported decreased temperatures on the left during verbal tasks and on the right during spatial tasks. Brain metabolic rate is so great that entering blood does tend to be cooler,[24] and although both the hypothalamus and the temporal lobe are very near the measurement site, about half-way to the midsagittal plane, the internal carotid artery is even closer, separated by a thin and sometimes incomplete bony lamella and is a formidable potential heat source or sink. Therefore, I tend to share the expectations of Meiners and Dabbs, but in my own brief explorations (with two subjects), I could make sense of the data only if I assumed the direction depended on baseline overall level. Instrumentation improvements (e.g., infrared sensing rather than direct tympanic contact and individual ear molds) may help, and further validation efforts are in progress (Arlette Swift, personal communication). Given the very gross regionality of activation likely to be reflected in carotid flow, it does not appear a promising method for localization within hemispheres, but gross left/right differences might be of interest in some applications, for example, long-term monitoring of gross hemispheric shifts in recovery from unilateral stroke.

For greater regional specificity and more reliable quantification, rheoencephalography and transcranial Doppler sonography have more immediate applicability.

Rheoencephalography

Also known as cerebral electrical impedance or impedance plethysmography, this approach, which is based on the impedance difference between blood and surrounding tissues, with blood flow changes reflected in changes of form or magnitude of impedance waves recorded when low intensity alternating current is passed through the head, has been studied for over 40 years, without gaining wide clinical acceptance. Slow development of improvements in instrumentation or analysis may account for some of the neglect, but more may be due to the specific needs of clinical practitioners first attracted to it, which may not coincide with those of neuropsychological investigators.

Recent engineering studies have identified several technical improvements and alternative indices for specific aspects of blood flow.[25] Jacquy *et al.*[26] emphasized rheoencephalography's relatively poor spatial resolution but superior temporal resolution, on the order of ± 10 sec, comparing their findings of latencies between EEG desynchronization after visual stimulation and impedance changes with latencies between desynchronization and blood flow directly measured in animals, as reported by previous investigators.

I was more impressed with the contrast between what appeared to be large, sustained increases over at least 2-3 min during a visual attention test in contrast to the habituation evident within 1-2 min of simply looking at a picture[26] (pp. 344-345, 347). Although limited in spatial resolution, the technique may be able to differentiate between major regions, such as frontal, temporal, left versus right hemisphere homologous sites, etc.[27]

Colditz *et al.*[28] directly compare rheoencephalography and xenon clearance measures of cerebral blood flow in neonates and make the point that interpretation of results is difficult because "there is no single method of measuring blood flow which provides a standard for comparison of other techniques" (p. 462). They and other authors also emphasize the large measurement error of the clearance technique itself which can account for reductions in the correlation beyond more basic differences in what the measure may entail.

Colditz *et al.*[28] acknowledge that difficulties in quantitative estimations using rheoencephalography, differences in blood viscosity and other factors may make comparisons between subjects invalid,[25] but while these considerations may still justify the hesitance of clinicians to use the technique diagnostically, they should not keep us from exploiting its special advantages of noninvasiveness and good temporal resolution in monitoring changes within individuals or comparing direction or rate of change between individuals. Colditz et al.[29] used it precisely this way in a study that directly compared Doppler and cerebral electrical impedance measures: they closely agreed on latency and extent of blood flow changes with rapid as compared to gradual indomethacin infusions in neonates.

Transcranial Doppler Sonography

In contrast to the generally poor acceptance of rheoencephalography in clinical work, a variety of techniques based on the Doppler phenomenon are widely accepted and used, which means wide availability of instruments and opportunities for collaboration or consultation in their use for neuropsychological explorations. Other ultrasound techniques are also widely available, raising the possibility of noninvasive, relatively inexpensive and "portable" imaging techniques for coordinating blood flow findings with individual brain anatomies. Ultrasound Doppler recording of blood flow velocity in extracranial arteries, reported in 1965,[30] was extended to intraoperative recording of intracranial flow in adults[31] and recording through the open fontanels in infants.[32]

Using a lower frequency, less attenuated by mature skulls,[33] opened the way for rapid, "real-time" noninvasive monitoring of flow in middle, anterior, and posterior cerebral arteries in adults. In 1987, Aaslid[34] demonstrated its sensitivity, fine temporal resolution, and some regional specificity in detecting activation by crude visual stimuli: with 20-sec light on/light off periods, some response to light onset was evident in the posterior artery in 1 sec, half of the full response in 2-3 sec, and 90% of the full response within 4-6 sec, with some reduction (adaptation) in the last 10 sec—in contrast to a much smaller increase in the middle cerebral artery and practically no response in the anterior artery.

Comparisons of left and right middle cerebral artery flow during cognitive tasks were made soon after by Droste et al.[35,36] who claimed only modest success in finding anything other than bilateral increases with a series of putative left- and right-hemisphere tasks: greater left than right increase during "noun finding aloud" in one report,[36] and greater right increase in three right-hemisphere tasks in other report.[35] Their proposals to improve left-right comparisons in future studies include simultaneous measurements of right and left arteries or quickly alternating measurements, and measurements in more distal branches of the arteries. Both improvements would no doubt be useful, but my impression is that their analysis of the data already obtained may have been too conservative and did not take full advantage of the temporal resolution they document in their descriptions and several of their figures.

Each task had a 90-sec duration but within this period, for each task, a peak response was seen at about 8 sec, decreasing variably afterwards (ca. 8-20 sec), then increasing to an apparent steady state during the last half of the period (from about 42 sec on). It is interesting that a small peak is also seen at the onset of rest periods, especially on the right, and that in two of the three tasks shown in one report[35] and all three shown in the other report,[36] the early peak during the task performance was greater on the right—all but one of which would seem a good "left-hemisphere" task. Habituation was also reported[35] to be greatest on the right. I suggest that the Right Time for looking at left/right differences is not during the full 90 sec of the task assignment but during the steady state period—in these procedures and at this level of subject training and habituation, during the last 48 sec of the 90-sec task, but possibly during somewhat different periods with different tasks, subjects, or amount of practice.

To include values from the initial 42 sec obscures the left/right differences in two ways: it excessively weights the right-sided values, making it deceptively easy to find right increases during right-hemisphere tasks and hard-to-find left increases during left-hemisphere tasks, and the statistical reliability of either finding is greatly compromised by the excessively large standard error undoubtedly resulting from the extreme increases and decreases evident in the first 20 sec or so. Of course, this is post hoc, but cross validation should readily test my argument and perhaps help develop a powerful new strategy.

That is, designated right- or left-hemisphere cognitive tasks are used to validate our indices of brain activation, but these indices can then be used to validate our tasks and to dissect them, separating the intended from the actual tasks—we tell the subject to do one thing, but the subject may do something else unprescribed and perhaps undescribed, either at the onset of the task (as I have argued happened in Droste *et al.*) or at some point during it. Years ago, I suggested (private communication) that some of the hypofrontality of schizophrenic subjects might be due to their failure to obey instructions to keep their eyes closed—that is, hyperposteriority and thus relative hypofrontality. Subsequent improvements in experimental control may have eliminated this as a very general possibility, but the possibility remains that schizophrenic subjects do something else in the course of a study—not so obvious as opening their eyes when told not to—that detracts from relative frontal activation. Hallucinatory intrusions, obsessive preoccupations, and hypervigilant diversion of attention to non-task auditory or visual events are obvious possibilities.

Without a moment-by-moment monitoring of some index of activation (e.g., rheoencephalographic or Doppler measures of blood flow), we cannot separate a *tonic* hypofrontality (or hyperfrontality, for that matter), either as a *trait* manifested chronically in a given patient group or as a *state* manifest in specified tasks or conditions, from a *phasic* hypofrontality. If a given patient is capable of good frontal activation at times, but cannot maintain it throughout tasks of the length convenient for our slower recording methods, the brief periods of activation and inactivation will, when averaged over these longer time bases, look exactly the same as an overall weakness in activation; but the two different ways of achieving hypofrontality are surely different in their theoretical implications, and perhaps in the practical prescriptions they may suggest.

Left/right specialization studies could benefit greatly if we could reliably identify the point in a series of trials at which a subject will reliably go quickly into the appropriate hemispheric activation after some initial floundering around (cf. the old learning set or "learning to learn" literature), or the point at which a novel task becomes routine and dominant activity shifts from right to left hemisphere.[37] Despite their crude spatial resolutions, techniques with good temporal resolution can advance the cause of more comprehensive and fine-grained brain mapping by selecting optimal onset times for (e.g.) PET or SPECT time-exposures.

Further Examples of the Right Time

Sanada *et al.*[38] cited prior cCBF and PET evidence of increased cortical blood flow or metabolism "during" absence seizures, and other PET evidence of decreased metabolism during absence status; but because of the long exposure times (10 min), it wasn't clear to what extent these results reflected changes during seizures and to what extent they included post-ictal changes. Using transcranial Doppler recordings of the middle cerebral artery in one patient whose seizures lasted typically 8 sec, they found that velocity started to decrease approximately 7 sec after seizure onset, returned to pre-ictal level approximately 17 sec later and increased slightly, with stable normal values re-established about 48 sec after the seizure's end.

In another patient, with absence seizures ranging from 8-26 sec, velocity for seizures lasting more than 15 sec was greater than for shorter seizures, but the latencies of velocity changes were similar for short and long attacks, i.e., about 7-9 sec. The generality of these findings and the functional implications are unclear at this point, but one obvious possibility is that the functional disturbance of what appears electrophysiologically to be, for example, an 8-sec absence might well last 2-3 times that long.

Stefan et al.[39] report impressive attempts to select the right time for SPECT mapping of ictal changes in focal seizures of frontal and frontocerebral onset. With one patient, whose ictal and interictal EEG focus was inferior mesial left temporal lobe, injection of the SPECT tracer was late—720 sec after onset—and "ictal" hyperperfusion was seen in the *right* temporal region. With injection 140 sec after a second seizure, SPECT showed bitemporal hyperperfusion. Only when injection was initiated 73 sec after seizure onset was hyperperfusion localized to the left temporal site determined by ictal and interictal EEG.

Using the earlier injection time, one patient was found to have hyperperfusion in the same locus both ictally and interictally. Was this true anomaly, or could it be that for this particular patient the earlier injection was not early enough? Another patient had bilateral EEG signs but right hyperperfusion according to SPECT. With slightly later injection time (either absolutely or relative to some individual characteristics of this patient), might not EEG and SPECT have agreed, erroneously?

To get measures at the right place at the right time, it would seem useful to select likely targets by means of rCBF, SPECT, or PET—or perhaps EEG—and then aiming roughly at these targets with rheoencephalography or Doppler, determine significant times at which to aim subsequent exposures with rCBF, SPECT, or PET.

This is perhaps a good context in which to remind the reader of a metabolic technique, based on PET principles, but sacrificing comprehensive brain mapping in favor of finer temporal resolution and greater freedom for repetitive testing: the simplified two-detector system described by Bice (Part II, this volume), a good candidate for verifying some of the spatial and temporal targets and quantifying activity at the right place at the right time.

TONIC/DIFFUSE AROUSAL vs. PHASIC/FOCUSED AROUSAL: 40-Hz EEG

For over a decade, Gevins (this volume) has argued the importance of finer temporal resolution to more precise and meaningful spatial localization of functions, citing rapid shifts of activity and involvement of several brain areas even within a very brief (1.2 sec) visuomotor task.[40] Gevins et al.[41] suggested that "the rapid change in the side of localized process may account for conflicting reports of lateralization in studies which lacked adequate spatial and temporal resolution" and that "advanced radiological methods reveal relative localization and lateralization, but cannot resolve temporal sequencing because of the long time required for observation. Studies of ongoing, background electrical activity do not reveal split-second changes in neurocognitive patterns . . ." (p. 97).

More recently, Gevins *et al.*[42] conclude, "The measurement of event-related covariances is currently the only practical means of identifying narrow-band, fraction-of-a-second patterns of wave shape similarity and timing differences between event-related signals recorded from different scalp sites. Measurements of spectral coherence, as are conventionally estimated from smoothed periodograms or autoregressive models, have not yet achieved a similar degree of temporal and frequency resolution . . . By definition, topographic maps of potential or metabolic activity do not show this type of information" (p. 72).

These split-second shifts have been revealed in a technique which is based on recording of event-related potentials (ERP) with latencies on the order of 300 msec or less and comparably small durations, so in EEG terms the focus has been on very low frequencies: "Our primary interest was in event-related wave forms in the delta and theta bands"[43] (p. 177), but in a very recent report, Gevins *et al.*[44] point out that ". . . there is a wealth of data in other frequency regions and their accompanying time intervals that has yet to be explored" (p. 158).

For over two decades, Sheer has been studying EEG bursts in a higher frequency region, nominally 40 Hz, but ranging from 35-85 Hz, depending on species and locus[45] (p. 343). He also emphasizes the value of very fine temporal resolution and has recently said that he and others are "trying to demonstrate momentary electrophysiological connectivity between sensory and motor cortex by a coherent lock-in of 40 Hz at significant behavioral times during a 1-sec task in humans."[46]

He made this remark in commenting on a research news summary[47] of a different line of work which emphasized temporal synchrony as a possible mechanism for unifying widespread neurons in a coherent response to a specific visual object, and in which it was suggested that "one of the features that makes the 40-hertz oscillations attractive as a mediator of visual awareness . . . is that their time scale corresponds with that of attention flitting from one object to another. The neurons typically stay phase-locked for several hundred milliseconds, which would allow them to make and break their liaisons in roughly the same period that a person's attention moves from one subject to the next" (p. 857).

I found it difficult to research 40-Hz studies, because 40 Hz did not appear as a major descriptor in my indexing source, and the catch-all "beta" included either too wide an undefined range of "high" frequencies (usually of tonic activity) or a band truncated at too low a frequency. Many studies that did specify 40 Hz appeared to be describing photic or auditory driving by stimulus trains at this frequency.

However, this may best be understood as augmenting a middle-latency evoked potential occurring naturally at this frequency, and as Sheer[45] points out, while the "forcing function" of 40-Hz ERPs elicited by 40-Hz stimulation is more stable and constant, 20-Hz stimulation produces a more variable 40-Hz response that is "more sensitive to changes in focused arousal, as affected by relevant state conditions, behavioral contingencies, and brain impairments" (p. 348).

Sheer differentiates focused arousal in specific sensory systems from that which is more loosely coupled to complex multisensory systems[45] (pp. 344-345). In an example with cats bar-pressing for milk reward during 10-sec periods signaled by 4-per-second light flashes, bursts of 40-Hz activity were recorded from the lateral geniculate nucleus for each flash, allowing investigators to average 40 samples over each 10-sec period. However, Sheer points out that they could have measured the number of rectified oscillations (80 peaks per sec) above a pre-set amplitude threshold, over the 10-sec period, and that this latter approach would be appropriate for more complex contingent events that did not allow response averaging—"stimulus sets and, in humans, instructional sets and problem solving."

The difficulty in distinguishing between diffuse and/or tonic arousal and focused arousal or momentary local activation using traditional "EEG desynchronization" is analogous to the difficulty I have already pointed out in using EEG or nonspecific autonomic activity to identify the kind of sensory detection and sensory (or higher perceptual) discrimination implicit in the orienting reflex, as indexed by phasic cardiac deceleration. In one study,[48] decreased latencies of 40-Hz bursts, evident within 150-300 msec of presenting auditory or visual shape stimuli to be discriminated, were directly coordinated to cardiac deceleration indices of orienting reflexes—occurring, of course, seconds later. In other words, 40-Hz recordings may give us a much earlier look at the orienting reflex and allow much finer temporal precision in identifying relevant stimulus events.

In some exploratory human clinical applications, groups have been compared simply in terms of the "amount" of 40-Hz activity: for example, in contrast to patients with Alzheimer's dementia, depressed and normal subjects were both found to show increased activation during cognitive tasks,[49] but its potential applications go far beyond this. For example, children with learning disability (LD) characterized by impaired reading had less 40-Hz *left*-hemisphere activity during a verbal task (listening to sentences to be repeated) than either control subjects or children whose LD was characterized by impaired arithmetic; however, during a nonverbal task (looking at faces to be recognized), children with arithmetic LD had less *right*-hemisphere 40-Hz activity than children with reading LD, whose right hemisphere activations in this task was normal.[50]

Provocative as demonstrations of lateralized 40-Hz activity in specified cognitive tasks are (further examples in Sheer[45]), they do not fully exploit the temporal resolution possible with this measure. Bursts of 40-Hz activity lasting 100-200 msec are usual, and although 50 msec may be too brief a period in which to identify 40-Hz activity reliably, 100 msec is probably sufficient in many contexts (Sheer, personal communication). This suggests to me that even if 40-Hz activity never proves capable of paralleling the multichannel covariance analysis of Gevins *et al.*, 40-Hz recording is possible within a realm of temporal resolution that would allow us to target specific times and places (during brief cognitive tasks) at which the work of Gevins *et al.* indicates something special is happening. In specific cases, failure to confirm expected activity might upon further investigation reveal two possible types of deviation: (1) delayed completion of a normal sequence of regional activation, or (2) aberrant sequences. Gevins *et al.*[51] describe a change in pattern and/or sequence in normal subjects whose performance was impaired following prolonged mental work, and it would be interesting to see if similar changes occur in particular pathological conditions even at the beginning of work.

In any case, regional 40-Hz recording is a good candidate for some of the longer-period monitoring and probes within periods discussed earlier in this paper. For example, if normal subjects show activity 90% of the time in, for example, the left frontal area during a few minutes of a given task, how does this compare with the proportion of time such activity is seen in members of a given diagnostic group and how is activity distributed through this period? This is yet one more way to approach the question of "weak" versus "variable" frontal activation in schizophrenia as the underlying basis of what appears to be "hypofrontality" in some longer "time exposure" views, and within this context the work of Gevins *et al.*[44] suggests a specific target for a more closely timed look. They found a difference between early and late P3 peaks depending on type of feedback, with notification of inaccurate responses increasing the late peak relative to the early peak, but notification of accurate responses decreasing it relative to the early peak; they cite prior work suggesting that the late P3 is related to use of feedback in reinforcing or revising the behavioral response.

At what points during, for example, the Wisconsin Card Sorting Test might frontal activation in schizophrenic subjects be especially lacking—might it be at precisely the points at which they receive the feedback needed to guide their next sort? Reaction to feedback in other patient groups, such as those with right-hemisphere stroke,[52] might also be interesting to study in this way.

REFERENCES

1. HALPERIN, J. M. 1991. The clinical assessment of attention. Int. J. Neurosci. In press.
2. BROUGHTON, R. 1982. Human consciousness and sleep/walking rhythms: A review and some neuropsychological considerations. J. Clin. Exp. Neuropsychol. **4:** 193-218.
3. ARMITAGE, R. & R. KLEIN. 1979. Rhythms in human performance: 1½-hour oscillations in cognitive style. Science **204:** 1326-1328.
4. LEFEVER, F. F. 1986. What can coma patients hear? Exploratory evaluations using the cardiac deceleration response (abstract). J. Clin. Exp. Neuropsychol. **8:** 141-142.
5. CHASE, T. N., L. MORETTI & A. L. PRENSKY. 1968. Clinical and electroencephalographic manifestations of vascular lesions of the pons. Neurology **18:** 357-368.
6. HAWKES, C. H. & L. BRYAN-SMYTH. 1974. The electroencephalogram in the "locked-in" syndrome. Neurology **24:** 1015-1018.
7. WEBER, P. L. 1984. Sensorimotor therapy: Its effect on encephalograms of acute comatose patients. Arch. Phys. Med. Rehabil. **65:** 457-462.
8. SHIMUZU, H. 1978. Reliable and precise identification of R-waves in the EKG with a simple peak detector. Psychophysiology **15:** 499-501.
9. STOTTS, L. J. & W. M. PORTNOY. 1979. Digital beat-to-beat cardiotachometer. Am. J. Phys. Med. **58:** 86-90.
10. GERBER, S. E., A. MULAC & B. J. SWAIN. 1976. Idiosyncratic cardiovascular response of human neonates to acoustic stimuli. J. Am. Audiol. Soc. **1:** 185-191.
11. YOKOYAMA, K., R. JENNINGS, P. ACKLES, P. HOOD & F. BOLLER. 1987. Lack of heart rate changes during an attention-demanding tack after right hemisphere lesions. Neurology **37:** 624-630.
12. BRAND, E. & H. VAN DER VLUGT. 1986. Electrocardiac recording during a continuous performance task in hyperactive boys and two control groups (abstract). J. Clin. Exp. Neuropsychol. **8:** 122.
13. FOX, N. A. & S. W. PORGES. 1985. The relation between neonatal heart period patterns and developmental outcome. Child Dev. **56:** 28-37.
14. PORGES, S. W., P. M. MCCABE & B. G. YONGUE. 1982. Respiratory heart rate interactions: Psychophysiological implications for pathophysiology and behavior. *In* Perspectives in Cardiovascular Pathophysiology. J. T. Cacioppo & R. E. Petty, Eds.: 223-264. Guilford. New York, NY.
15. MILLER, P. S., J. S. RICHARDSON, C. A. JYU, J. S. LEMAY, M. HISCOCK & D. L. KEEGAN. 1988. Association of low serum anticholinergic levels and cognitive impairment in elderly presurgical patients. Am. J. Psychiatry **145:** 342-345.
16. TANDON, R. & J. F. GREDEN. 1989. Cholinergic hyperactivity and negative schizophrenic symptoms. Arch. Gen. Psychiatry **46:** 745-753.
17. SAIJA, A., R. L. HAYES, B. G. LYETH, C. E. DIXON, T. YAMAMOTO & S. E. ROBINSON. 1988. The effect of concussive head injury on central cholinergic neurons. Brain Res. **452:** 303-311.
18. KLØVE, H. 1987. Activation, arousal, and neuropsychological rehabilitation. J. Clin. Exp. Neuropsychol. **9:** 297-309.
19. CANNON, T. D., M. FUHRMAN, S. A. MEDNICK, R. A. MACHON, J. PARNAS & F. SCHULSINGER. 1988. Third ventricle enlargement and reduced electrodermal responsiveness. Psychophysiology **25:** 153-156.
20. CONTE, R. & M. KINSBOURNE. 1988. Electrodermal lability predicts presentation rate effects and stimulant drug effects on paired associate learning in hyperactive children. Psychophysiology **25:** 64-70.
21. PRUNĂ, S. 1990. Improved technique for testing autonomic dysfunction: Evaluation of transient behavior of the autonomic response. Med. & Biol. Eng. & Comput. **28:** 119-126.

22. SWIFT, A. B. & M. B. PERLMAN. 1985. A noninvasive index of hemispheric activity. Percept. Mot. Skills **60:** 515-524.

23. MEINERS, M. L. & J. M. DABBS, JR. 1977. Ear temperature and brain blood flow: Laterality effects. Bull. Psychon. Soc. **10:** 194-196.

24. HAYWARD, J. N., E. SMITH & D. G. STEWART. 1966. Temperature gradients between arterial blood and brain in the monkey. Proc. Soc. Exp. Biol. Med. **121:** 547-551.

25. JEVNING, R., G. FERNANDO & A. F. WILSON. 1989. Evaluation of consistency among different electrical impedance indices of relative cerebral blood flow in normal resting individuals. J. Biomed. Eng. **11:** 53-56.

26. JACQUY, J., P. CHARLES, A. PIRAUX & G. NOËL. 1980. Relationship between the electroencephalogram and the rheoencephalogram in the normal young adult. Neuropsychobiology **6:** 341-348.

27. JACQUY, J. & P. SQUELART. 1984. Right hemispheric activation on chronognosia: A preliminary study by rheoencephalograpy. Neuropsychobiology **11:** 3-6.

28. COLDITZ, P., G. GREISEN & O. PRYDS. 1988. Comparison of electrical impedance and ^{133}xenon clearance for the assessment of cerebral blood flow in the newborn infant. Pediatr. Res. **24:** 461-464.

29. COLDITZ, P., D. MURPHY, P. ROLFE & A. T. WILKINSON. 1989. Effect of infusion rate of indomethacin on cerebrovascular responses in preterm neonates. Arch. Dis. Child. **64** (1 Spec. No.): 8-12.

30. MIYAZAKI, M. & K. KATO. 1965. Measurement of cerebral blood flow by Doppler technique. JPN. Circ. J. **29:** 375-382.

31. NORNES, H., A. GRIP & P. WIKEBY. 1979. Intraoperative evaluation of cerebral hemodynamics using directional Doppler technique: Part 1. Arteriovenous malformations. J. Neurosurg. **50:** 145-151.

32. MUCHAIDZE, Y. A. & E. V. SYUTKINA. 1979. Determination of the linear velocity of the cerebral blood flow in premature infants. Hum. Physiol. **5:** 595-599.

33. AASLID, R., T.-W. MARKWALDER & H. NORNES. 1982. Noninvasive transcranial Doppler ultrasound recording of flow velocity in basal cerebral arteries. J. Neurosurg. **57:** 769-774.

34. AASLID, R. 1987. Visually evoked dynamic blood flow response of the human cerebral circulation. Stroke **18:** 771-775.

35. DROSTE, D. W., A. G. HARDERS & E. RASTOGI. 1989. A transcranial Doppler study of blood flow velocity in the middle cerebral arteries performed at rest and during mental activities. Stroke **20:** 1005-1011.

36. DROSTE, D. W., A. G. HARDERS & E. RASTOGI. 1989. Two transcranial Doppler studies on blood flow velocity in both middle cerebral arteries during rest and the performance of cognitive tasks. Neuropsychologia **27:** 1221-30.

37. GOLDBERG, E. & L. D. COSTA. 1981. Hemisphere differences in the acquisition and use of descriptive systems. Brain Lang. **14:** 144-173.

38. SANADA, S., N. MURAKAMI & S. OHTAHARA. 1988. Changes in blood flow of the middle cerebral artery during absence seizures. Pediatr. Neurol. **4:** 158-161.

39. STEFAN, H., J. BAUER, H. FEISTEL, H. SCHULEMANN, U. NEUBAUER, B. WENZEL, F. WOLF, B. NEUNDORFER & W.-J. HUK. 1990. Regional cerebral blood flow during focal seizures of temporal and frontocentral onset. Ann. Neurol. **27:** 162-166.

40. GEVINS, A. S., J. C. DOYLE, B. A. CUTILLO, R. E. SCHAFFER, R. S. TANNEHILL, J. H. GHANNHAM, V. A. GILCREASE & C. L. YEAGER. 1981. Electrical potentials in human brain during cognition: New method reveals dynamic patterns of correlation. Science **213:** 918-922.

41. GEVINS, A. S., R. E. SCHAFFER, J. C. DOYLE, B. A. CUTILLO, R. S. TANNEHILL & S. L. BRESSLER. 1983. Shadows of thought: Shifting lateralization of human brain electrical patterns during brief visuomotor task. Science **220:** 97-99.

42. GEVINS, A. S., S. L. BRESSLER, N. H. MORGAN, B. A. CUTILLO, R. M. WHITE, D. S. GREER & J. ILLES. 1989. Event-related covariances during a bimanual visuomotor task. I. Methods and analysis of stimulus- and response-locked data. Electroencephalogr. Clin. Neurophysiol. **74:** 58-75.

43. GEVINS, A. S., N. H. MORGAN, S. L. BRESSLER, J. C. DOYLE & B. A. CUTILLO. 1986. Improved event-related potential estimation using statistical pattern classification. Electroencephalogr. Clin. Neurophysiol. **64:** 177-186.

44. GEVINS, A. S., B. A. CUTILLO, S. L. BRESSLER, N. H. MORGAN, R. M. WHITE, J. ILLES & D. S. GREER. 1989. Event-related covariances during a bimanual visuomotor task. II. Preparation and feedback. Electroencephalogr. Clin. Neurophysiol. **74:** 147-160.
45. SHEER, D. E. 1989. Sensory and cognitive 40-Hz event-related potentials: behavioral correlates, brain function, and clinical application. *In* Brain Dynamics. E. Başar & T. H. Bullock, Eds.: 339-374. Springer-Verlag, New York, NY.
46. SHEER, D. E. 1990. Letter submitted to Editor, Science.
47. BARINAGA, M. 1990. The mind revealed? Science **249:** 856-858.
48. VARNER, J. L., J. W. ROHRBAUGH, S. R. PAIGE & R. J. ELLINGSON. 1984. Attention-related changes in a computer-extracted 40-Hz EEG rhythm. Biomed. Sci. Instrum. **20:** 81-83.
49. KELLER, W. J. 1989. Forty Hertz EEG activity in depressed elderly (abstract). J. Clin. Exp. Neuropsychol. **11:** 95.
50. MATTSON, A. J., D. E. SHEER & J. M. FLETCHER. 1989. 40 Hertz EEG activity in LD and normal children (abstract). J. Clin. Exp. Neuropsychol. **11:** 32.
51. GEVINS, A. S., S. L. BRESSLER, B. A. CUTILLO, J. ILLES & R. M. FOWLER-WHITE. Effects of prolonged mental work on functional brain topography. Electroencephalogr. Clin. Neurophysiol. In press. As cited by Gevins, A. S. *et al.,* 1989. Brain Topogr. **2:** 37-56.
52. LEFEVER, F. F. 1989. Hemispatial neglect (letter). Neurology **39:** 1006.

Autonomic Activity

PETER H. VENABLES

Department of Psychology
University of York
Heslington, York YO1 5DD
United Kingdom

INTRODUCTION

The use of measurement of autonomic activity is perhaps one of the more unlikely methods of creating a window on the brain, and it is therefore necessary to attempt some justification for this approach at the outset. The methods used are essentially old-fashioned and, in comparison with, for instance, computerized axial tomography, magnetic resonance imaging, positron emission tomography, neuromagnetic field resonance, and even topographical EEG and ERP mapping, may appear to be in the horse-and-buggy era. While many of these more recently introduced methods have the aim of pinpointing activity or dysfunction in particular localized areas of the brain, findings using these methods do not necessarily give information about the functioning of the structure studied, nor how it is integrated with the totality of brain function. It may therefore be important to consider the role of a "window on the brain" as providing a window on its relatively global function rather than being an index relating to the more detailed structural status of a particular system. With this in mind it may often be relevant to relate autonomic activity to more global aspects of behavior as indicators of higher nervous system activity.

Measurement of autonomic activity has some advantages and if the accompanying disadvantages are also clearly recognized, benefits may be seen to accrue. The main advantages are those of relative simplicity and comparatively low cost; the noninvasiveness of the techniques, both psychologically and physiologically; and the ability to deal with the effects of single stimuli, with no averaging required and information being gathered from each response.

The main disadvantage of the use of autonomic measures is that they are indirect indices of higher activity—the activity of the brain, which is the prime purpose of measurement in the context of this book. The measures have possible multiplicity of determination, and they involve systems with multiple functions.

Let us consider these aspects in more detail. One of the disadvantages of the "heavy machinery" methods of gaining information on cortical activity is that they are psychologically invasive. If the patient, or even the normal control, has to put his head in a large probe, it must have an effect on the subject's psychological state and hence the cortical activity which the investigator is trying to measure. Even completing the attachment of a large array of EEG electrodes is not without its disturbing effect. In consequence, measures which involve the placement of few electrodes or even only involve the subject putting a finger in a photoplethysmograph cuff are to be considered as desirable. Also, in general, apart from the possible slight abrasion of the skin to obtain a better electrical contact, the measures used are physiologically noninvasive. In comparison there is, for example, the necessity to expose the subject to radioactive materials in order to use some of the other methods mentioned above.

One particular advantage to be considered is the ability of autonomic measures to provide current indices of the subject's state, either as a tonic measure of his ongoing activity or as a phasic measure of his response to an individual stimulus. This should be compared with, for instance, measures of averaged cortical activity which are necessary to provide an evoked-response waveform in which the relation of that activity to an individual stimulus rather than to a train of stimuli is obtained only with difficulty by, for instance, template matching or "Woody filtering."[1]

Perhaps the main disadvantage of the measurement of autonomic activity as a "window on the brain" rather than as a measure in its own right is that of indirectness. Electrodermal activity measured at the palm of the hand is a long way from the amygdala or hippocampus which may be the prime seat of the activity that is the point of interest with many intervening stages involved.

Furthermore, the indices that are being measured are not, in the main, conveniently provided as windows of some higher activity, but are main indicators of some vital function. Thus, although the investigator may be interested in cardiac activity because he thinks that it provides some measure of the subject's attentional stance, the prime function of the heart is the maintenance of vital function, and other activity is superadded to that in a peripheral fashion. In particular, if cardiac activity is taken as an example, we are faced with the difficulty imposed by dual innervation. Heart rate is, of course, at any time determined by the balance of sympathetic and parasympathetic activity, the assessment of which at any one time presents difficulties.

These issues will arise again as more specific details of measures of autonomic activity are considered. The remainder of the paper will concentrate on two particular measures—first, the electrical activity of the skin and second, cardiovascular activity— not because these are the sole measures that are of value, but rather because most work in the past has concentrated on these two areas and hence most is known about them. In addition they present different and contrasting problems to the investigator which serve to illustrate issues of relevance to the present discussion.

ELECTRODERMAL ACTIVITY

The electrical activity of the skin takes two forms: endosomatic and exosomatic. In the measurement of endosomatic activity one electrode is placed on the palm of the hand and the other of an electrically indifferent site, such as a lightly abraded area of the forearm, and a potential difference may be recorded between the two electrodes. If physiological levels of electrolyte are used, this potential will range from $+10$ mV to -70 mV, the polarity being that at the palmar site. This potential is designated skin potential level (SPL). If the subject is presented with a stimulus, such as a tone, a skin potential response (SPR) will be elicited. The form of the response is usually initially negative going, followed by a larger positive deflection. Because it is impossible to separate the contribution to the final waveform of the mechanisms responsible for the positive and negative elements, it is not usual to attempt to quantify the SPR. Rather its existence is used in an all-or-none fashion to indicate the presence or absence of a response. Skin potential activity is designated as endosomatic, as no external source of potential is applied across the skin. It is to be contrasted to exosomatic activity where a potential difference is imposed across two electrodes, a current flows between them, and the index measured is the resistance (or the conductance) of the electrical pathway between the two electrodes. In this instance skin conductance level (SCL) is the term given to the tonic level of electrodermal activity and skin conductance response (SCR) to the phasic activity. In contrast to the SPR, the SCR is uniphasic, being a temporary increase in skin conductance with a latency of about 2 sec and a maximum amplitude of some 2-3 microsiemens. An idealized diagram representing the SCR is presented in FIGURE 1. Two magnitude measures of skin conductance activity—SCL and SCR amplitude—are shown. In addition there are three temporal measures: latency, the time from stimulus onset to the point of inflection of the SCR waveform; rise time, the time taken to reach peak amplitude; and half recovery time, the time taken for the exponentially decaying response to reach half amplitude value. TABLE 1 shows typical interrelations between these aspects of skin conductance. While amplitude and level are related and found to be so in all studies, and rise time and recovery time are also

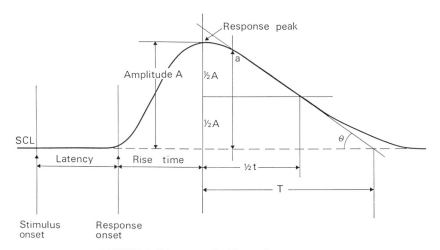

FIGURE 1. Diagrammatic skin conductance response.

related, there is relative independence of the other measures from each other, suggesting a possible independence of underlying mechanisms. The SCR was traditionally known and still sometimes appears in the literature as the GSR (galvanic skin response). The newer term, however, provides a clearer indication of the form of measurement and is preferable.

Peripheral Mechanisms

Understanding of the peripheral mechanisms underlying electrodermal activity is essential in order to make use of the measure as an indicant of higher activity. The main peripheral mechanisms of the system are the eccrine sweat glands, which are

TABLE 1. Interrelations between Skin Conductance Variables

| | Skin conductance response | | | |
	Amplitude	Latency	Rise Time	Recovery Time
Skin conductance level	0.33	−0.14	−0.01	−0.12
Amplitude		−0.12	−0.17	0.12
Latency			0.25	0.18
Rise time				0.54

found in dense distribution on the palms of the hands and the soles of the feet. Sweating in these sites does not have the primary function of temperature regulation which is the main purpose of sweating in other sites where it involves apocrine as well as eccrine glands. The function of palmar and plantar sweating is somewhat obscure but it has been suggested that sweat at these sites has a protective function and makes the sites less vulnerable to injury in addition to increasing grip.[2] Sweat glands may be viewed as conducting paths in parallel. It is therefore appropriate to think of populations of sweat glands becoming active or losing their activity as being represented by changes in conductance rather than by changes in resistance. This argument is presented in more detail in Venables and Christie.[3] The skin and the sweat glands are however more than just a set of conducting pathways that may be switched in and out. A more complete model of the skin is presented by Fowles[4] and is shown in FIGURE 2, aligned with a diagrammatic sketch of the structure of the skin.

In this model, which is that of a single sweat gland and surrounding tissue, the skin may be thought of as possessing characteristic sites of resistance (or conductance) and sources of potential. In some instances the source of potential is a junction potential created by applying a peripheral electrolyte in order to connect the electrode to the body surface. That potential varies with the concentration of the external electrolyte in accordance with the Nernst equation.[5] Alternatively, it may be shown that resting SPL, measured with a constant value of external potassium chloride electrolyte, varies with values of extracellular potassium calculated from the electrocardiogram T-wave. Papadimitriou et al.[6] reported a correlation between plasma K^+ and the amplitude of the EKG T-wave to be $+.68$; Christie and Venables[7] showed that the correlation between the amplitude of the T-wave and resting, nonsudorific skin potential was $−.69$. This potential is labeled E3 in FIGURE 2 and is shown independently in the experiment alluded to when the values of E1 and E2 are minimal because sweat gland activity is attenuated in the resting subject. The human sweat duct (but not, for instance, that of the cat, thereby invalidating some electrodermal work using these subjects) has two sodium reabsorption mechanisms in the dermal and epidermal parts of the duct and the potentials associated with these mechanisms are indicated by E1 and E2 in FIGURE 2. These potentials are associated with duct filling and are therefore present when the subject is in an active state. These three potentials in dynamic combination make up the value of skin potential at any one time; variations in this potential due to duct filling and emptying and the extent of sodium reabsorption under hormonal control determine the extent and the shape of the skin potential response. To some extent the systems that determine the measured values of skin conductance are simpler and therefore more interpretable. R1 and R3 are respectively the resistances of the epidermal and the dermal duct as determined by the extent to which they are filled with sweat. R3 is the resistance of the epidermal duct wall associated with E2 and R4 the resistance of the dermal duct wall associated with E1. R5 represents the resistance of the stratum corneum (the outer dead layer of skin, which is capable of being hydrated by sweat emitted from the sweat glands), and R6 represents a fairly fixed resistance across an epidermal barrier layer (possibly the stratum lucidum). The main determination of SCL is thus the hydration of the stratum corneum, which to some extent represents the immediate past history of the activation of the subject and the extent to which sweat glands are full and how many of them are thus activated. The determination of the amplitude of the SCR is by the extent of duct filling and the numbers of ducts involved. The determination of the temporal variables of SCR is poorly understood. Latency of SCR varies with skin temperature (the correlation between latency and temperature has a typical value of $-.30$). Latency also varies positively with age and is roughly proportional to the length of the arm, thus suggesting that it can be a direct reflection of the speed of nervous transmission in sympathetic fibers. There is some suggestion that the recovery limb of the SCR is a reflection of the rate of absorption of sodium in the sweat ducts under the influence of the activity of mineralocorticoids such as aldosterone. Reabsorption does not appear to occur without triggering; the factors involved here are sodium concentration in sweat and ductal hydrostatic pressure. One possible candidate for the control of hydrostatic pressure is ductal myoepithelial contraction which has been suggested to be adrenergically controlled and may thus be independent of the secretory mechanisms of the eccrine sweat glands which, although innervated by the sympathetic nervous system, have a cholinergically controlled final pathway.

One of the main advantages of the electrodermal system as an indicator of higher function is that it is singly innervated. Work initiated by Hagbarth and colleagues[8,9] has shown a direct and strong relationship between the burst amplitude of sympathetic nerve activity recorded from the median nerve and the amplitude of the skin resistance response recorded from the hand. Thus, provided that suitable techniques are used in the recording of electrodermal activity and methods adopted to eliminate artifacts,[10] it

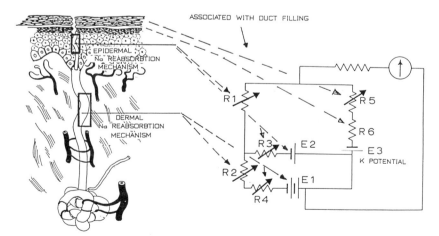

FIGURE 2. Sweat gland ductal mechanisms and their electrical representation.

can be stated with some confidence that the amplitude of the skin conductance response can be used as a measure of sympathetic activity.

Central Mechanisms

Knowledge of higher levels of control of electrodermal activity is derived from a variety of rather disparate sources. Care must be taken in the interpretation of the available material as it is derived from a variety of animal species, and there is lack of commonality in the final peripheral mechanisms between species. Thus, while it may be legitimate to use data on amplitude measures from both cats and monkeys, because cats do not have a double ductal reabsorption system it is probably only legitimate to use data from monkeys when considering recovery of the SCR. Additionally, data in certain instances are derived from animals under heavy anesthesia. Thus under these conditions a different pattern of levels of hierarchical control is likely to be found than when data are derived from nonanesthetized animals.

Pools of sympathetic neurones controlling sweat gland secretion are to be found in the ipsilateral venterolateral horn of the spinal cord. These pools are not structurally connected and only act in synchronized fashion when under control from higher centers. Thus, in the spinal cat spontaneous electrodermal activity in each limb is desynchronized.[11]

The next level of control is from the ventromedial bulbar reticular formation. There is considerable evidence that this structure has an inhibitory effect on electrodermal activity. Wang[12] stated that "intercollicular decerebration—that is, removal of the forebrain, the interbrain, and the rostral half of the midbrain—causes a sharp fall in the intensity of the galvanic skin reflex." In the intact animal the inhibitory influence of the bulbar reticular formation is normally overcome by the excitatory influence of other structures at a higher level. This finding is extended by Roy et al.[13] who showed that SPRs elicited by stimulation of the mesencephalic reticular formation are inhibited by simultaneous stimulation of the bulbar reticular formation. This work is of particular importance as the authors showed that inhibition of SPR due to bulbar reticular stimulation was accompanied by evidence of strong cortical arousal. Thus SPR inhibition was not a result of diffuse depression of the mesencephalic reticular formation. A further study[14] from the same laboratory using kittens as subjects showed that these effects were apparent from birth.

The definitive work on the next level of control is that of Bloch and Bonvallet.[15] They showed that the brainstem reticular formation, which in their experiments is the region extending between the bulbar reticular formation and the posterior hypothalamus, had a uniform and low threshold for the elicitation of electrodermal responses. The only region outside the brainstem reticular formation from which they were able to evoke electrodermal responses was a limited portion of the anterior hypothalamus. In 1973, Venables and Christie[3] suggested that the finding that the anterior hypothalamus was an excitatory site for electrodermal activity was in accord with earlier work cited by Darrow.[16] However, because this area is involved in thermoregulatory control and because even palmar and plantar areas are involved in temperature regulation above certain temperatures, it was suggested that the anterior hypothalamus was not a major site for the regulation of the other roles of electrodermal activity. These authors stated that "this may be too simplistic a point of view and does not do justice to the role of the hypothalamus as a mediator and coordinator of the activity of other centers." Recent unpublished material by Furhmann et al.[17] examining data from human subjects who have CAT scan evidence of third ventricular enlargement, which the authors suggest would involve the anterior hypothalamus, shows that those subjects who show such enlargement exhibited smaller skin conductance responses. If these findings are replicated then it may be justifiable to include the anterior hypothalamus as an important area controlling non-thermoregulatory electrodermal activity.

At a higher level there are data indicating the involvement of the limbic system. Yokota et al.[18] examined the effect of stimulation of the hippocampus, fornix, amygdala, and preoptic area. Stimulation of the hippocampus produced inhibition of the SPR, and that of the fornix produced greater inhibition of the SPR and depression of SPL. Stimulation of the amygdala produced facilitation of the SPR. Lang et al.[19] also showed that the amygdala appears to have an excitatory effect upon electrodermal activity. Bagshaw et al.[20] showed that amygdalectomy in monkeys produced a marked diminution in or even an absence of electrodermal responses, while ablation of the hippocampus appeared to have no effect. Re-analysis of the data on a finer time base, however, showed that hippocampectomy appeared to have the effect of decreasing response habituation.[21] More interesting, these data are the only source available to show that the limbic system appears to be involved in the determination of the recovery time of the SCR. The rate of recovery is faster among those animals undergoing hippocampectomy than among controls. Recent work employing the injection of 6-hydroxydopamine (6-OHDA) throws further light on the involvement of the limbic system in the determination of electrodermal activity. Yamamoto et al.[22] administered 6-OHDA intraventricularly to cats. 6-OHDA is a neurotoxin that selectively destroys catecholamine nerve terminals and induces compensatory denervation supersensitivity. After treatment, concentrations of noradrenaline were decreased (in comparison to controls) in the frontal cortex, hippocampus, nucleus accumbens, hypothalamus, and amygdala. There was a decrease in dopamine in nucleus caudatus and nucleus accumbens. The experimental cats all showed an elimination of habituation of the SCR to 100 dB auditory stimuli. Workers from the same laboratory[23] carried out a similar experiment on rats. In this instance, failure of habituation was also reported; however, it was also found that some rats exhibited electrodermal nonresponsivity. The authors point out that the findings on rats and cats are, however, not contradictory insofar as the experiment on rats used less intense auditory stimuli. Additional work indicated that with a stronger stimulus the rats tended to be nonhabituators and with a weaker stimulus some of the cats tended to show nonresponsivity. The importance of the findings lies in the demonstration of the involvement of the limbic system and the hippocampus in electrodermal activity, and in particular that this selective pharmacological intervention can produce a pattern of electrodermal activity which is very similar to that found in schizophrenic patients.[24]

It is inappropriate to attempt to outline any simple involvement of the cortex in electrodermal activity. In a discussion of this area Wang[25] makes the case for viewing the central mechanisms that control electrodermal activity in terms of Fulton's[26] principles of "long circuiting"; that is, that there is a tendency for electrodermal reflexes to involve control by the highest centers unless otherwise prevented. An example of this is given by the work of Zihl et al.,[27] which showed that it was possible to elicit an electrodermal response to the presentation of a stimulus to a blind part of the visual field in patients with damage to the geniculostriate pathway. The authors suggest that in these subjects the electrodermal response involves the retinotectal pathway.

Two areas of the cortex may be specially involved in electrodermal activity. Darrow[16] makes the case for an association between electrodermal activity and motor activity. He cites as an example the finding that lesions of the pre-motor cortex which result in a loss of inhibitory control of motor movement and hence result in "forced grasping" also involve lack of inhibition of secretory control and hence profuse sweating. This finding is in line with the suggestion of Edelberg[2] referred to above that palmar sweating is associated with the protection of the skin and increase in grip required by the hands. The other cortical area that may be of particular importance is that of the frontal lobes. Kimble et al.,[28] for instance, showed that in monkeys with lesions of the frontal cortex there were diminished SCRs to initial or novel presentations of stimuli, that is, stimuli that had signal or meaningful value.

An aspect of electrodermal activity that would be of particular value would be its use as an indication of extent of lateral hemispheric involvement of the brain. The existence of two hands and the usual contralateral connections that are found would suggest a simple state of affairs. However, unfortunately this is not the case. The first work in the area was that of Sourek.[29] In reporting on the effect of hemispheric lesions, he suggested that there was increased activity on the hand that was ipsilateral to the intact hemisphere; however, he also suggested that what might be responsible for this finding was a loss of contralateral inhibition. Most of the work since then has been involved in the decision between these two possible alternatives; the data do not appear to be interpretable in terms of other alternatives such as contralateral excitation. One of the most important of the more recent studies attempting to produce a definitive answer is that of Lacroix and Comper.[30] They used a paradigm that has been employed in later studies, namely, using a task of a particular kind in an attempt to engage an individual hemisphere and then examining the electrodermal activity from both hands. The first experiment of Lacroix and Comper examined the effect of the subject performing either a verbal task to engage the left hemisphere or a spatial task to engage the right. Responses were measured to stimuli consisting of questions having verbal or spatial relevance. SCRs were larger on the left hand than on the right hand during the verbal task and larger on the right hand than on the left hand during the spatial task. The authors interpret their results in terms of contralateral inhibition. It is also worth noting that the subjects in this experiment were female and in other contexts it is reported that less lateral differentiation occurs in females than in males. A recent study[31] has indeed reported that males display more asymmetry between the hands than do females. Three recent reviews of the area provide an equivocal picture. Freixa i Baque et al.[32] posed the questions, "Is EDA control ipsilateral or contralateral? Is its nature excitation or inhibition?" Their conclusion was that "these issues remain unresolved." Hugdahl[33] in the same vein suggested that "bilateral differences in EDA are small and easily distorted." Finally Miossec et al.[34] say in relation to the findings in the area that "the unknown factors are far more numerous than the certitudes." They suggest that this state of affairs is due to methodological difficulties which they classify under inadequate specification of the stimulating task, inadequate selection of subjects, and in many cases the use of nonstandard recording techniques. A recent study employing techniques that avoid such difficulties does appear to produce less equivocal data. The study by Rippon[35] used an EEG brain imager to ascertain that a task that was supposed to differentially engage the hemispheres did in fact do so. The study employed a tachistoscopically presented letter-matching task where the letters were to be matched nominally or according to their physical characteristics, with the intention of respectively engaging the left and right hemispheres. Activity in the EEG beta waveband provides clear-cut demonstration of hemispheric engagement (this was not evident in alpha blocking). When there was clear evidence of cortical engagement then there was also evidence of a diminution of electrodermal activity in the hand contralateral to the engaged cortical hemisphere. This appears to be strong support for the contralateral inhibitory theory. If this study is replicated, then it would appear that the aim of using electrodermal activity as a measure of hemispheric involvement may be on a sounder footing.

CARDIOVASCULAR ACTIVITY

While electrodermal activity has the advantage of being an index of the activity of only one branch of the autonomic nervous system, it has the disadvantage of being influenced by conditions such as electrolyte concentration at the recording site. In contrast electrocardiac activity is capable of being measured by any system that makes reasonable contact with the body surface or even, if cardiac rate measurements only are required, by simple photoplethysmographic techniques that merely involve the subject placing a finger in a cuff. The disadvantage of cardiac activity is that it is under control of both branches of the autonomic nervous system and in consequence it is not possible, without additional controls, to determine at any one time whether it is the sympathetic or parasympathetic branches which are responsible for the current measurement.

Much of the work undertaken by psychologists is only concerned with cardiac rate as an appropriate index, and little attention is paid to any other aspects of the electrocardiogram. Cardiac rate is measured either as heart rate (HR) expressed in beats per minute or as heart period (HP) or interbeat-interval (IBI) expressed in milliseconds.

Some attempts have been made to evolve an index of sympathetic activity from measurement of aspects of the cardiovascular system. Furedy and Heselgrave[36] have used the fact that there is little or no parasympathetic influence on the ventricular myocardium to suggest that the EKG T-wave may provide an index of ventricular repolarization and hence a measure of sympathetic activity. An increase in sympathetic activity is indicated by a decrease in T-wave amplitude. Another measure has been proposed by Obrist et al.[37] This involves measurement of the rate of change of pressure when blood is ejected from the heart. As left ventricular activity is under sympathetic control, rate of change of pressure may be considered to be an index of sympathetic activity. Measurement can be made conveniently and relatively noninvasively by a piezoelectric transducer placed over the carotid artery. Hence the measurement is referred to as carotid dP/dt. As a neck collar has to be worn in order to achieve good recordings, this does involve some disturbance to subjects that other measures may not introduce.

As stated above, however, the bulk of work done in this area uses only heart rate or period. Measures of tonic activity are relatively straightforward; complications arise, however, with the measurement of phasic responsivity. It is a characteristic of the system that changes in heart rate are a function of the tonic level from which those changes started; in other words, this is a classic instance of the "law of initial values." Although this is always cited as a complication of cardiac rate measurement, it is in fact no different from the consideration that has to be made in the measurement of SCR where the influence of SCL has to be taken into account. Depending on the context of the study, analysis of covariance or an appropriate multivariate technique may be used to take account of the tonic/phasic association.

More complex and difficult to deal with is the decision in any cardiac rate measurement on whether to base the rate on real time or physiological time. Changes in HR or HP may be expressed as changes occurring at particular times or particular beats. If the intention is to use cardiac rate activity alongside some other measure which is measured against real time, then clearly the former is to be preferred. On the other hand it may be convenient to take an HR measure which may be directly read from a cardiotachometer, rather than having to measure individual IBIs, in which case the data are inevitably in terms of physiological time. As the time at which a stimulus is presented is usually random with respect to the ongoing heart period, the start of a real time period must fall inconveniently between beats. FIGURE 3 shows the appropriate calculations that have to be made to derive a figure for an IBI to be set against a real-time period. The half-second real-time period which is shown provides a useful baseline. Graham[38] has reviewed the issue of the type of data to be used in the presentation of phasic heart rate changes. Her recommendation is that when real-time units are used as the time base then cardiac rate should be in terms of HR; on the other hand when cardiac time (beats) is used as the time base then it is appropriate to use IBIs as the unit of measurement.

When measuring changes in heart rate, consideration must be given to the nature of the baseline from which these changes are made. A large number of studies take the mean heart rate in a pre-stimulus period as the baseline. This pre-stimulus period must be large enough to encompass the cyclical fluctuations in heart rate, which are associated with the respiratory cycle and are known as sinus arrhythmia. This method of measurement, however, takes no account of the fact that the sinus arrhythmia would

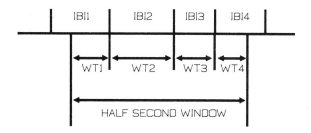

IBI =(IBI1∗WT1 + IBI2∗WT2 + IBI3∗WT3 + IBI4∗WT4)/500

FIGURE 3. Calculation of average interbeat-interval in real-time window.

have continued had there not been a stimulus to elicit a heart rate response. One method of coping with this dilemma is to use as a control for the elicited response a period of heart rate activity in which a stimulus has not been presented and which therefore contains the unmodified sinus arrhythmia. The selection of such a control recording however presents difficulties. Another means that has been employed is to model the post-stimulus heart rate on the basis of the pre-stimulus pattern. A first order auto regressive model for accomplishing this was proposed by Jones et al.[39] In this $D_t + AD_{t-1} + E_t$ where A is the auto correlation at lag 1 and D_t is the deviation from the mean at time t. The value of each point is predicted from the previous point and the overall autocorrelation between successive points. Lobstein,[40] arguing that a single-order autoregressive model was inadequate, suggested the use of a higher-order model. This model, for which there is a computer program using up to a seventh-order model, is of the form

$$D_t = AD_{t-1} + BD_{t-2} + CD_{t-3} + \ldots\ldots + E_t$$

where D is the deviation from the mean at time t, A is the autocorrelation at lag 1, and B, C, etc., are the partial autocorrelations at lags 2, 3, etc. E_t is the residual error at time t. Pre-stimulus data are used to generate a model in which each data point is predicted by the preceding, for instance, four or five points. Each post-stimulus point is predicted from the model on the basis of the observed data up to that point, and the differences between the observed and expected values are standardized with respect to the residual error. These standardized differences can be regarded as data from which cyclical or nontransient components have been removed. There has not been sufficient use of this analysis system and its comparison with the simple subtraction of the mean pre-stimulus baseline to say that its usefulness has been established. It does, however, appear to provide a useful resolution of the difficulty of coping with sinus arrhythmia. One doubt that can be raised is the extent to which the presentation of a stimulus evokes a change in respiratory pattern and hence a change in sinus arrhythmia so that the model predicted from pre-stimulus data is inaccurate.

As has been stated above, the heart receives both sympathetic and parasympathetic innervation. The basic rate of the heart is controlled by the pacemaker; in humans this has been estimated to have an intrinsic rate of between 100 and 120 beats per min. However, in a sample of young adults we might expect a resting level of heart rate to range between 40 to 80 beats per min. It follows therefore that the heart is normally under considerable parasympathetic or vagal restraint. Administration of an agent such as atropine which blocks vagal activity can result in an increase in heart rate of some 40 beats per min. At resting levels it is thus likely that the heart may reflect the extent to which the parasympathetic system is active. If the subject is exposed to nonstressful exercise while oxygen consumption is being measured, then there is a close linear relationship between oxygen consumption and heart rate.[41] Thus under normal conditions heart rate may be predicted from oxygen consumption. If the subject is exposed to conditions that are stressful as well as being physically demanding (such as parachute jumping or taking part in an assault course), then the heart rate exceeds that which is predicted by oxygen consumption. This "additional heart rate"[42] is probably a reflection of the extent to which sympathetic activity predominates in the control of heart rate. In summary the tonic level of heart rate may, depending on the circumstances under which the measurements are made, reflect the predominance of either the sympathetic or parasympathetic branches of the autonomic nervous system (ANS).

The identification of which branch of the ANS is responsible for phasic heart rate activity may be slightly easier to determine. Warner and Cox[43] provided data to show that the time constant of the parasympathetic nervous system was of the order of 1 sec while that of the sympathetic nervous system was about 8 sec. Obrist et al.[44] reported data on the heart rate response of subjects with and without vagal blockade to an intense stimulus. The normal pattern of phasic HR response to an intense stimulus is one of initial HR acceleration followed by a subsequent deceleration. FIGURE 4, which is adapted from Obrist et al.,[44] shows this pattern of response in the intact subjects, but in the case of those with vagal blockade there is no initial acceleration, and the late acceleration which might result from the expected mobilization of the sympathetic nervous system peaks at about 9 sec. Thus, it would appear that the early HR acceleration to an intense stimulus is due to a decrease in parasympathetic activity rather than to an increase in sympathetic activity.

A further attempt to measure separately activity in one of the branches of the autonomic nervous system influencing cardiac activity has been made by Porges et al.[45] These authors have devised a measure of vagal tone by assessing the extent to which increases and decreases in heart rate covary with respiration. The measure is based on the fact that during inspiration the stretch receptors in the lungs are prepotent in inhibiting the vagal efferents to the heart, resulting in HR acceleration, while during expiration the vagal influence on the heart is increased resulting in cardiac deceleration. The amplitude of this respiratory sinus arrhythmia is thus suggested to be related to vagal tone. The estimate of vagal tone is made by calculating the dependence of spectral density of the heart rate on the frequency of breathing and is calculated by cross-spectral analysis of the two variables.

As suggested in the introduction, a valid way of relating autonomic activity to higher nervous function is by means of behavioral indices. A strong and productive area of work is that which relates changes in heart rate to aspects of attention. If a subject is presented with a low-intensity tone or an interesting visual image which evokes an orienting response, the typical pattern of heart rate response is of initial deceleration, followed by acceleration and a subsequent secondary deceleration.[46] FIG-URE 5 shows such a pattern of phasic HR changes. Although current work in this area probably dates from a seminal chapter by Lacey,[47] these phenomena were reported at the turn of the century. Darrow[48] reports that Mentz observed a slowing of the pulse during "voluntary attention" and Lehmann (1899) observed a quickening of the pulse in the "concentration of attention" and a slowing of the pulse after the presentation of sensory stimuli. This distinction is now designated by the concepts of "open" and "closed" attentional stance. Thus for instance Edwards and Alsip,[49] using male under-graduates as subjects, showed that when they were presented with the picture of an attractive girl they showed HR deceleration; on the other hand when given an anagram to solve, and where "attention" had to be "concentrated" and be "closed" to external distraction, then HR acceleration was shown. Although initial HR deceleration is generally considered to be part of the orienting response and to be associated with openness to the environment, there are several slightly different concepts associated with HR acceleration. The idea of closed attentional stance in order to be able to deal

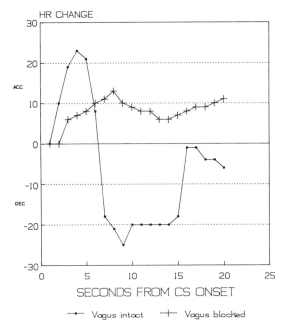

FIGURE 4. Second-by-second HR changes in subjects with and without vagal blockade. Adapted from Obrist et al.[44]

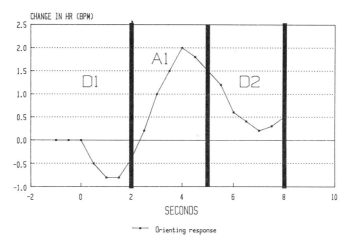

FIGURE 5. Temporal HR windows for a typical orienting response.

with the internal manipulation of material is elaborated in the work of Coles and Duncan-Johnson[50] and is suggested to involve information processing. A slightly different view is that derived from Russian work,[51] where HR acceleration is associated with the presence of the "defensive" response. The function of such a response is to protect the organism from overstimulation from external sources. It is generally recorded as a response to intense stimulation but is also seen in conditions where the psychological content of the stimulation is deemed to be threatening to the subject. Thus, Hare and Blevings[52] showed that spider phobic subjects showed heart-rate acceleratory responses to pictures of spiders, whereas to neutral scenes they showed deceleratory responses.

Two different theories of the mechanisms underlying these phenomena are current. That of Lacey[47] involves the pressure-sensitive receptors in the carotid sinus and aortic arch. The prime function of these receptors is the homeostatic control of blood pressure; however, it is Lacey's contention that "inhibitory control of higher levels of the nervous system is vested in this same visceral pathway." Bonvallet et al.[53] showed that distention of the carotid sinus produced a decrease in electrocortical activity. Also in this context Bonvallet and Allen[54] describe an ascending bulbar inhibitory mechanism which exerts inhibitory control of cortical, autonomic, and muscular activities. The potential difficulty with this theoretical mechanism is that while it can reasonably be seen to account for the defensive aspect of the acceleratory HR response and for the increase in sensory sensitivity required for the orienting deceleratory response, it is less easy to accommodate the idea of increased information processing which Coles and Duncan-Johnson[50] report as accompanying HR acceleration. The alternative theory is that of Obrist and his colleagues.[55] The view of these workers is that the changes in heart rate should be viewed as part of the totality of somatic changes. This cardiac-somatic coupling view suggests that HR deceleration is part of general somatic "quietening" and is accompanied by a decrease in general muscle tension and eye blinking. Thus improved receptivity of external stimuli may be brought about by an improvement in signal/noise ratio where the signal is the neural event stimulated by the external stimulus and the noise is the background of ongoing neural activity.

Whichever of these theories is correct, the empirical findings which they aim to explain appear to be well founded and in the present context are important in that they are a further indication that measures of autonomic function are capable of providing access to higher activity.

SUMMARY

A review such as this can do no more than provide an indication of the issues involved in using autonomic activity as a means of providing "a window on the brain."

Several points arise. One of the most important is that of careful and appropriate use of techniques available. One well-known textbook of experimental psychology published some time ago advocated the use of two dimes applied to the palm of the hand for the measurement of electrodermal activity. It was this sort of recommendation that led to the use of psychophysiological measurement falling into disrepute. As indicated in the second section, it is important to understand fully the peripheral mechanisms involved before measurement of electrodermal activity can be usefully carried out. Appropriate use of silver/silver chloride electrodes and physiologically appropriate levels of saline in the electrolyte medium can lead to accurate and repeatable measurement where artefact is not carelessly introduced.

Equally important is the context in which studies are carried out. The psychological invasiveness of the technique is important to recognize, and it is here that measurement of autonomic activity probably scores over other methods that are available insofar as very little restriction of the subject is required and the number of transducers that must be applied is minimal.

The measurement of autonomic activity within the totality of the experimental context is all important. As an example Dawson and Schell[56] investigated the SCR to words which had previously been associated with shock. When these words were presented to the ear to which attention was not directed in a dichotic listening paradigm, an SCR could be elicited although the subject was unaware of the presentation of the stimulus. The importance of the Dawson and Schell study was the care that they took to make sure that the subject really was unaware of the critical stimulus and had not momentarily switched attention from the attended ear. More important, their experiment, in contrast to some which had gone before, used a balanced design in which the critical stimuli were presented on different occasions to each ear. As a result of this it was found that critical stimuli, which were presented to the left ear, right hemisphere, gave rise to SCRs, even when the subject was not aware of their presentation, whereas stimuli presented to the right ear, left hemisphere elicited no response. Thus although the important response in this experiment is an autonomic one, because of the experimental design that is employed, the eventual finding is that which supports the idea of the right hemisphere being the site of pre-attentive processing.

Finally, another of the outcomes of the review is the suggestion that by appropriate processing of the signal or the measurement of a critical portion of it, it may be possible to provide a wanted index which would not be evident in the gross recording.

Thus, it may be suggested that the measurement of autonomic activity can stand on its own, or preferably in conjunction with other measures reviewed in this book, to provide valuable insights into brain function.

REFERENCES

1. WOODY, C. D. 1967. Characterization of an adaptive filter for the analysis of variable latency neuroelectric signals. Med. Biol. Eng. **5:** 539-553.

2. EDELBERG, R. 1971. Electrical properties of the skin. *In* A treatise on the skin. Vol. 1. H. R. Elden, Ed.: 513-550. Wiley. New York, NY.

3. VENABLES, P. H. & M. J. CHRISTIE. 1973. Mechanisms, instrumentation, recording techniques and quantification of responses. *In* Electrodermal Activity in Psychological Research. W. F. Prokasy & D. C. Raskin, Eds.: 1-124. Academic Press. New York, NY.

4. FOWLES, D. C. 1973. Mechanisms of electrodermal activity. *In* Methods in physiological psychology. Vol 1: Bioelectric recording techniques, Part C, Receptor and Effector Processes. R. F. Thompson & M. M. Patterson, Eds.: 232-271. Academic Press. New York, NY.

5. CHRISTIE, M. J. & P. H. VENABLES. 1971. Effects on "basal" skin potential level of varying the concentration of an external electrolyte. J. Psychosom. Res. **15:** 343-348.

6. PAPADIMITRIOU, M., R. R. ROY & M. VARKARAKIS. 1970. Electrocardiographic changes and plasma potassium levels in patients on regular dialysis. Br. Med. J. **2:** 268-269.

7. CHRISTIE, M. J. & P. H. VENABLES. 1971. Basal palmar skin potential and the electrocardiogram T-wave. Psychophysiology **8:** 779-786.

8. HAGBARTH, K-E., R. G. HALLIN, A. HONGELL, H. TOREBJORK & B. G. WALLIN. 1972. General characteristics of sympathetic activity in human nerves. Acta Physiol. Scand. **84:** 164-176.

9. LIDBERG, L. & B. G. WALLIN. 1981. Sympathetic nerve discharges in relation to amplitude of skin resistance responses. Psychophysiology **18:** *268-270.*

10. VENABLES, P. H. & M. J. CHRISTIE. 1980. Electrodermal activity. *In* Techniques in Psychophysiology. I. Martin & P. H. Venables, Eds.: 3-67. Wiley. Chichester.

11. LADPLI, R. & G. H. WANG. 1960. Spontaneous variations of skin potentials in foot pads of normal striatal and spinal cats. J. Neurophysiol. **23:** 448-452.

12. WANG, G. H. 1958. The galvanic skin reflex. A review of old and recent works from a physiologic point of view. Part I. Am. J. Phys. Med. **36:** 295-320; Part II. **37:** 35-37.

13. ROY, J. C., B. DELERM & L. GRANGER. 1974. L'inhibition bulbaire de l'activite electrodermale chez le chat. Electroencephalogr. Clin. Neurophysiol. **37:** 621-632.

14. DELERM, B., M. DELSAUT & J. C. ROY. 1982. Mesencephalic and bulbar reticular control of skin potential responses in kittens. Exp. Brain Res. **46:** 209-214.

15. BLOCH, V. & M. BONVALLET. 1960. Le declenchment des responses electodermales a partir du systeme reticulaire facilitateur. J. Physiol. (Paris) **52:** 25-26.

16. DARROW, C. W. 1937. Neural mechanisms controlling the palmar galvanic skin reflex and palmar sweating. Arch. Neurol. Psychiatry **37:** 641-663.

17. FURHMANN, M., T. D. CANNON & S. A. MEDNICK. 1987. The neuroanatomical mediators of skin conductance. Personal communication.

18. YOKOTA, T., A. SATO & B. FUJIMORI. 1963. Analysis of inhibitory influence of bulbar reticular formation upon sudomotor activity. Jpn. J. Physiol. **13:** 145-154.

19. LANG, A. H., T. TUOVINEN & P. VALLEALA. 1964. Amygdaloid after-discharge and galvanic skin response. Electroencephalogr. Clin. Neurophysiol. **16:** 366-374.

20. BAGSHAW, M. H., D. P. KIMBLE & K. H. PRIBRAM. 1965. The GSR of monkeys during orienting and habituation and after ablation of the amygdala, hippocampus and inferotemporal cortex. Neuropsychologia **3:** 111-119.

21. PRIBRAM, K. H. & D. McGUINNESS. 1975. Arousal activation and effort in the control of attention. Psychol. Rev. **82:** 116-149.

22. YAMAMOTO, K., K. HAGINO, T. MOROJI & T. ISHII. 1984. Habituation failure of skin conductance response after intraventricular administration of 6-hydroxydopamine in cats. Experientia **40:** 344-345.

23. YAMAMOTO, K., H. KIYOSUMI, K. YAMAGUCHI & T. MOROJI. 1985. Two types of changes in skin conductance activity after intraventricular administration of 6-hydroxydopamine in rats. Prog. Neuro-Psychopharmacol. Biol. Psychiatry **9:** 245-250.

24. VENABLES, P. H. 1980. Peripheral measures of schizophrenia. *In* Handbook of Biological Psychiatry. Part II. Brain Mechanisms and Abnormal Behavior—Psychophysiology. H. M. Van Praag, H. M. Lader, O. J. Rafaelson & E. J. Sachar, Eds.: 79-96. Marcel Dekker. New York, NY.

25. WANG, G. H. 1964. Neural Control of Sweating. University of Wisconsin Press. Madison, WI.

26. FULTON, J. F. 1926. Muscular Contraction and the Reflex Control of Movement. Williams & Wilkins. Baltimore, MD.

27. ZIHL, J., F. TRETTER & W. SINGER. 1980. Phasic electrodermal responses after visual stimulation in the cortically blind hemifield. Behav. Brain Res. 1: 197-203.

28. KIMBLE, D. P., M. H. BAGSHAW & K. H. PRIBRAM. 1965. The GSR of monkeys during orienting and habituation after selective ablations of cingulate and frontal cortex. Neuropsychologia 3: 121-128.

29. SOUREK, K. 1965. The nervous control of skin potential in man. Proceedings of the National Academy of Czechoslovakia. Prague.

30. LACROIX, J. M. & P. COMPER. 1979. Lateralization in the electrodermal system as a function of cognitive/hemispheric manipulations. Psychophysiology 16: 116-129.

31. MARTINEZ-SELVA, J. M., F. ROMAN, F. A. GARCIA-SANCHEZ & J. GOMEZ-AMOR. 1987. Sex differences and the asymmetry of specific and non-specific electrodermal responses. Int. J. Psychophysiol. 5: 155-160.

32. FREIXA I BAQUE, E., M. C. CATTAEU, Y. MIOSSEC & J. C. ROY. 1984. Asymmetry of electrodermal activity: A review. Biol. Psychol. 18: 219-239.

33. HUGDAHL, K. 1984. Hemispheric asymmetry and bilateral electrodermal recordings: A review of the evidence. Psychophysiology 21: 371-393.

34. MIOSSEC, Y., M. C. CATTEAU, E. FREIXA I BAQUE & J. C. ROY. 1985. Methodological problems in bilateral electrodermal research. Int. J. Psychophysiol. 2: 247-256.

35. RIPPON, G. M. J. 1987. Topographical mapping and bilateral electrodermal research: An attempt to resolve methodological issues. Paper presented at the meeting of the Society for Psychophysiological Research. Oct. 17. Amsterdam.

36. FUREDY, J. J. & R. J. HESLEGRAVE. 1983. A consideration of recent criticisms of the T-wave amplitude index of myocardial sympathetic activity. Psychophysiology 20: 204-221.

37. OBRIST, P. A., J. E. LAWLER, J. L. HOWARD, K. W. SMITHSON, P. L. MARTIN & J. MANNING. 1974. Sympathetic influences on cardiac rate and contractility during acute stress in humans. Psychophysiology 11: 405-427.

38. GRAHAM, F. K. 1978. Constraints on measuring heart rate and period sequentially through real and cardiac time. Psychophysiology 15: 492-495.

39. JONES, R. H., D. H. CROWELL & L. E. KAPUNIAI. 1969. Change detection model for serially correlated data. Psychol. Bull. 71: 352-358.

40. LOBSTEIN, T. 1978. Detection of transient responses in adult heart rate. Psychophysiology 15: 380-381.

41. ASTRAND, I. 1960. Aerobic work capacity in men and women with special reference to age. Acta Physiologica Scand. Suppl. 49: 169.

42. BLIX, A. S., S. B. STROMME & H. URSIN. 1974. Additional heart rate—an indicator of psychological activation. Aerosp. Med. 45: 1219-1222.

43. WARNER, H. R. & A. COX. 1962. A mathematical model of heart rate control by sympathetic and vagus efferent information. J. Appl. Physiol. 17: 349-352.

44. OBRIST, P. A., D. M. WOOD & M. PEREZ-REYES. 1965. Heart rate during conditioning in humans: Effect of UCS intensity, vagal blockade and adrenergic block of vasomotor activity. J. Exp. Psychol. 70: 32-42.

45. PORGES, S. W., R. E. BOHRER, G. KEREN, M. N. CHEUNG, G. J. FRANKS & F. DRASGOW. 1981. The influence of methylphenidate on spontaneous autonomic activity and behavior in children diagnosed as hyperactive. Psychophysiology, 18: 42-48.

46. GRAHAM, F. K. & R. K. CLIFTON. 1966. Heart rate change as a component of the orienting response. Psychol. Bull. 65: 305-320.

47. LACEY, J. I. 1967. Somatic response patterning and stress: Some revision of activation theory. *In* Psychological Stress: Issues in Research. M. H. Appley & R. Trumbull, Eds.: 14-37. Appleton-Century. New York, NY.

48. DARROW, C. W. 1929. Differences in the physiological reactions to sensory and ideational stimuli. Psychol. Bull. **26:** 185-201.
49. EDWARDS, D. C. & J. E. ALSIP. 1969. Intake-rejection, verbalization and affect effects on heart rate and skin conductance. Psychophysiology **6:** 6-12.
50. COLES, M. G. H. & C. C. DUNCAN-JOHNSON. 1975. Cardiac activity and information processing: The effects of stimulus significance, and detection and response requirements. J. Exp. Psychol. Hum. Percept. Perform. **1:** 418-428.
51. SOKOLOV, E. N. 1963. Perception and the Conditioned Reflex. Pergamon. Oxford.
52. HARE, R. D. & G. BLEVINGS. 1975. Defensive responses to phobic stimuli. Biol. Psychol. **3:** 1-13.
53. BONVALLET, M., P. DELL & G. HIEBEL. 1954. Tonus sympathique et activite electrique corticale. Electroencephalogr. Clin. Neurophysiol. **6:** 119-144.
54. BONVALLET, M. & M. B. ALLEN. 1963. Prolonged spontaneous and evoked reticular activation following discrete bulbar lesions. Electroencephalogr. Clin. Neurophysiol. **15:** 969-988.
55. OBRIST, P. A., R. A. WEBB, J. R. SUTTERER & J. L. HOWARD. 1970. Cardiac deceleration and reaction time: An evaluation of two hypotheses. Psychophysiology **6:** 695-706.
56. DAWSON, M. E. & A. M. SCHELL. 1982. Electrodermal responses to attended and nonattended significant stimuli during dichotic listening. J. Exp. Psychol. Hum. Percept. Perform. **8:** 315-324.

Application of Psychophysiology in Clinical Neuropsychology

MAUREEN J. LEVINE [a,b] AND M. GUERAMY [c]

[a]Department of Psychology
Central Michigan University
Mt. Pleasant, Michigan 48859
[c]Neuroscience Division
Mid-Michigan Regional Medical Center
Midland, Michigan 48870

Psychophysiological studies of information processing in humans with cortical and subcortical brain damage are few. Investigations to date have primarily examined the relationship of behavior to neural physiological systems in hypoxia, hemorrhage, ablations, transplants, anesthesia, and pharmacological treatments in animals.[1] However, a voluminous body of psychophysiological literature exists that provides evidence that physiological responses in humans are associated with ability to orient to, process, organize, and recall information obtained through the sensory channels.[2] Deficits in these functions are among the salient problems reported for most patients with central nervous system (CNS) damage.[3,4] Therefore, a fruitful approach to understanding the functional losses in patients with brain damage would be one that incorporates psychophysiological techniques in the application of clinical neuropsychology. In this paper, a discussion of the assumptions of psychophysiology relevant to central nervous system disorders is presented. In light of these assumptions, studies utilizing psychophysiological techniques with neurological patient populations are reviewed, and the integration of psychophysiology in the neuropsychological assessment and treatment of neurological disorders is discussed.

PSYCHOPHYSIOLOGICAL PARAMETERS

Sokolov[5] developed a theoretical model to explain the results of studies on the nature of the orienting reflex (OR) introduced by Pavlov. He found that stimuli that produce the OR could also yield a defense reflex (DR). The OR responds to stimuli in low- and moderate-range intensities, and the DR responds to stimuli at higher levels of intensity. A third classification of reflex parameters, the startle reflex (SR), was introduced by Fleshler[6] to account for rat behavior and was extended to human responses by Hatton, Berg, and Graham.[7]

[b]To whom correspondence should be sent.

Sokolov associated a variety of responses by the autonomic nervous system (ANS) with the OR and the DR. Subsequent studies[8] suggested that the most robust ANS measure associated with these reflexes appears to be changes in heart rate (HR). Deceleration of heart rate corresponds to OR whereas acceleration is found with DR and SR. The latter two reflexes can be distinguished from each other by the response latency; SR occurs earlier than two sec after the onset of a stimulus and DR occurs after two seconds.[9]

An important feature of the various responses is the rate of habituation. Indeed, the differences in habituation rates were critical for Sokolov's interpretation of the experimental findings in terms of OR and DR. The habituation of OR was relatively rapid when compared to that of DR. Rapid habituation was also observed for SR.[10] The descriptive reflex names, that is, orienting, defense, and startle and their respective habituation patterns are consistent with evolutionary theory.

Most of the disagreements with the Sokolov model found in the literature are what would be expected in a field with a rapid increase in instrumental sophistication and analytic capabilities. Koepke and Pribram[11] replicated the experiments of Sokolov which elucidated the concept of the OR and essentially agreed with the earlier results. Graham's[12] excellent reviews generally support the Sokolov model of OR and DR with the inclusion of SR and additional ANS responses. However, these reviews did not include the more recent work of Turpin and Siddle.[13] Therefore, we discuss their contributions in more detail.

Turpin[14] reviewed the evidence for the support of the Sokolov model and carried out experiments which studied the effects of the intensity of auditory stimuli on autonomic responses. Turpin found that the literature failed to support reliably Sokolov's results on the peripheral vascular responses. He also found some discrepancies between the work of some authors and those of Sokolov on the habituation paradigm. He ascribed part of the problems in the literature to the range of audio stimuli intensities that overlap the boundary between the OR and DR proposed by Sokolov. Turpin claimed that additional discrepancies are the results of faulty experimental designs, for example, a within-subject rather than a between-subject analysis. Another problem according to Turpin was the use of auditory stimuli with instantaneous rise time. These had been shown by Graham[10] to elicit SR rather than DR. Graham had concluded that rapid habituation observed for DR was due to the mistaken belief that a DR was being observed rather than an actual SR.

Despite the improved equipment and experimental design, Turpin and Siddle[15] are in general agreement with Graham and Clifton,[9] Graham and Slaby,[10] and Graham.[12] They obtained HR acceleration and HR deceleration at low and high intensities, respectively, and also observed the SR peak. They did not obtain reciprocal vasoconstriction-vasodilation for OR as reported by Sokolov. Instead they obtained vasoconstriction at both sites. They also obtained the reciprocal effect for the SR. Electrodermal conductance agreed with most of the literature findings, increasing with onset and habituating with continued stimuli. The orienting HR habituated as expected. However, because it was biphasic, exhibiting an increase at long-range latency (LRL), habituation judgments in the accelerating portion were difficult to establish. For digital pulse amplitude (DPA), the positive component habituated, but masked possible habituation of the negative component. For the intensity levels, 45, 60, 75, and 105 dB, only the 75-dB level did not exhibit HR habituation. It would appear that the anomalous behavior at 75 dB might be due to it being the boundary between OR- and DR-stimulation-intensity levels. The major discrepancies found were in the vasodilation at the higher intensity stimuli which according to Sokolov should characterize a DR response. Also, significant habituation was obtained at the high-intensity levels even when the response direction was consistent with the DR profile. Turpin[14] interprets these results as indicating that the presence of SR is more prevalent than previously indicated. Turpin goes further by stating that HR acceleration should be considered as SR and that the distinction between SR and DR should be avoided. In a subsequent study, Turpin and Siddle[16] used a high-intensity stimulus, 110 dB. They observed on HR a short latency response (SLR) corresponding to SR, which was followed by LRL acceleration. Concomitant vasodilation on the forearm was found. Its main difference from the classical DR was the rapid habituation. Turpin and Siddle identify the LRL as a fight/flight response previously reported in a number of studies, and they proposed that the DR of Sokolov is a variation of the fight/flight response. The incongruence of the rapid habituation is believed to result from the energy exhaustion of the receptors.

Obrist[17] presents results of his own work and those of others to support his position that ANS responses are inadequate measures of behavioral states. His analysis does not differentiate among different types of stimuli such as for onset of tasks, for conditioning experiments, or for ANS responses to meaningless signals. Pavlov had originally expressed the view that OR had to habituate before conditioning could occur. Sokolov had distinguished the differing effects of signal and nonsignal stimuli. Obrist's experimental results that question the validity of indexing behavioral states are part of an ongoing controversy whose resolution will provide a framework for new experimental designs. Obrist also presents philosophical arguments that the major functions of the ANS were maintenance and responding to somatic changes. Sympathetic and parasympathetic changes could only be small perturbations of magnitude of the ANS measures and therefore would have large inherent errors. These criticisms may not apply universally. Reproducible small differences are being measured routinely in science. In any event, experiments designed to distinguish ANS components originating from the sympathetic and parasympathetic systems from those of somatic and autonomous origins are clearly needed.

A good example of the validity of HR change as a measure of a behavioral state is afforded by the work of Miller and Morse[18] in which a hearing discrimination test was used with 3- to 4-month-old infants. Two stimuli—[dae] and [gae]—which are in different phonetic categories corresponding to the positioning of the tongue were utilized. Artificially produced phonetic stimuli based on a three-formant mode were used. A within-category change of the same stimulus was obtained by minor variations of the element of its formants. A between-category change replaced the [dae] by [gae] and vice versa. A 20/20 paradigm was used. Twenty repetitions of a stimulus were followed by another 20 of the same or within-category, or between-category change to give the control group (C), within group (W), or between group (B) experimental conditions, respectively. All three conditions exhibited a HR deceleration indicating an OR. Habituation was observed for all conditions starting at 6.5 sec poststimulus for the first set of 20 stimuli. After onset of the second set, complete habituation of HR at the base level was found for conditions C and W. However, deceleration that was followed by habituation starting at 2.5 sec after stimulus onset was observed for condition B. The authors interpret these results as an indication of stimuli discrimination for condition B. They explain the finding by postulating that OR occurred after the discriminated stimulus of the second set. However, earlier onset of habituation in the 2.5 sec rather than 6.5 sec in the first set may indicate that dishabituation took place. This study is a good example of the HR responses for a noncorrelated OR. For infants of this age readying of the somatic system for possible action is obviously not necessary. Similar experimental designs in the study of nonverbal neurological populations would underscore the benefits of the interface of psychophysiology and neuropsychology. Some preliminary work in this direction has been carried out by LeFever[19] with comatose patients, the details of which are given in the following discussion.

PSYCHOPHYSIOLOGICAL STUDIES IN CNS DAMAGE

Most studies of patient populations with CNS damage have investigated orienting and/or habituation variables. Oscar-Berman and Gade[20] examined orienting and habituation of skin conductance and pulse volume in a group of normal subjects and patient groups with Korsakoff's syndrome, Parkinson's disease, Huntington's chorea, and aphasia. Hyporeactivity was reported for the patients with Korsakoff's syndrome and those with Huntington's chorea. Patients with Parkinson's disease and aphasia responded similarly to the normal control groups. The authors proposed that the findings are due to the generalized functional impairments observed for the patient groups with Korsakoff's syndrome and Huntington's disease. Rogozea and Florea-Ciocoiu[21] also examined the orienting reflex and its habituation in patients with late post-traumatic encephalic syndrome (LPTES). They reported that auditory stimuli elicited an increased intensity and resistance to habituation of the EEG components of the orienting reflex in 184 patients with LPTES. According to Rogozea and Florea-Ciocoiu, the findings were the results of hyperreactivity induced by a post-traumatic, cicatrix lesion. Heilman, Schwartz, and Watson[22] found hyperreactivity in patients with left hemisphere damage and hyporeactivity in right hemisphere damage. Holloway and Parsons[23] proposed that there is not generalized autonomic change as a result of brain damage and that some areas of damage may produce a significant decrease or increase in acceleration whereas others will have no effect.

Based on the premise that hemispheric tumor processes may cause psychophysiological disturbances—specifically, alteration in habituation of the orienting response— Rogazea, Florea-Ciocoiu, and Constantinovici[24] examined resistance to habituation of somatic (EMG), autonomic, and EEG components of the orienting response to repetitive auditory stimuli in 41 patients with epileptogenic cerebral tumors (ECT) and in three control groups composed of 43 normal control subjects, 36 patients with non-epileptogenic cerebral tumors (NCT), and 49 patients with partial generalized seizures of unknown etiology (SUE groups). The effects of tumor size, histology, and site of lesion were also examined. Resistance to habituation was greater for patients with epileptogenic cerebral tumors. An increased resistance to habituation was also observed in the NCT and SUE groups compared to that of the normal control group. Significant increases in resistance to habituation of the orienting response were reported in patients with temporal epileptogenic tumors, as well as in patients with central, parietal tumors, frontal, and occipital tumors. Increased resistance to habituation correlated with increased hemispheric tumor size (> 6 cm). Patients with ECT and generalized seizures showed the most resistance to habituation whereas in the NCT groups resistance was less than in the ECT and SUE groups. The authors proposed that alteration in activity of neural pathways involved in control and alterations of repetitive sensory measures are affected more because cerebral pathology impacts on surrounding parenchyma. They further proposed that the observed differences for sites with more disturbance in the temporal-central regions are related to the morphofunctional dimensions of the site. These areas may be more involved in the control of general excitability.

Habituation has also been studied for a group of patients with Gilles de la Tourette's syndrome. Bock and Goldberger[25] explored the issue that Gilles de la Tourette's syndrome involves a disruption in arousal modulation and inhibition resulting in a poorly controlled startle response. In this study, 20 patients with Gilles de la Tourette's syndrome were compared to 20 patients with chronic medical illnesses using parameters of skin conductance level to auditory and visual stimuli. The findings indicated no disturbance in habituation or arousal for the patient group with Gilles de la Tourette's syndrome. Less change in tonic arousal level over time was present in the Tourette's group than in the control group. The authors proposed that the patients with Tourette's may have made more effort to stay alert, and the presence of the observer influenced the Tourette's patient group. In a recent study, Bartfai and colleagues[26] examined computer tomography scans, neuropsychology test performance, habituation of heart rate, and bilateral skin conductance (SC) in 18 schizophrenic patients. They reported the nonhabituators comprising 28% of the group had commenting voices and an inability to feel. The nonhabituators also tended to have wider third ventricles than habituators, who comprised 39% of the group. The authors propose that nonhabituators may be an important subgroup among schizophrenic populations. A number of studies have also explored habituation in depressed populations in comparison to normal subjects. As a group, depressed patients show a failure to dishabituate.[27] Overall these findings are relevant in the differential diagnosis of functional organic etiologies in neuropsychology, for example, psychosis versus brain damage or depression versus dementia.

To date investigations have primarily examined orienting and habituation parameters in patient populations with central nervous system disorders. There are few investigations of physiological responses associated with attentional, cognitive, or retrieval functions of information processing. An exception is the Brouwer and van Wolffelaar[28] study of sustained attention and sustained effort utilizing vigilance and heart rate parameters in a group of eight patients with closed head injury (CHI) and a control group of eight normal subjects. The groups were examined at two intervals, three months apart, within six months post-trauma time. Performance on a low event rate vigilance task and recordings of heart rate variability were analyzed. The authors reported no evidence of impairment in sustained effort in the patients with closed head injury. Difference in response latencies and in discrimination of small differences in loudness, especially in early recovery period, were observed. These findings provide evidence that the current view that closed head injury patients experience impaired sustained attention and effort in task performance may be questionable.

In a recent study Levine, Gueramy, and Friedrich[29] compared the physiological parameters involved in the processing of bisensory memory tasks and their recall in a group of 30 patients with closed head injury and a group of 29 normal controls. Continuous recording of heart rate, galvanic skin responses, and respiration were carried out on an automatic computerized system during the presentation and recall of four intersensory (auditory and visual) experimental conditions. Physiological responses that occurred with the simultaneous presentation and recall of bisensory tasks were different for patients with closed head injury than for the normal control group.

The results indicated that the magnitude of heart rate decelerations and accelerations of the CHI group were lower than those of the control group (Wilcoxon, $p < 0.001$). Significant differences in mean heart rate were found for tasks ($p < 0.001$), and a significant interaction ($p < 0.001$) was found for task $\times$ groups. Mean heart rate across tasks for control and head-injured groups is shown in FIGURE 1.

Significant differences between the groups for heart rate variance were not found, but significant differences ($p < 0.001$) were obtained for tasks and periods. Significant differences between groups for galvanic skin response were also not found, although differences were obtained for tasks $\times$ periods ($p < 0.001$). Mean galvanic skin response during preperiod, stimulus, and recall periods across tasks for head-injured and control groups is shown in FIGURE 2.

For the CHI group, the respiration variance was significantly different between tasks ($p < 0.01$). The performance of the CHI group on each task for each error type was worse than that found for the control group (Wilcoxon, $p < 0.001$).

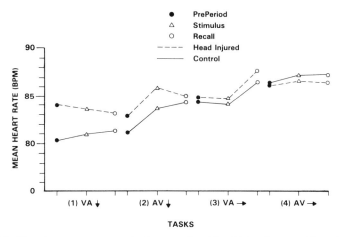

FIGURE 1. Mean heart rate across tasks for control and head-injured groups. V = visual; A = auditory; ↓ = paired recall; → = serial recall.

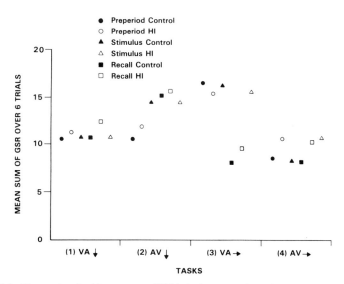

FIGURE 2. Mean galvanic skin response (GSR) during preperiod, stimulus, and recall periods across tasks for head-injured and control groups.

More effective adjustment of the physiological response was associated with the more efficient performance of the normal control groups. The authors proposed that the results are in accord with Babkin's[30] antagonistic-synergistic model of the autonomic nervous system. It is suggested that head injury impacts on the balanced set of inhibitory and activating signals controlling the autonomic system, and this balanced control is needed for effective processing.

Closed head injury has been the focus of a number of studies in recent years. In spite of this few investigations of patients in coma and vegetative states have been carried out. Long-term survival from catastrophic closed head injury associated with a vegetative state is rare. Jennett and Teasdale's[4] data and those of Levy, Jones, and Plum[31] indicate that only 1-2% of all patients in coma from traumatic head injury or medical illness survive in vegetative state. Nevertheless, this condition represents a serious problem in terms of the numbers of patients involved and the effect on family survivors.

LeFever[19] discusses the importance of attempting to establish communication with comatose patients. He examined the cardiac component of the orienting response to differential acoustical and semantic stimuli in two comatose patients. Stimuli included words and pure tones for 500 and 1000 Hz at 85 dB, presented at bedside through earphones to one patient and ambiently in an acoustic chamber to the other. Twenty repetitions of the same word were followed by 20 repetitions of another. Cardiac deceleration was observed in one patient in 7 of 8 transitions between different words (p < 0.02). Delayed data retrieval limited further study of stimulus parameters. The preliminary work undertaken to date suggests that patients in comatose states represent a population whose study would clearly benefit from psychophysiological applications.

INTEGRATION OF PSYCHOPHYSIOLOGY IN ASSESSMENT
AND TREATMENT

Significant scientific study is under way to further our understanding of the process in the recovery from brain damage. Donald Stein,[32] in a master lecture series on clinical neuropsychology, describes his challenging research on factors that promote recovery from brain damage, such as hormonal effects, age at injury, type of injury, and contextual variables. Stein describes the specific temporal sequence of primary and secondary biochemical and morphological events that occur after traumatic brain injury. The brain response to injury is rapid, orderly, and complex. In spite of the increased ability of medical science to enhance survival in the face of brain damage, neuropsychology has yet to meet the challenge of functional survival. Efforts are clearly under way to develop neurorehabiliation treatments, and this movement would be enhanced by an integration of psychophysiological techniques at the point of assessment as well as in intervention programs.

In this paper studies were reviewed that point out the benefit of psychophysiological designs in the area of differential diagnoses of patient populations served by clinical neuropsychology. Extensive additions to this work are needed; nevertheless, the efforts reported to date are very promising. The studies have shown that nonverbal populations including infants, children, and adults can be assessed. Utilizing psychophysiological designs, the effects of treatments may also be monitored. At this time little is known regarding the effects of stimulation provided to patients in the recovery phase after brain trauma. Animal and human studies provide evidence that factors such as intensity, context, nutrition, hormonal states, and sex differences are extremely important, but these are as yet unexplored topics in human neurorehabilitation. The increasing efficacy of psychophysiological methodology for the diagnosis and treatment of neurological disorders is growing in importance and has great promise.

ACKNOWLEDGMENTS

The authors are indebted to Patricia Wolfgram, Director of Midland Hospital Center Library, for her valuable assistance with the literature search. We wish to express our appreciation to Mary Jane Cashen of Central Michigan University for her assistance in assembling and typing the manuscript.

REFERENCES

1. BUTTERS, N., J. J. ROSEN & D. G. STEIN. 1974. Recovery of behavioral functions after sequential ablation of the frontal lobes of monkeys. *In* Plasticity and Recovery of Functions in the Central Nervous System. D. G. Stein, J. J. Rosen & N. Butters, Eds.: 429-466. Academic Press. New York, NY.
2. OHMAN, A. 1979. The orienting response, attention and learning: An information processing perspective. *In* The Orienting Reflex in Humans. H. D. Kimmel, E. H. van Olst & J. F. Orlebeke, Eds.: 443-471. Lawrence Erlbaum Associates. Hillsdale, NJ.
3. LEVIN, H., A. L. BENTON & R. GROSSMAN. 1982. Neurobehavioral Consequences of Head Injury. Oxford University Press. New York, NY.
4. JENNETT, B. & G. TEASDALE. 1981. Management of Head Injuries. F. A. Davis Company. Philadelphia, PA.
5. SOKOLOV, E. N. 1963. Perception and the Conditioned Reflex. Pergamon Press. Oxford.
6. FLESHLER, M. 1965. Adequate acoustic stimulus for startle reaction in the rat. J. Comp. Physiol. Psychol. **61:** 200-207.
7. HATTON, H. M., W. K. BERG & F. K. GRAHAM. 1970. Effects of acoustic rise on heart rate response. Psychon. Sci. **19:** 101-103.
8. LACEY, J. I., J. KAGAN, B. C. LACEY & H. A. MOSS. 1963. The visceral level: Situational determinants and behavioral correlates of autonomic response pattern. *In* Expression of the Emotion in Man. P. H. Knapp, Ed. International University Press. New York, NY.
9. GRAHAM, F. K. & R. K. CLIFTON. 1966. Heart rate change as a component of the orienting response. Psychol. Bull. **65:** 305-320.
10. GRAHAM, F. K. & D. A. SLABY. 1973. Differential heart rate changes to equally intense white noise and tone. Psychophysiology **10:** 347-362.
11. KOEPKE, J. E. & K. H. PRIBRAM. 1967. Habituation of the vasoconstriction response as a function of stimulus duration and anxiety. J. Comp. Physiol. Psychol. **64:** 502-504.
12. GRAHAM, F. K. 1979. Distinguishing among orienting, defense and startle reflexes. *In* The Orienting Reflex in Humans. H. D. Kimmel, E. H. van Olst & J. F. Orlebeke, Eds.: 137-167. Lawrence Erlbaum Associates. Hillsdale, NJ.
13. TURPIN, G. & D. A. T. SIDDLE. 1979. Effects of stimulus intensity on electrodermal activity. Psychophysiology **16:** 582-591.
14. TURPIN, G. 1986. Effects of stimulus intensity on autonomic responding: The problem of differentiating orienting and defense reflexes. Psychophysiology **23(1):** 1-14.
15. TURPIN, G. & D. A. T. SIDDLE. 1983. Effects of stimulus intensity on cardiovascular activity. Psychophysiology **20:** 611-624.

16. TURPIN, G. & D. A. T. SIDDLE. 1978. Cardiac and forearm plethysmographic responses to high intensity auditory stimuli. Biol. Psychol. **6:** 267-282.
17. OBRIST, P. A. 1982. Cardiac-behavioral interactions: A critical appraisal. *In* Perspectives in Cardiovascular Psychophysiology. J. J. Cacioppo & R. E. Perry, Eds.: 265-295. The Guilford Press. New York, NY.
18. MILLER, C. L. & P. A. MORSE. 1976. The "heart" of categorical speech discrimination in young infants. J. Speech and Hear. Res. **19:** 578-589.
19. LEFEVER, F. F. 1985. Sensory or semantic discrimination in coma and locked in syndromes: Assessments using cardiac deceleration response. Paper presented at the Fifth Annual Meeting of The National Academy of Neuropsychologists. October 15. Philadelphia, PA.
20. OSCAR-BERMAN, M. & A. GADE. 1979. Electrodermal messages of arousal in humans with cortical and subcortical brain damage. *In* The Orienting Reflex in Humans. H. D. Kimmel, E. H. van Olst & J. F. Orlebeke, Eds.: 665-676. Lawrence Erlbaum Associates. Hillsdale, NJ.
21. ROGOZEA, R. & V. FLOREA-CIOCOIU. 1974. Nervous reactivity disturbance in patients with late post traumatic encephalic syndromes. Appl. Neurophysiol. **42:** 224-233.
22. HEILMAN, K. M., H. D. SCHWARTZ & R. T. WATSON. 1978. Hypoarousal in patients with neglect syndrome and emotional indifference. Neurology **28:** 229-232.
23. HOLLOWAY, F. A. & O. A. PARSONS. 1971. Habituation of the orienting reflex in brain damage patients. Psychophysiology **8(5):** 623-634.
24. ROGOZEA, R., V. FLOREA-CIOCOIU & A. CONSTANTINOVICI. 1983. Habituation of the orienting reaction in patients with epileptogenic cerebral tumors. Biol. Psychol. **16:** 65-84.
25. BOCK, R. D. & L. GOLDBERGER. 1985. Tonic phasic and cortical arousal in Gilles de la Tourette's Syndrome. J. Neurol. Neurosurg. Psychiatry. **48:** 535-544.
26. BARTFAI, A., S. E. LEVANDER, H. NYBACH & D. SCHALLING. 1987. Skin conductance nonresponding and nonhabituation in schizophrenic patients. Acta Psychiatr. Scand. **75:** 321-329.
27. REUS, V. I., H. S. PEEKE & C. MINER. 1985. Habituation and cortisol dysregulation in depression. Biol. Psychiatry **20:** 980-989.
28. BROUWER, W. H. & P. C. VAN WOLFFELAAR. 1985. Sustained attention and sustained effort after closed head injury: Detection and 0.10 Hz heart rate variability in a low event rate vigilance task. Cortex **21:** 111-119.
29. LEVINE, M. J., M. GUERAMY & D. FRIEDRICH. 1987. Psychophysiological responses in closed head injury. Brain Injury **1(2):** 171-181.
30. BABKIN, B. P. 1946. Antagonistic and synergistic phenomena in the automatic nervous system. Trans. R. Soc. Can. **40(5):** 1-25.
31. LEVY, D. E., R. P. JONES & F. PLUM. 1978. The vegetative state and its prognosis following nontraumatic coma. Ann. N. Y. Acad. Sci. **315:** 293-306.
32. STEIN, D. G. 1988. In pursuit of new strategies for understanding recovery from brain damage: Problems and perspectives. *In* Clinical Neuropsychology and Brain Functions: Research, Measurement and Practice. T. Boll & B. K. Bryant, Eds.: 13-55. American Psychological Association. Washington, DC.

Dichotic Listening: New Developments and Applications in Clinical Research[a]

GERARD E. BRUDER[b]

New York State Psychiatric Institute, and
Department of Psychiatry
Columbia University College of Physicians and Surgeons
New York, New York 10032

Several years ago, Teng[1] published an article entitled "Dichotic Ear Difference Is a Poor Index for the Functional Asymmetry between the Cerebral Hemispheres." Although this article may have had a chilling effect on the application of dichotic listening in clinical neuropsychological contexts, dichotic listening research has continued on several important fronts. A recent book entitled *Handbook of Dichotic Listening: Theory, Methods and Research*[2] gives ample evidence that the title of Teng's article is not justified on either empirical or theoretical grounds. This paper gives an overview of the dichotic listening tests available to both researchers and clinicians, discusses some methodological issues that are important for proper use of these techniques, and illustrates the current application of dichotic tests to study both lateralization of emotions in normal subjects and alterations of lateralization in patients with emotional disorders. No attempt is made to give a comprehensive review of these areas because this is available elsewhere.[3,4] Rather, the most recent studies in these areas are presented in some detail so as to illustrate how dichotic listening tests can be used to obtain reliable and theoretically meaningful findings in both normal and clinical populations.

VERBAL DICHOTIC TESTS

The dichotic listening tests used in the pioneering studies of Broadbent[5] and Kimura[6,7] were understandably rather crude in design. Strings of different digits were presented via earphones to the right and left ears. The subject's task was to recall the digits heard in each ear. The digits presented to the two ears had relatively little acoustic overlap, and subjects could therefore potentially perceive and report the digits from each ear. Kimura[6] observed that normal adults have a mean right-ear advantage on this dichotic digit task, which she attributed to left-hemisphere dominance for language. Support for the validity of this test in assessing language lateralization was provided by Kimura[7] in a study with epileptic patients, in which sodium amytal was administered to determine the hemisphere dominant for speech. Patients with left-hemisphere domi-

[a] Supported, in part, by grant MH36295 from the National Institute of Mental Health.
[b] Address correspondence to Dr. Gerard Bruder, Department of Biopsychology, New York State Psychiatric Institute, 722 West 168 Street, New York, NY 10032.

nance showed greater mean accuracy in the right ear, whereas patients with right-hemisphere dominance showed greater mean accuracy in the left ear. The magnitude of the right-ear advantage for dichotic digits is, however, generally small (5-10%), and the test-retest reliability has been reported to be very low, i.e., r = .36 and r = −.11.[1] Also, the interpretation of ear advantages on the dichotic digit test is problematic because memory loss, attentional bias, and order of reporting digits can all contribute substantially to laterality effects.

An important methodological advance was the development of dichotic tasks using nonsense syllables. Only a single pair of nonsense syllables is presented on each trial, thus reducing memory load to a minimum. Also, the nonsense syllables that are presented to two ears are more closely aligned, resulting in greater competition of input. In the most frequently used nonsense syllable task, a different consonant-vowel syllable (ba, da, ga, pa, ta, ka) is presented simultaneously to the two ears and the subject checks off the two syllables on a mutiple-choice answer sheet.[8] Since the syllables are recorded in natural speech, there is only partial fusion of input to the two ears and subjects can, on some trials, correctly perceive the syllables in both ears. This task has consistently yielded a mean right-ear (left-hemisphere) advantage of 10 to 15% in children and adults.[8,9] The test-retest reliability of this consonant-vowel test has been found to be between .60 and .80 for both normal adults and psychiatric patients.[3,9,10]

Other nonsense syllable tests have been constructed using both synthesized speech and natural speech, modified by computer to yield dichotic pairs that are "perfectly fused." The different syllables presented to the two ears fuse to form a single percept, and the subject is thereby required to report only one syllable per trial. For instance, Wexler and Heninger[11] used a fused vowel-consonant-vowel (VCV) nonsense syllable test, in which a stop consonant (b, d, p, t, g, or k) was preceded and followed by the vowel "a". This test was found to yield very high test-retest reliability in both normal subjects (r = .91) and in psychiatric patients (r = .89). Moreover, the frequency of individuals showing a right-ear advantage was comparable to the incidence of left-hemisphere dominance for speech derived from neurological samples. When only subjects with statistically significant ear advantages were considered, 93% of right-handers had right-ear (left-hemisphere) dominance.[12]

Another test using "perfectly fused" dichotic pairs is the fused-rhymed words test.[13] This test consists of presenting single-syllable word pairs that differ only in the initial consonant (e.g., coat in the right ear and goat in the left ear). The pair fuse to form a single image and subjects use a multiple-choice answer sheet to indicate the word they heard. All words begin with a stop consonant (b, d, p, t, g, or k) and are digitized natural speech. The fused-rhymed words test was reported to have a test-retest reliability of .85. Also, when only subjects with significant ear advantages were considered, 98% of right-handers had a right-ear (left-hemisphere) advantage.

A different form of dichotic word test was developed by Geffen and her associates.[14,15] In their dichotic monitoring task, a series of dichotically presented word pairs is presented and the subject is asked to press a response button when a specific target word is heard. Target words (e.g., black) occur infrequently among nontarget words consisting of semantically unrelated words, some of which are phonemic foils (e.g., track). The words are digitized natural speech and only some of the items are fusable word pairs. The percentage of correct detections of targets (hits) and incorrect responses to phonemic foils (false alarms) in each ear permits the calculation of separate signal detection accuracy measures for the right and left ear. This task has yielded relatively large mean right-ear (left-hemisphere) advantages of 15 to 20% in children and adults, and the test-retest reliability was found to be .81. Geffen and Caudrey[16] have also reported strong evidence for the validity of the dichotic monitoring test in measuring hemispheric lateralization for speech. They tested individuals whose hemispheric dominance was determined during sodium amytal tests or unilateral electroconvulsive treatment. Twenty-seven of the 28 individuals with left-hemisphere dominance had a right-ear advantage, whereas four of the seven individuals with right-hemisphere dominance had a left-ear advantage.

NONVERBAL DICHOTIC TESTS

Many studies have demonstrated a mean left-ear (right-hemisphere) advantage for dichotically presented nonverbal material such as melodies,[17] musical chords,[18] environmental sounds,[19] tone contours,[20] and complex tones.[21] Kimura's dichotic melodies test typifies early efforts to measure hemispheric dominance for musical stimuli. A different musical passage is played simultaneously to each ear, followed by four binaurally presented musical passages—two making up the dichotic pair and the other two, foils. The subject is required to choose the two passages that were heard in the dichotic pair. Although Kimura observed mean left-ear (right-hemisphere) advantage for dichotic melodies, test-retest reliability has been found to be only .46.[22] Also, musicians have been reported to have a mean right-ear (left-hemisphere) advantage for dichotic melodies.[23]

Sidtis[21] developed the Complex Tone Test that gives evidence of being more reliable than the dichotic melodies test. In this test, a different complex tone is presented simultaneously to the two ears and this is followed by a binaurally presented probe tone. The probe tone is either the same as one member of the dichotic pair or is different from both. Subjects use a nonverbal response to indicate whether or not the probe tone matched one of the dichotic stimuli. The complex tones consist of square waves with different fundamental frequencies. This test was found to yield a mean left-ear (right-hemisphere) advantage in adults, and it has a reliability coefficient of .50 to .70.[3,21]

Evidence for the validity of the Complex Tone Test has come in studies of neurological patients with unilateral cerebral lesions. If the right hemisphere is superior for complex pitch processing, then lesions in the auditory cortex on the right side should disrupt performance on the Complex Tone Test. Sidtis and Volpe[24] tested 28 patients who had unilateral strokes. The right-hemisphere lesioned group had impaired performance for dichotic complex tones but not for dichotic consonant vowels, whereas the left-hemisphere lesioned group had impaired performance for dichotic consonant vowels but not dichotic complex tones. In a study by Zatorre,[25] patients who had a unilateral temporal lobectomy were tested on a task requiring the discrimination of a missing fundamental frequency in binaural complex tones. Patients who showed a deficit on this task were those with a lesion involving Heschl's gyrus in the right hemisphere. Zatorre concluded that the right auditory cortex plays a critical role in perceiving the pitch of complex tones.

Dichotic listening techniques can also be used to study hemispheric lateralization for auditory spatial perception. When a click stimulus is presented to one ear via earphones, followed after a brief delay of 0.1 to 1.0 ms by a click stimulus to the other ear, the subject perceives a single "fused" click localized toward the ear that receives the lead click. By manipulating the interaural delay, one can vary the location in which the click is perceived. Studies in neurological patients indicate that disturbance of localization of sounds in either dichotic listening or free-field tasks is primarily associated with damage to posterior regions of the right brain.[26,27] It has also been suggested that the right hemisphere is dominant for auditory spatial perception.[28] If this is the case, it might be expected that normal subjects would be better at making fine spatial discriminations when sounds are perceived to be in the left hemispace than in the right hemispace. There are reports that localization of sound in space tends to be biased toward the left hemispace and that accuracy is somewhat better in the left than in the right space.[29]

We used a dichotic click paradigm to further investigate whether there are hemispatial differences in localization of sounds.[30] The task involved discriminating a small difference in apparent location of a standard stimulus and a comparison stimulus. The location of stimuli was manipulated by varying the interaural delay between dichotically presented click stimuli. The subject's task was to press a response button if the comparison stimulus was in a different location than the standard stimulus. A total of 30 right-handed subjects (half males and half females) were tested on this task. Although there was an overall advantage for spatial discrimination in the left hemispace compared to the right hemispace, this effect was primarily present in male subjects. Males showed a 14.5% mean left-hemispace advantage, whereas females showed little or no mean asymmetry. In terms of frequency, 87% of males had a left-hemispace advantage and 47% of females had a left-hemispace advantage ($\chi^2 = 8.24$, p < 0.02). Studies that have found sex differences in tasks involving visual spatial perception (e.g., dot localization or enumeration, line orientation, or perception of faces) have similarly found greater left-hemispace advantages in males than in females.[31,32,33,34] Test-retest reliability of hemispatial advantages for the dichotic localization task was .50, with 87% of subjects having the same direction of asymmetry in the initial and retest sessions.

USING MULTIPLE DICHOTIC TESTS

The variety of verbal dichotic tasks available today raises a question as to which test to select for a given study. The most frequently used verbal tasks include dichotic digit tests, nonsense syllable tests, fused-word tests, and the dichotic monitoring test. The issue of which test to use is an important one because there is no evidence that the various verbal dichotic tests measure the same underlying hemispheric lateralization. In fact, dichotic digit, nonsense-syllable, and word tests show very low intertest correlations.[1,35] This may be attributable to the very different content of these tests. They differ in memory load, meaningfulness of items, in the use of natural versus synthetic speech, in the extent of fusion or competition of dichotic pairs, and in susceptibility to attentional bias. It is probably safe to assume that the various verbal dichotic tests measure somewhat different aspects of information processing and thereby reflect laterality for different functional systems in the brain.

The findings of Wexler and associates[35-37] point to a research strategy of using both fused-nonsense-syllable and fused-word tests to provide data for mapping cerebral functions. Despite the similarity of characteristics of the fused-nonsense-syllable and fused-word tests, as well as their good reliability, ear asymmetry scores for these tests did not correlate. Evidence that these tests tap different aspects of cerebral function was evident in the differential relation of asymmetry scores on these tests to the field dependence index on the Wexler Adult Intelligence Scale (WAIS). Right-ear advantages on the nonsense syllable task were positively correlated with field dependence, whereas ear advantages on the fused-word test were not. The field dependence index of the WAIS includes the object assembly and block design subtests, which are affected by right hemisphere lesions. Wexler and Halwes[35] suggest that association areas in the right hemisphere may be involved in processing of dichotic nonsense syllables, and this contributes to the difference in ear advantages between nonsense syllables and words. Further evidence that different functional systems are involved in processing dichotic nonsense syllables and words was apparent in the opposite changes of ear advantages for these two tests during clinical recovery from acute psychotic episodes.[36] In a diagnostically mixed group of psychotic patients, recovery was accompanied by an increase in right-ear advantage for nonsense syllables, but a decrease in right-ear advantage for words. Wexler postulated that the physiological system involved in processing meaningful stimuli has an inhibitory relationship with the physiological system that processes nonsense. The balance of activation of these two systems is altered in opposite directions during an acute psychotic episode and recovery, which results in the different changes in ear advantage observed for dichotic nonsense syllables and words. Although further research is needed to evaluate this theoretical formulation, the comparison of ear advantages on different verbal dichotic tests would appear to be a useful approach for studying alterations of cerebral function in psychiatric disorders.

Another approach for using multiple dichotic tests in the same study stresses the importance of comparing findings for verbal and nonverbal dichotic tasks. This provides converging evidence to aid in the theoretical interpretation of dichotic listening findings. For instance, a number of studies have found abnormally large right-ear advantages for dichotic words in at least a subgroup of psychotic patients.[38–41] The interpretation of this finding is a problem because it could stem from left-hemisphere hyperactivation, right-hemisphere dysfunction, or an interhemispheric transfer deficit. The availability of data for a nonverbal dichotic test can help rule out at least one of these alternative interpretations. A deficit of interhemispheric transfer would be expected to result in an abnormally large right-ear advantage for verbal tests and an abnormally large left-ear advantage for nonverbal tests. This was clearly not found in studies that have tested psychotic patients on verbal and nonverbal dichotic tests.[40,42] Before giving an illustration of the application of both verbal and nonverbal dichotic tests in a study of cerebral laterality in depressed patients, another methodological issue should be addressed.

ACCURACY AND ASYMMETRY SCORES

The difference in accuracy for material presented to the right and left ears provides a measure of dichotic listening asymmetry. The use of this measure, however, has been criticized because difference scores are correlated with overall performance level. Differences in asymmetry scores between groups or individuals will therefore be difficult to interpret if they also differ in performance level. A number of "accuracy-adjusted" indices of asymmetry has been used to deal with this problem. This raises the question as to which asymmetry index is best for a given study. Perhaps the most widely used index has been the percent of correct (POC) index, in which the difference in accuracy for the right and left ear is simply divided by the overall accuracy [(R − L)/ (R + L)]. Harshman and Lundy[43] present a number of logical considerations that argue in favor of the use of POC as the one "natural" method for assessing asymmetry. However, some have cited evidence that POC does not adequately correct for differences in accuracy when overall performance is above 50%.[44,45] Similarly, an alternate index of asymmetry, referred to as percent of error (POE), is constrained at accuracy levels less than 50%. This led Repp[45] to recommend the use of the asymmetry index e, which entails the use of POC $[(R - L)/(R + L)]$ for accuracy scores less than 50% and POE $[(R - L)/(2 - R - L)]$ for accuracy scores greater than 50%. Even the index e may not be immune to the influence of performance level, and the use of this or other "accuracy-adjusted" asymmetry scores can in some cases lead to misleading results.[46,47] Bryden and Sprott[48] proposed yet another asymmetry index, λ, that has the advantage of providing significance tests for individual data. This index appears to have similar properties to the index e and they are highly correlated.[44]

It would appear that there is no one ideal index of asymmetry, although some indices (e.g., e or λ) may be better in certain cases for correcting asymmetry scores for differences in performance levels. Whatever "accuracy-adjusted" asymmetry index one selects, it alone cannot provide a complete account of the data for a dichotic listening test. Another important, and often neglected, step is to report the absolute accuracy scores for each ear. Indeed, when comparing dichotic listening performance for different groups or different sessions, absolute accuracy scores may prove to be more useful than asymmetry scores. There are three good reasons for using accuracy scores. First, asymmetry scores are inherently limited because they give information only about the relative difference in scores for the right and left side. If one group has a larger right-ear advantage than another, the question remains as to whether this was because of better right-ear accuracy, poorer left-ear accuracy, or a combination of both. Only a comparison of absolute accuracy scores between groups can address this question. Second, it is important to know whether there are differences in overall accuracy $(R + L)$. Do clinical groups and controls differ in overall accuracy for specific dichotic tests? Or, does clinical improvement result in improved accuracy on one dichotic test but not another? Third, absolute accuracy scores are generally more reliable than asymmetry scores and may reveal differences between groups or test sessions that are not evident for asymmetry scores.

In the next section, the dichotic listening data for depressed patients and control subjects are analyzed using absolute accuracy scores. ANOVAs are performed to assess the significance of differences in accuracy between groups, ears, and test sessions. Since groups did not differ in overall accuracy, the use of an "accuracy-adjusted" asymmetry index would add little additional information. Actually, differences in ear advantages between patient and control groups were essentially the same when we considered both accuracy scores and asymmetry (e index) scores.[49]

DICHOTIC LISTENING IN DEPRESSED PATIENTS

Dichotic listening studies have found abnormal ear advantages in depressed patients.[3] The most consistent finding has been the failure of groups of depressed patients to show a mean left-ear (right-hemisphere) advantage for nonverbal dichotic tasks. There are, however, marked individual differences in ear advantages among depressed patients, and some depressed patients show the normal direction of ear advantage on nonverbal dichotic tests. Bruder[50] reviewed evidence suggesting that these individual differences are, in part, related to differences in the clinical features of patients, e.g., their diagnostic subtype or symptom features. A study was therefore conducted to further examine differences in dichotic ear advantages among diagnostic subtypes of depression. A second purpose was to test patients before and after treatment with antidepressants so as to examine whether alterations of dichotic asymmetry in depressed patients persist or disappear after clinical recovery. Although a detailed account of the pretreatment findings of his study is available elsewhere,[49] pre- versus post-treatment comparisons are presented here for the first time.

Two diagnostic dimensions were examined in the study. First, we compared the dichotic asymmetry of bipolar depressed patients with a history of hypomania (bipolar II) and unipolar depressed patients without such a history. We had previously found a difference between bipolar and unipolar subtypes in threshold asymmetries for a dichotic click detection task,[51] but no comparable data existed for standard dichotic listening tasks. Second, the bipolar versus unipolar comparison was made in tandem with a comparison of melancholia versus atypical depression. The criteria for a diagnosis of melancholia (as defined by DSM-III)[52] include features associated with endogenous depression (e.g., depression worse in morning, weight loss or anorexia, psychomotor retardation, or agitation) and the essential features of anhedonia and nonreactivity of mood to pleasurable events. We chose to examine melancholia because of suggestions that "endogenomorphic depression" with pervasive anhedonia and nonreactivity of mood is associated with a CNS disorder.[53] A nonmelancholia contrast group consisted of atypical depressed patients who had symptoms that are in some respects polar opposites of melancholia. The criteria for atypical depression include the essential feature of reactivity of mood with preserved pleasure capacity and associated features such as hypersomnia, overeating, and rejection sensitivity.[54]

This study used a verbal dichotic test, in which consonant-vowel syllables were spoken in natural speech,[8] and a nonverbal dichotic test, i.e., the Complex Tone Test.[21] We also used two visual tachistoscopic tasks, but these data will not be dealt with here. Patients were tested after a minimum drug-free period of 7-10 days, during which they received a placebo (single-blind). Patients who did not respond to the placebo were then treated with, in most cases, a standard tricyclic antidepressant (imipramine) or a monoamine oxidase inhibitor (MAOI) antidepressant (phenelzine). Data are presented below for 35 patients with major depressive disorders who were retested after approximately six weeks of treatment and also for 22 normal controls who were retested at comparable test-retest intervals.

There were significant differences in dichotic ear advantages between melancholia and atypical depression, but not between bipolar and unipolar depression.[49] This report will therefore focus on the pre- and post-treatment data for the melancholic, atypical depression, and normal control groups. A $3 \times 2 \times 2$ (Group $\times$ Ear $\times$ Session) ANOVA was performed on the accuracy data for the nonsense syllable task and for the Complex Tone Test. There were significant Group $\times$ Ear interactions for both the nonsense syllable task, $F (2,54) = 5.69$, $p = 0.006$, and the Complex Tone Test, $F (2,54) = 4.47$, $p = 0.016$. The nature of these interactions is evident in FIGURE 1. Melancholic depressives had an abnormally large right-ear advantage for nonsense syllables, whereas atypical depressives had the same right-ear advantage as normal controls. Most importantly, the larger right-ear advantage in melancholic depressives was clearly due to their poorer left-ear accuracy for identifying nonsense syllables. Analyses of simple effects revealed a significant difference among groups in left-ear accuracy, $F (2,54) = 3.84$, $p = 0.028$, but not in right-ear accuracy. Melancholic depressives also showed a right-ear advantage for complex tones, which is opposite the direction of ear advantage seen for atypical depressives and normal controls. Although there is a suggestion in FIGURE 1 that accuracy for complex tones in the right ear was better in melancholic patients than in the other groups, there was no significant difference in accuracy among groups for either ear.

Comparison of pre- versus post-treatment accuracy scores in FIGURE 1 revealed only one significant change across sessions. Melancholic patients showed a significant improvement in left-ear accuracy for consonant-vowel identification during treatment ($p < 0.01$). Thirteen of the 16 melancholic patients who were treated with a tricyclic

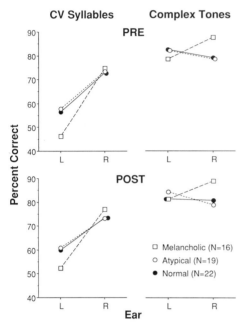

FIGURE 1. Accuracy scores for CV syllables (*left*) and complex tones (*right*) for each group in pre- and post-treatment sessions.

or MAOI antidepressant were rated by psychiatrists to be clinical responders, as evidenced by a marked amelioration of symptomatology. Despite this clinical improvement and the increase in left-ear accuracy, melancholic patients continued to show an abnormally large right-ear advantage for syllables in the post-treatment session. Also, the abnormal direction of ear advantage for complex tones in melancholic patients was still present during the post-treatment session. Comparison of pre- versus post-treatment asymmetry (e index) scores did not reveal a significant change in ear advantages for any of the groups on either test. Another issue is whether or not pre- versus post-treatment changes in accuracy on the dichotic listening tests were related to changes in clinical state. Clinical improvement, as measured by pre- to post-treatment reductions in Clinical Global Impression (CGI) ratings, was associated with increases in left-ear accuracy for nonsense syllables ($r = -.38$, $p = 0.03$), but not with right-ear accuracy ($r = -.09$, NS).

The use of both verbal and nonverbal dichotic listening tests, as well as absolute accuracy scores, can provide some clues as to the mechanisms that might underlie alterations of perceptual asymmetry in melancholia. The abnormally large right-ear advantage for melancholic patients could have resulted from one of several sources. Their right-ear advantage for complex tones would appear to rule out an interhemispheric transfer deficit, since this model would have predicted not only a large right-ear advantage for nonsense syllables, but also, a large left-ear advantage for complex tones.[55] Alternatively, overactivation of the left-hemisphere and resulting attentional bias toward the right hemispace could account for the enhanced right-ear advantage in melancholic patients.[56] This model might, however, have predicted better right-ear accuracy in melancholic patients than in the other groups, but this was not the case. The finding that the large right-ear advantage for nonsense syllables in melancholic patients was due to poor left-ear accuracy is more consistent with an hypothesis of right hemisphere dysfunction.[40,57] The presence of a right-ear advantage for complex tones in melancholic patients also lends support for this hypothesis.[55]

Melancholic patients showed some improvement during treatment in left-ear accuracy for the verbal task. This could reflect improvement in right-hemisphere function, which agrees with prior findings of improved performance on visuospatial tests of right-hemisphere function during treatment with antidepressants.[58,59] Despite this improvement, abnormalities of dichotic ear advantages in melancholic patients did persist following antidepressant treatment. This suggests that a state-independent (trait) characteristic could, at least in part, underlie the abnormal dichotic asymmetry in melancholia.

The difference in dichotic asymmetry between melancholia and atypical depression is of interest from a clinical perspective. These diagnostic subtypes appear to be differentially related to outcome of treatment with antidepressants. Melancholia generally responds favorably to standard tricyclic antidepressants, whereas atypical depression responds preferentially to MAOI antidepressants.[54] This suggested to us the possibility that tricyclic antidepressants might work best in depressed patients who, like melancholic patients, display abnormal dichotic asymmetry. A preliminary evaluation of this possibility was, therefore, conducted by comparing dichotic asymmetry of subgroups formed on the basis of their clinical response to a tricyclic or MAOI antidepressant.[60] The depressed patients were participants in ongoing drug studies, in which they were treated, in most cases double-blind, with either a tricyclic or MAOI antidepressant. An important design feature of this study is that patients received an initial 10-day placebo washout (single-blind) that enabled us to exclude at least some patients who respond to a placebo. Patients were judged to be treatment responders or nonresponders on the basis of a psychiatrist's CGI ratings. Treatment responders were those rated to be much improved or very much improved at the end of about six weeks of treatment with a tricyclic or MAOI antidepressant. The subgroups of treatment responders and nonresponders did not differ in demographic characteristics or handedness. Also, although treatment responder and nonresponder subgroups did not differ in ratings of severity of depression in the pretreatment session, responders showed significantly lower ratings of depression than nonresponders in the post-treatment session.

Patients who responded to a tricyclic antidepressant differed significantly from tricyclic nonresponders in ear advantages for dichotic complex tones, but not for nonsense syllables.[60] FIGURE 2 shows the accuracy scores on the Complex Tone Test for tricyclic responders (TCA-R) and nonresponders (TCA-NR) who were retested

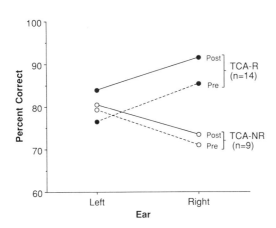

FIGURE 2. Accuracy scores for complex tones for tricyclic responders (TCA-R) and nonresponders (TCA-NR) in pre- and post-treatment sessions.

after approximately six weeks of treatment. A 2 × 2 × 2 (Group × Ear × Session) ANOVA of these accuracy scores revealed a highly significant Group × Ear interaction, $F (1,21) = 13.5$, $p = 0.001$. Responders showed an abnormal direction of asymmetry for complex tones, i.e., a mean right-ear advantage, whereas nonresponders showed the normal direction of asymmetry, i.e., a mean left-ear (right-hemisphere) advantage. As can be seen in FIGURE 2, the opposite direction of ear advantage for tricyclic responders and nonresponders was equally present in the pre- and post-treatment sessions. Although more tricyclic responders had melancholic depressions than did tricyclic nonresponders, this difference was not solely responsible for the difference in dichotic asymmetry between these subgroups. The opposite ear advantage for complex tones in tricyclic responders and nonresponders was still present when we analyzed the pretreatment accuracy data for only nonmelancholic patients, $F (1,23) = 4.4$, $p = 0.048$.

The difference in dichotic asymmetry between treatment responders and nonresponders was specific to tricyclic antidepressants in that analyses of pre- and post-treatment data for MAOI responders and nonresponders did not reveal significant differences in ear advantages for these subgroups. Since the difference in dichotic asymmetry was present both before and after treatment, it appears to represent a state-independent characteristic. The exact nature of the difference and its possible clinical utility as a predictor of treatment outcome should be further investigated using multiple dichotic tests, as well as more direct measures of hemispheric asymmetry, e.g., event-related brain potentials or measures of regional cerebral activity.

LATERALIZATION OF EMOTIONAL PERCEPTION IN NORMAL SUBJECTS

Dichotic listening tests have also provided evidence in normal subjects of right-hemisphere advantage for the perception of emotional stimuli.[4] Studies using dichotically presented nonverbal stimuli with different emotional qualities (crying, laughing, moans, etc.) have observed a left-ear advantage in normal adults.[61,62] In these studies, however, it is not possible to determine whether laterality effects are attributable to emotional processing, or arise simply from the nonverbal nature of the processing. Two techniques have recently been developed that use verbal stimuli to study lateralization of emotion. One technique manipulates the intonation or prosody of dichotic speech;[63] the other manipulates the emotional content of dichotic fused-words.[64] Not surprisingly, rather different findings have been reported for these two techniques.

Bryden and MacRae[63] introduced a dichotic monitoring task that provides a separate estimate of ear advantage when subjects attend to the verbal content or to the affective tone of words. In this task, dichotic two-syllable words differing only in the initial consonant were spoken in happy, sad, angry, or neutral tones. The subject's task in one block of trials was to indicate, as rapidly as possible, whether a specific target word was present, and, in a second block, to indicate whether a specific emotional tone was present. The data for 32 normal right-handed subjects showed a highly significant task-by-ear interaction, in which there was a right-ear advantage for target words, but a left-ear advantage for target emotions. This is a replication of prior findings by Ley and Bryden.[65] However, the findings differed from those of the earlier study in an important respect. Bryden and MacRae found a larger left-ear advantage for angry and sad targets than for happy targets, whereas Ley and Bryden found no difference as a function of the valence of emotions. There were two differences in the procedures of these studies that could have contributed to the difference in findings. First, one study required the detection of target emotions, whereas the other required categorization of different emotions. Focusing on a specific target emotion may have produced a priming or activation associated with this emotion, and this might not be found when categorizing emotions. Second, one study required divided attention to both ears, whereas the other required focused attention to either the right or the left ear. Further study of the effects of divided versus focused attention on dichotic asymmetry for emotional stimuli is needed to evaluate the importance of this factor.

Wexler et al.[64] used a fused-rhymed words task, with words that were reported to produce positive, negative, or neutral emotional responses. The dichotic stimuli consisted of word pairs of four different types: neutral-neutral (gill, dill), positive-neutral (hug, tug), negative-neutral (died, bide), and positive-negative (pie, die). Each pair fused to form a single percept, and the subject reported the word that was heard using a multiple-choice answer sheet that contained the dichotic pair and two foils. The subjects were 40 right-handers who were classified on the basis of self-report personality questionnaires to be in one of three groups: true low anxious, true high anxious, or repressive.

Although all four types of word pairs produced a mean right-ear advantage, the presence of emotionally positive words was associated with a larger right-ear advantage. In contrast, emotionally negative words did not differ from neutral words in ear advantage. Wexler et al. cite other studies finding evidence of an association of left-hemisphere activation and positive affect,[66,67] and they suggest that the two most likely explanations of the larger right-ear advantage for positive affect are (1) facilitation of left-hemisphere auditory receptive function, and (2) increased sensitivity of left-hemisphere frontal attentional centers to stimulus-specific arousal.

Wexler et al. also found differences among personality groups. High-anxious subjects and repressive subjects showed increased right-ear advantages for emotional words, whereas low-anxious subjects showed a nonsignificant decrease in right-ear advantage for emotional words. The three groups also differed in asymmetry scores for neutral words, with low-anxious subjects having higher asymmetry scores compared to high-anxious subjects and repressors. Thus, the different effects of emotional content on the asymmetry scores for these groups could be a byproduct of their differences in baseline asymmetry scores.

The findings for the above studies can be summarized in the following way. Negative affect was more effective than positive affect in inducing a left-ear advantage for the detection of emotional tone,[63] whereas positive affect was more effective than negative affect in altering the right-ear advantage for dichotic fused-words.[64] These different findings are likely the result of task differences. In the Bryden and MacRae study,[63] subjects were instructed to attend to a specific emotional tone, without any need to attend to verbal content. It is therefore not surprising that a left-ear advantage was obtained for this task. The greater left-ear advantage for negative emotional tone than positive emotional tone could reflect greater involvement of the right hemisphere with negative emotions. Alternatively, it could merely be more difficult to evoke positive emotions. In the Wexler et al. study,[64] the subject's task was to identify dichotically presented fused words; emotion enters only secondarily in terms of the meaning of the words. Understandably, a right-ear advantage is obtained for all conditions in this verbal task. The greater enhancement of right-ear advantage for positive affect than for negative affect could reflect the greater involvement of the left hemisphere with positive emotions.[66,67] Why words with negative emotional content did not result in some reduction of right-ear advantage is still a mystery. It would appear that further study is needed to establish more definitely whether positive and negative emotions do indeed differentially alter hemispheric processing of dichotic stimuli.

CONCLUSIONS

Dichotic listening tests can provide valid data concerning hemispheric lateralization for processing a variety of different types of verbal stimuli, nonverbal stimuli, and emotionally-laden stimuli. New techniques developed over the last several years have improved the reliability of dichotic asymmetry measures and have reduced or eliminated some methodological problems that arise from the lack of input competition, heavy memory load, or use of mutiple responses. The most reliable and valid verbal dichotic tests use fused words or nonsense syllables and dichotic monitoring techniques. These tests have the advantage of requiring only a single multiple-choice or detection response on each trial and are therefore ideal for use with clinical populations. The fused words and dichotic monitoring techniques can not only provide measures of lateralization for verbal processing, but have also been adapted for measuring lateralization of affect. Progress has also been made in the development of nonverbal dichotic tests. One of the best appears to be the Complex Tone Test, which provides a measure of right-hemisphere advantage for complex pitch perception.

The variety of dichotic listening tests available today has led to a new research strategy. This involves the use of multiple dichotic tests that can provide information about different cerebral functional systems. The use of fused words and nonsense syllable tests in psychotic patients has provided information on recovery-related changes in the different functional systems that process auditory stimuli as meaningful or as nonsense. Moreover, the use of both verbal and nonverbal dichotic tests has yielded evidence supporting the hypothesis of right hemisphere dysfunction in depressive disorders. The role of the right hemisphere in processing emotional stimuli, and in particular negative affect, received further support by having normal subjects engage in different tasks, i.e., detection of words or emotional tone, with the same dichotic stimuli.

Further application of recently developed dichotic listening tests in neurological and psychiatric populations would seem to be worthwhile. In particular, dichotic monitoring tasks could be used to study lateralization for both cognitive and emotional processing in psychiatric patients with different types of affective disorders. In normal subjects, further study of the relationship of individual differences in dichotic listening performance to personality variables would be of interest. The findings of Wexler et al.[64] indicate that ear advantages for dichotic fused words can differ markedly in low-anxious and high-anxious subjects.

Studies in normal and clinical populations would also benefit by obtaining more direct measures of hemispheric activity while subjects engage in dichotic listening tests. For instance, Molfese and Adams[68] have called for more studies in which brain event-related potentials are recorded during standard dichotic presentation of stimuli. Since event-related potentials are time-locked to dichotic stimuli, these data might help clarify the stages of information processing at which hemispheric asymmetries are present and might thereby also facilitate the interpretation of abnormalities of dichotic listening in clinical groups. A recent study by Coffey et al.[69] illustrates the value of measuring regional cerebral blood flow (rCBF) during dichotic listening tests. Measurements of rCBF were obtained in a resting baseline condition and during a two-tone pitch discrimination task that yields a left-ear (right-hemisphere) advantage in about 75% of normal right-handed subjects. Subjects with a significant left-ear advantage (N = 9) showed an increase in rCBF in the right posterior temporal lobe during this dichotic task, whereas subjects with a right-ear advantage (N = 5) showed an increase in rCBF in the left posterior temporal lobe. Although confirmation is needed in larger samples, these findings are important for two reasons: (1) they provide additional validation for the use of dichotic tests as measures of functional asymmetries, and (2) they indicate that individual differences in dichotic ear advantages are related to differences in regional cerebral activity.

Finally, a number of recent findings point to a potential application of dichotic listening tests for dealing with the clinical and biological heterogeneity of affective disorders. We have found evidence that individual differences in dichotic asymmetry among depressed patients are related to their diagnostic subtype and even to their clinical response to a standard antidepressant. Wexler et al.[70] divided patients having affective disorders into two subgroups on the basis of their difference in right-ear advantage for fused-word and nonsense syllable tests. These subgroups differed in their serum testosterone level and in their relationship between testosterone level and symptom severity. The above findings illustrate the value of using dichotic listening asymmetry to form subtypes of affective disorder, which can then be compared for differences in clinical features, in biochemical or physiological alterations, and in responsiveness to specific forms of treatment.

ACKNOWLEDGMENT

I thank Martina Voglmaier for assisting with the preparation of this manuscript.

REFERENCES

1. TENG, E. L. 1981. Dichotic ear difference is a poor index for functional asymmetry between the cerebral hemispheres. Neuropsychologia 19: 235-240.
2. HUGDAHL, K., Ed. 1988. Handbook of Dichotic Listening: Theory, Methods and Research. John Wiley. New York, NY.
3. BRUDER, G. E. 1988. Dichotic listening in psychiatric patients. In Handbook of Dichotic Listening: Theory, Methods and Research. K. Hugdahl, Ed. John Wiley. New York, NY.
4. BRYDEN, M. P. 1988. Dichotic studies of the lateralization of affect in normal subjects. In Handbook of Dichotic Listening: Theory, Methods and Research. K. Hugdahl, Ed. John Wiley. New York, NY.
5. BROADBENT, D. E. 1954. Perception and Communication. Pergamon Press. New York, NY.
6. KIMURA, D. 1961. Cerebral dominance and the perception of verbal stimuli. Can. J. Psychol. 15: 166-171.
7. KIMURA, D. 1961. Some effects of temporal lobe damage on auditory perception. Can. J. Psychol. 15: 156-165.
8. BERLIN, C. I., L. F. HUGHES, S. S. LOWE-BELL & H. L. BERLIN. 1973. Dichotic right-ear advantage in children 5 to 13. Cortex 9: 393-401.
9. SPEAKS, C., N. NICCUM & E. CARNEY. 1982. Statistical properties of responses to dichotic listening with CV nonsense syllables. J. Acoust. Soc. Am. 72: 1185-1194.
10. RYAN, W. J. & M. MCNEIL. 1974. Listener reliability for a dichotic task. J. Acoust. Soc. Am. 56: 1922-1923.
11. WEXLER, B. E. & G. R. HENINGER. 1979. Alterations in cerebral laterality during acute psychotic illness. Arch. Gen. Psychiatry. 36: 278-284.

12. WEXLER, B. E., T. HALWES & G. R. HENINGER. 1981. Use of a statistical significance criterion in drawing inferences over hemispheric dominance for language function from dichotic listening data. Brain Lang. **13:** 13-18.

13. WEXLER, B. E. & T. HALWES. 1983. Increasing the power of dichotic methods: The fused rhymed words test. Neuropsychologia **21:** 59-66.

14. SEXTON, M. A. & G. GEFFEN. 1981. Phonological fusion in dichotic monitoring. J. Exp. Psychol. (Hum. Percept.) **7:** 422-429.

15. CLARK, C. R., L. B. GEFFEN & G. GEFFEN. 1989. Invariant properties of auditory perceptual asymmetry assessed by dichotic monitoring. In Handbook of Dichotic Listening: Theory, Methods and Research. K. Hugdahl, Ed. John Wiley. New York, NY.

16. GEFFEN, G. & D. CAUDREY. 1981. Reliability and validity of the dichotic monitoring test for language laterality. Neuropsychologia **19:** 413-423.

17. KIMURA, D. 1964. Left-right differences in the perception of melodies. Q. J. Exp. Psychol. **16:** 355-358.

18. GORDON, H. W. 1980. Degree of ear asymmetry for perception of dichotic chords and for illusory chord localization in musicians of different levels of competence. J. Exp. Psychol. (Hum. Percept.) **6:** 516-527.

19. CURRY, F. K. W. 1967. A comparison of left-handed and right-handed subjects on verbal and nonverbal dichotic listening tasks. Cortex **3:** 343-352.

20. COLBOURN, C. J. & W. A. LISHMAN. 1979. Lateralization of function and psychotic illness: A left hemisphere deficit? In Hemispheric Asymmetries of Function and Psychopathology. J. Gruzelier & P. Flor-Henry, Eds.: 539-559. Elsevier. Amsterdam.

21. SIDTIS, J. J. 1981. The complex tone test: Implications for the assessment of auditory laterality effects. Neuropsychologia **19:** 103-112.

22. BLUMSTEIN, S., H. GOODGLASS & V. TARTTER. 1975. The reliability of ear advantage in dichotic listening. Brain Lang. **2:** 226-236.

23. BEVER, T. & R. CHIARELLO. 1974. Cerebral dominance in musicians. Science **185:** 537-539.

24. SIDTIS, J. J. & B. T. VOLPE. 1988. Selective loss of complex-pitch or speech discrimination after unilateral cerebral lesion. Brain Lang. **34:** 235-245.

25. ZATORRE, R. J. 1988. Pitch perception of complex tones and human temporal lobe function. J. Acoust. Soc. Am. **84:** 566-572.

26. BISIACH, E., L. CORNACCHIA, R. STERZI & G. VALLAR. 1984. Disorders of perceived auditory lateralization after lesions of the right hemisphere. Brain **107:** 37-52.

27. RUFF, R. M., N. A. HERSH & H. PRIBRAM. 1981. Auditory spatial deficits in the personal and intrapersonal frames of reference due to cortical lesions. Neuropsychologia **19:** 435-443.

28. ALTMAN, J. A., L. J. BALANOV & V. L. DEGLIN. 1979. Effects of unilateral disorder of the brain hemisphere function in man on directional hearing. Neuropsychologia **17:** 295-301.

29. HARTMANN, W. M. 1983. Localization of sound in rooms. J. Acoust. Soc. Am. **74(5):** 1380-1391.

30. BRUDER, G. E., S. SUTTON & P. JASIUKAITIS. 1986. Hemispheric lateralization for auditory temporal and spatial perception: Familial handedness and sex effects. Paper presented at the Eastern Psychological Association meetings. April. New York, NY.

31. KIMURA, D. 1969. Spatial location in left and right visual fields. Can. J. Psychol. **23:** 445-458.

32. MCGEE, M. G. 1979. Human Spatial Abilities: Sources of Sex Differences. Praeger. New York, NY.

33. MCGLONE, J. 1980. Sex differences in human brain asymmetry: A critical survey. Behav. Brain Sci. **3:** 215-263.

34. NICHELLI, P., A. MANNI & P. FAGLIONI. 1983. Relationships between speed, accuracy of performance and hemispheric superiorities for visuo-spatial pattern processing in the two sexes. Neuropsychologia **21:** 625-632.

35. WEXLER, B. E. & T. HALWES. 1985. Dichotic listening tests in studying brain-behavior relationships. Neuropsychologia **23:** 545-559.

36. WEXLER, B. E. 1986. Alterations in cerebral laterality during acute psychotic illness. Br. J. Psychiatry **149:** 202-209.

37. WEXLER, B. E. 1988. Dichotic presentation as a method for single hemisphere stimulation studies. In Handbook of Dichotic Listening: Theory, Methods and Research, K. Hugdahl, Ed. John Wiley. New York, NY.

38. LERNER, J., I. NACHSHON & A. CARMON. 1977. Responses of paranoid and nonparanoid schizophrenics in a dichotic listening task. J. Nerv. Ment. Dis. 164: 247-252.

39. LISHMAN, W. A., B. K. TOONE, C. J. COLBOURN, E. R. L. McMEEKAN & R. M. MANCE. 1978. Dichotic listening in psychiatric patients. Br. J. Psychiatry 132: 333-341.

40. YOZAWITZ, A., G. BRUDER, S. SUTTON, L. SHARPE, B. GURLAND, J. FLEISS & L. COSTA. 1979. Dichotic perception: Evidence for right hemisphere dysfunction in affective psychosis. Br. J. Psychiatry 135: 224-237.

41. GRUZELIER, J. H. & N. V. HAMMOND. 1980. Lateralized deficits and drug influences on the dichotic listening of schizophrenic patients. Biol. Psychiatry 15: 759-779.

42. JOHNSON, O. & D. CROCKETT. 1982. Changes in perceptual asymmetries with clinical improvement of depression and schizophrenia. J. Abnorm. Psychol. 91: 45-54.

43. HARSHMAN, R. A. & M. E. LUNDY. 1988. Can dichotic listening measure "degree of lateralization"? In Handbook of Dichotic Listening: Theory, Methods and Research. K. Hugdahl, Ed. John Wiley. New York, NY.

44. BRYDEN, M. P. 1982. Laterality: Functional Asymmetry in the Intact Brain. Academic Press. New York, NY.

45. REPP, B. H. 1977. Measuring laterality effects in dichotic listening. J. Acoust. Soc. Am. 62: 720-737.

46. BRADSHAW, J. L., V. BURDEN & N. C. NETTLETON. 1986. Dichotic and dichhaptic techniques. Neuropsychologia 24: 79-90.

47. JONES, B. 1983. Measuring degree of cerebral lateralization in children as a function of age. Dev. Psychol. 19: 237-242.

48. BRYDEN, M. P. & D. A. SPROTT. 1981. Statistical determination of degree of laterality. Neuropsychologia 19: 571-581.

49. BRUDER, G. E., F. M. QUITKIN, J. W. STEWART, C. MARTIN, M. M. VOGLMAIER & W. M. HARRISON. 1989. Cerebral laterality and depression: Differences in perceptual asymmetry among diagnostic subtypes. J. Abnorm. Psychol. 98: 177-186.

50. BRUDER, G. E. 1983. Cerebral laterality and psychopathology: A review of dichotic listening studies. Schizophr. Bull. 9: 134-151.

51. BRUDER, G. E., S. SUTTON, P. BERGER-GROSS, F. QUITKIN & S. DAVIES. 1981. Lateralized auditory processing in depression: Dichotic click detection. Psychiatry Res. 4: 243-266.

52. AMERICAN PSYCHIATRIC ASSOCIATION. 1980. Diagnostic and Statistical Manual of Mental Disorders. 3rd edit. Washington, DC.

53. KLEIN, D. F., R. GITTELMAN, F. QUITKIN & A. L. RIFKIN. 1980. Diagnosis and drug treatment of psychiatric disorders: Adults and children. 2nd edit. Williams & Wilkins. Baltimore, MD.

54. LIEBOWITZ, M. R., F. M. QUITKIN, P. J. STEWART, P. McGRATH, W. HARRISON, J. S. MARKOWITZ, J. RABKIN, E. TRICAMO, D. M. GOETZ & D. F. KLEIN. 1988. Antidepressant specificity in atypical depression. Arch. Gen. Psychiatry 45: 129-137.

55. SIDTIS, J. J. 1988. Dichotic listening after commissurotomy. In Handbook of Dichotic Listening: Theory, Methods and Research. K. Hugdahl, Ed. John Wiley. New York, NY.

56. KINSBOURNE, M. 1970. The cerebral basis of lateral asymmetries in attention. Acta Psychol. 33: 193-201.

57. FLOR-HENRY, P. 1976. Lateralized temporal-limbic dysfunction and psychopathology. Ann. N. Y. Acad. Sci. 280: 777-795.

58. FROMM, D. & D. SCHOPFLOCHER. 1984. Neuropsychological test performance in depressed patients before and after drug therapy. Biol. Psychiatry. 19: 55-71.

59. STATON, R. D., H. WILSON & R. A. BRUMBACK. 1981. Cognitive improvement associated with tricyclic antidepressant treatment of psychotic major depressive illness. Percept. Mot. Skills 53: 219-234.

60. BRUDER, G. E., J. W. STEWART, M. M. VOGLMAIER, W. M. HARRISON, P. McGRATH, E. TRICAMO & F. M. QUITKIN. 1990. Cerebral laterality and depression: Relations of perceptual asymmetry to outcome of treatment with tricyclic antidepressants. Neuropsychopharmacology 3: 1-10.

61. KING, F. L. & D. KIMURA. 1972. Left-ear superiority in dichotic perception of vocal nonverbal sounds. Can. J. Psychol. 26: 111-116.

62. CARMON, A. & I. NACHSHON. 1973. Ear asymmetry in perception of emotional non-verbal stimuli. Acta Psychol. 37: 351-357.

63. BRYDEN, M. P. & L. MACRAE. 1989. Dichotic laterality effects obtained with emotional words. Neuropsychiatr. Neuropsychol. Behav. Neurol. 1(3): 171-176.
64. WEXLER, B. E., G. SCHWARTZ, S. WARRENBURG, M. SERVIS & I. TARLATZIS. 1986. Effects of emotion on perceptual asymmetry: Interactions with personality. Neuropsychologia 24: 699-710.
65. LEY, R. G. & M. P. BRYDEN. 1982. A dissociation of right and left hemispheric effects for recognizing emotional tone and verbal content. Brain Cognition 1: 8-9.
66. DAVIDSON, R. J. & N. A. FOX. 1982. Asymmetrical brain activity discriminates between positive and negative affective stimuli in human infants. Science 218: 1235-1237.
67. SACKEIM, H. A., M. G. GREENBERG, M. A. WEIMAN, R. C. GUR, J. P. HUNGERBUHLER & N. GESCHWIND. 1982. Hemispheric asymmetry in the expression of positive and negative emotions. Arch. Neurol. 39: 210-218.
68. MOLFESE, D. L. & C. L. ADAMS. 1988. Auditory evoked responses as an index of laterality: Findings from studies of speech perception. In Handbook of Dichotic Listening: Theory, Methods and Research. K. Hugdahl, Ed. John Wiley. New York, NY.
69. COFFEY, C. E., M. P. BRYDEN, E. S. SCHROERING, W. H. WILSON & R. J. MATHEW. 1989. Regional cerebral blood flow correlates of a dichotic listening task. J. Neuropsychiatry 1: 46-52.
70. WEXLER, B. E., J. W. MASON & E. L. GILLER. 1989. Possible subtypes of affective disorder suggested by differences in cerebral laterality and testosterone: A preliminary report. Arch. Gen. Psychiatry 46: 429-433.

The Staggered Spondaic Word Test

A Ten-Minute Look at the Central Nervous System through the Ears

JACK KATZ[a,b] AND PAULA S. SMITH[c]

[a]Department of Communicative Disorders and Sciences
University at Buffalo
State University of New York
Buffalo, New York 14260
[c]Niagara County Speech, Hearing and Language Center
Lockport, New York 14094

The Staggered Spondaic Word (SSW) test was developed 30 years ago to assess the integrity of the central auditory system.[1] It followed from the "sensitized speech" concept of Bocca et al.[2] and from the binaural approach that was demonstrated by Matzker.[3] The SSW was contemporary with other early dichotic procedures of Feldmann[4] and Kimura.[5]

There are two major applications of the SSW. It is used (1) in locating brain abnormalities resulting from tumors, strokes or degenerative conditions, and (2) in the evaluation of auditory-processing problems associated with learning and other disabilities.

BACKGROUND

The SSW was first reported in 1962. It employed competing messages in a complex presentation mode. Since that time it has been widely used as a research tool, as well as with clients or pupils who received audiological services. The test has been used with a variety of special populations including the mentally retarded,[6] autistic,[7] emotionally disturbed,[8] hearing impaired, and the elderly.[9,10] The SSW has also been adapted for use in other languages.[11,12]

The earliest SSW studies evaluated the test's ability to differentiate pathological states from normal ones. It was found that skull-trauma cases with significant involvement of the temporal region showed a contralateral effect. That is, the ear opposite the brain lesion was shown to have a major deficit. In 1963, Katz et al.[13] reported that peripheral hearing loss cases could not be readily differentiated from central ones. This was remedied by the use of a correction factor to account for errors due to peripheral

[b]Address correspondence to Professor Jack Katz, Department of Communicative Disorders and Sciences, University at Buffalo, 109 Park Hall, Buffalo, NY 14260.

hearing distortion. A follow-up report provided cut-off scores to differentiate two groups of brain lesion cases, peripherally hearing-impaired subjects and normal controls.[14]

Support for the identification-localization functions of the SSW came from several sources employing a variety of pathological groups. These include temporal lobectomy,[15] tumor,[16,17] stroke,[18] commissurotomy,[19] and degenerative disorders, such as Alzheimer's disease.[20]

In the late sixties and early seventies, attention turned to the auditory problems of learning-disabled individuals. One of the available procedures for this type of evaluation was the SSW. A number of papers described the test as being sensitive to the auditory-processing problems in those with learning difficulties.[21,22] Other reports followed.[23–25] The categorization that was used for site-of-lesion testing was neither appropriate nor sufficiently sensitive to evaluate the learning disabled. Therefore, a statistical standard was introduced and recently updated.[26,27]

THE SSW TEST

Procedures and C-SSW Scores

Descriptions of the SSW test and the standard scoring procedures are detailed elsewhere.[28,29] Briefly, the SSW test stimuli are familiar spondaic (compound) words. Spondees were chosen because they are moderately resistant to peripheral hearing distortion and, therefore, less likely to produce results that are confounded by hearing impairment. Each item of the test is preceded by the phrase, "Are you ready?" The listener is instructed to repeat all of the words after the introductory phrase. The test words are delivered to the listener via a tapeplayer and an audiometer at a comfortably loud level (50 dB SL). The corrected SSW (C-SSW) scores are utilized to evaluate the patient's performance. The first test item is shown in FIGURE 1.

The challenge to the central nervous system is based on the dichotic presentation (different words presented to each ear at the same time) and the complex, staggered mode of delivery. The C-SSW scores are utilized to evaluate the level of performance. The listener's verbatim responses are noted on a score sheet. Each test word of the

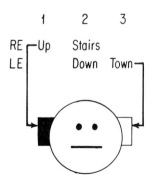

FIGURE 1. The first test item of the SSW test begins in the right ear (RE) and ends in the left (LE). The temporal sequence is shown at the top.

FIGURE 2. The second item of the SSW test begins in the left ear and ends in the right. In each item two words are noncompeting (NC), and two are competing (C).

	1 NC	2 C	3 NC
RIGHT EAR		in	law
LEFT EAR	out	side	

40-item procedure is scored as either correct or incorrect, regardless of response sequence. A correction factor based on the individual's word-recognition score is used to further offset the effects of peripheral auditory distortion. Odd-numbered items begin in the right ear and end in the left. Even-numbered items follow the reversed pattern, as shown in FIGURE 2.

Additional diagnostic information is obtained from reversals (variation in response order) and other "response biases." Certain test behaviors may also shed light on the auditory problem. These include characteristics such as quick and delayed responses.

Response Bias

Response biases such as Order Effects and Type A pattern are calculated from "eight cardinal numbers" (8 CNs). The latter numbers are the total error for the eight columns representing the four words in right-ear-first (REF) items followed by the four words in the left-ear-first (LEF) items (FIG. 3).

Two types of response bias are of particular interest. The first is Order Effects, which refers to a tendency to make more errors at the beginning of items (regardless of the ear) or at the end. An Order Effect high/low indicates significantly more errors on the first two words of the items than on the last two, and Order Effect low/high indicates the reverse situation. In brain lesion cases, each pattern is associated with different regions. For example, Order Effect, low/high is likely to be seen in Wernicke's aphasics and high/low in Broca's aphasics.[30-33] It should be noted that the test is sensitive to dysfunction in either hemisphere, with or without language impairment.[18,33]

The second response bias is the Type A pattern. The criterion for the Type A is based on the 8CNs. There must be more errors by a factor of 2 in column F (or B) than in each of the other seven columns, as well as a specified absolute difference based on the individual's age. This pattern is frequently seen in corpus callosum tumor cases, as well as in patients with lesions in other regions of the CNS.[34]

SSW FINDINGS IN SITE-OF-LESION CASES

The two major sources of information for locating cerebral lesions are (1) the severity of the score based on the percentage of C-SSW errors, and (2) the use of response bias. The severity of the score helps to differentiate lesions to the auditory reception (AR) centers versus lesions that spare these regions. Response bias has been found to be most useful in locating impairments in various parts of the cerebrum, based on asymmetrical patterns that are noted in the 8CNs.

Posterior Temporal Lesions

Auditory Reception and the Association Region

The AR center (primarily Brodmann's area 41) is embedded in Heschl's gyrus on the opercular surface of the middle-posterior portion of the temporal lobes.[35] They receive input directly from the auditory brainstem. The auditory cortex (primarily Brodmann's area 22) includes the middle and posterior portions of the superior gyrus of each temporal lobe.[36] Each receives input from the AR center for further analysis. Luria[37] points out that the auditory cortex serves as the phonemic zone of the brain. Auditory information is translated into recognizable speech sounds in this region, and

Right-Ear-First Items				Left-Ear-First Items			
RNC	RC	LC	LNC	LNC	LC	RC	RNC
up	stairs	down	town	out	side	in	law
day	light	lunch	time	wash	---	--	----
---	---	----	---	----	----	---	---
--	----	---	----	---	--	----	--
0	10	3	1	1	4	11	0
(A)	(B)	(C)	(D)	(E)	(F)	(G)	(H)

SUM*

FIGURE 3. SSW items: the total errors for the right-ear-first item conditions and the left-ear-first conditions yield eight important sums. These numbers are referred to as the eight cardinal numbers (8CNs). They are used in calculating both the SSW scores and response biases, such as Order Effects and Type A patterns. Sample results are shown which are considered symmetrical in that the two right noncompeting (RNC) scores (columns A and H) are similar, as are the right competing (RC) scores (columns B and G). Similar results are shown for left noncompeting (LNC) and left competing (LC) scores. SUM represents the eight cardinal numbers.

phonemic knowledge is stored there. Information that is processed in the auditory cortex is then available for further language processing.[38,39] Luria[40] noted that patients with lesions of the phonemic zone tended to miss the endings of (Russian) words. Similarly, Burns and Canter[41] noted that posterior temporal (PT) cases have more difficulty in comprehending the ends of sentences than the beginnings.

Baru and Karaseva[42] found that auditory cortex lesion cases were unique in their inability to process rapid auditory signals. In order to compensate for this deficit, it was necessary to increase the intensity level of the signals by 25 dB, whereas for normal subjects and patients with other cerebral lesions it required only 10 dB. When we consider the trading relationship between intensity and time,[43] this finding is consistent with the work of Tallal and Piercy[44,45] and Tallal[46] who studied the categorical perception in children with severe language impairment. They found recognition of consonant sounds to be faulty when the acoustic formant transitions were maintained at a normal 45 msec duration. However, when the transition durations were increased to 90 or 135 msec, the children performed as well as the normal control subjects.

Behaviorally, posterior temporal cases are somewhat slow in responding to speech and require even more time when the material is longer or complex. Damage to the auditory cortex on the left side can be expected to produce receptive difficulties for speech sounds as well as language, as noted in patients with Wernicke's aphasia. Even after recovering from the primary aphasic symptoms, Wernicke's cases may still need additional time to sort out their vague perceptions. Recently, Blumstein[47] presented supporting evidence for slow processing in Wernicke's aphasics. She was able to demonstrate improved performance using time-expanded speech.

Indications from the SSW Score

In 1963, Arthur Epstein, a neurologist at the Tulane School of Medicine noted that SSW results in brain lesion cases could be divided into two obvious subgroups. He pointed out that patients with damage to the AR and surrounding centers of either hemisphere exhibited many errors in the ear contralateral to the damage. However, in cerebral lesion cases in which the posterior half of the temporal lobe was spared, fewer errors were noted and the side of the disorder was often unrelated to the affected ear on the SSW. These observations have been supported in a number of investigations.[14,17,18,48-50]

For purposes of illustration, a group of 110 cases with well-localized lesions were studied. Seventy were assembled from previous investigations[14,18,30,34,49] and 40 cases were added to provide a sufficiently large database. FIGURE 4 shows the results for the 42 cases with lesions involving the right or left AR center. Means and standard deviations for the four conditions are displayed separately for those with right- and left-hemisphere involvement. Moderate or severe SSW scores are typically obtained in AR cases.[51] This requires, among other criteria, a condition error score of 26% or greater.[14] Forty-one (98%) of those with AR lesions had moderate or severe C-SSW scores. The contralateral effect is seen more clearly in the right hemisphere cases, as those with left-sided damage also had depressed performance in the left-competing condition. These results may be compared with the data for 46 non-auditory reception (NAR) cases (FIG. 5). The latter subjects had lesions of the cerebrum which did not involve Heschl's gyrus. In contrast to the AR group, only 11% of the NAR cases had moderate C-SSW scores and none had a severe score.

Indications from Response Bias

Additional diagnostic support for involvement of the posterior temporal region can be obtained from response bias information. The Order Effect low/high has been

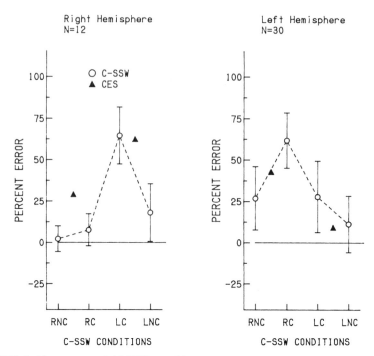

FIGURE 4. Mean corrected (C-SSW) condition scores and standard deviations for auditory reception (AR) lesion cases. The four conditions are right noncompeting (RNC), right competing (RC), left competing (LC), and left noncompeting (LNC). The competing environmental sound (CES) test means are displayed for each ear. Separate results are shown for right AR (*left panel*) and left AR (*right panel*) cases. Left panel: SDs for CES are right ear = 15, left ear = 20; right panel: right ear = 31, left ear = 9.

recognized as a common feature when there is a lesion of the PT lobe.[30,31] This finding of significantly more errors at the endings of test items than at the beginnings was recently replicated in a CT-scan cross-validation study.[49]

In the group of 110 verified cases, the incidence of Order Effect low/high was compared for the AR and NAR cases. Forty-three percent of the AR cases showed this PT response bias, whereas none of the NARs demonstrated the posterior pattern. Thus, only those with involvement of the region in and around Heschl's gyrus had a posterior Order Effect.

To summarize, the posterior portion of the temporal lobe is associated with phonemic identification and phonemic memory. The SSW findings in PT lesion cases, in either hemisphere, are exemplified by many errors overall and performance falling into the moderate or severe category. The major portion of the errors is found in the ear opposite the lesion, especially on the competing portion of the items. In addition, PT response bias is frequently noted. The Order Effect low/high is a strong indication of AR involvement in cerebral lesion cases. A person's slow or imprecise processing of speech could contribute to errors on the second halves of items.

Frontal and Anterior Temporal Lesions

Behavioral Characteristics

The frontal and anterior temporal lobes form the anterior cerebral (AC) region of the brain. They serve some unique but mostly similar or related behavioral functions. In the frontal lobe, the prefrontal cortex is the most anterior portion. Among other functions, it appears to provide for a differential response to each of two stimuli.[52] Broca's area, in the inferior frontal convolution, is the major expressive language center. It is located in the language-dominant hemisphere, usually the left.[53] The motor cortex is situated in the posterior frontal region, along the fissure of Rolando. Serving the motor cortex with higher-order motor planning and postural functions are the premotor and supplementary motor regions, which lie anterior to it.

The anterior temporal region contains two important structures, the hippocampus and the amygdala. The hippocampus runs the length of the temporal lobe, medially and inferiorly. It is well recognized as a vital memory-processing region.[54-56] The amygdala is situated superiorly at the anterior end of the hippocampus. It is associated with memory processing and behavior. Two recent animal studies help to elucidate its

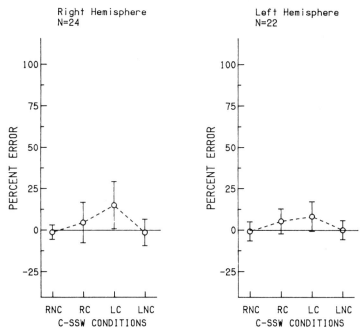

FIGURE 5. Mean corrected (C-SSW) condition scores and standard deviations for non-auditory reception (NAR) lesion cases. The four conditions are right noncompeting (RNC), right competing (RC), left competing (LC), and left noncompeting (LNC). Separate results are shown for right NAR (*left panel*) and left NAR (*right panel*) cases.

complex functions. The amygdala appears to have a direct auditory connection from the medial geniculate body. When this pathway is lesioned, there is a reduced bodily response to conditioned aversive stimuli; however, the response to the unconditioned stimulus remains unchanged.[57] With the introduction of norepinephrine into the amygdala, avoidance behavior to noxious stimuli may not be learned.[58] Fedio and Van Buren[59] stimulated the cerebral cortex in patients who were about to undergo brain surgery. They found different error patterns for words when the posterior temporal and the anterior temporal-frontal regions were stimulated. Posterior stimulation appeared to interfere with processing while stimulation of the anterior sites interfered with retrieval.

A wide variety of symptoms have been noted with damage to the anterior temporal or frontal regions. Struss and Benson[60] list nine behavioral characteristics concomitant with frontal lobe lesions. They are motor impairment (both hypo- and hyperkinetic), sensory and perceptual dysfunction (fixation on initial feature), attentional difficulties (inability to inhibit distractions), abnormal awareness (sensory neglect), perseveration (although not exclusively a frontal sign), sequence disturbances, memory failure (stored information is not readily accessible), personality changes (unrestrained, tactless, callous lack of concern, obstinate, childish), and intellectual changes (unimaginative, ineffective, careless working habits). McAllister and Price[61] note that because of the similarities in behavior, frontal lobe lesion cases may be misdiagnosed as schizophrenics.

Left and right AC lesions produce distinctly different impairments.[62] The effects of left-sided disorders will be reviewed here because they relate most specifically to langauge and academic learning. It is also worth noting that with the reduction in verbal skills there tends to be an improvement in visual abilities.

Removal of the anterior temporal lobe (including the amygdala and up to 2 cm of the hippocampus) reduces performance in immediate verbal recall, short-term and delayed recall, and produces an increase in the percentage of forgetting. Anterior-temporal lobectomy patients dropped from the normal memory category into the "handicapping" range. Diminished reasoning and problem-solving ability were also noted.[62]

Another important characteristic of those with anterior temporal lobe lesions is poor listening ability in a background of noise. A reduced "cocktail party" skill was noted in patients who had anterior-temporal lobectomies.[63] This may be associated with an impairment of the temporal-lobe enhancement mechanism that is thought to enable the listener to increase the prominence of a selected sound or the salience of a particular voice.[64]

Unlike the confined area of the brain that is identified as AR, the NAR region is any portion of the cerebrum other than the AR zones. The lesion is considered NAR only if the AR region is spared. AR lesions may involve any of the NAR areas, but must also include Heschl's gyrus. Thus, NAR cases exclude AR involvement, but AR cases include at least adjacent regions around Heschl's gyrus.

Indications from the SSW Score

The frontal and anterior temporal regions are defined as NAR, unless the lesion extends posteriorly to include the AR center.[31,32] We refer to this portion of the brain as the anterior cerebral region. It is probable, based on the results of parietal lobe cases, that the sensory strip can be included as AC because the SSW results are consistent with the performance of those having frontal and anterior temporal lesions.

In NAR cases, SSW performance overlaps the results of normal control and hearing-loss subjects.[14] More than one-half of the NAR cases with essentially normal hearing fall into the normal range for corrected SSW scores. The others are likely to have mild scores. The NAR cases that have mild SSW scores are similar in this respect to some of the hearing-loss subjects. If an individual has a mild score and no significant hearing loss, it can be taken as evidence of an NAR dysfunction. NAR cases with normal SSW scores can be differentiated from the normal population if they demonstrate significant response biases. Response bias also provides site-of-dysfunction information.

Of the 46 NAR cases mentioned previously, 38 had involvement of the AC region. Eleven percent of the AC cases had mild scores. The use of the error peak as a contralateral indicator in NAR cases is inappropriate.[14,18] Fifty-five percent of the NARs had contralateral error peaks, 40% ipsilateral, and 5% had equal scores bilaterally. Thus, it would be hazardous to suggest the side of lesion based on the error peak in NAR cases (especially if the peak is in the left ear). AR and NAR cases can be differentiated because the PT patients have poor scores (in the ear opposite the lesion). The NAR subjects have relatively good scores, but the results are devoid of side-of-dysfunction information.[14,18] When response bias information is employed, the hit rate for NAR cases increases.[31] Ignoring these SSW fundamentals is a major violation of the test.[50]

Indications from Response Bias

The Order Effect high/low is one of the three response biases that is associated with AC lesions. Among the AC cases, 38% had the Order Effect high/low. In the AR group, 22% had the same indicator. This is not felt to be evidence of false-positive results. It should be reiterated that all of the AR cases had involvement outside the small AR region. Damage usually extended anteriorly from Heschl's gyrus (e.g., stroke involving the temporal branches of the middle cerebral artery).

It is hypothesized that the greater number of errors on the first compound word of the items, as compared to errors on the second one, relates to poor memory. A rapidly fading memory is likely to show up in this fashion on the SSW. It is therefore not surprising that a group that has poor recall and difficulty in delayed-response tasks would have an Order Effect high/low. This is clearly differentiated from the purer AR patients, who have limited phonemic decoding skills. Patients with AR lesions do not perform as accurately on the second half of the items as on the first, presumably because of the time and effort spent on the initial words.

An observation that we have made over the years is that individuals with AC bias also tend to blurt out their responses immediately after the item is presented. Sometimes they begin to respond even before the item is completed. They often explain that this behavior is an attempt to avoid forgetting the words.

In summary, anterior cerebral cases tend to have limited skills for listening in noise and have poor auditory memories. On the SSW test, they have fewer errors than posterior temporal patients, with performance falling into the normal or mild C-SSW category. More than one-third of the ACs demonstrated an anterior Order Effect, which is just one of three anterior cerebral indicators. A rapidly fading memory could contribute to the poorer performance noted at the beginning of items.

Temporo-parieto-occipital Lesions

The anatomical point on the cortex at which the temporal, parietal, and occipital lobes meet is not clearly marked. Nevertheless, the functional contributions of this area are considerable. Just as geographical junctions between land masses have great strategic significance, this region of the brain, with its unique location, assumes important intercommunication functions.

The angular gyrus of the temporo-parieto-occipital (TPO) region is strategically situated between the auditory cortex of the temporal lobe and the visual cortex of the occipital lobe. It has long been recognized as a vital auditory-visual integration center.[65] In the left hemisphere, it is situated in close proximity to the language center, planum temporale.[66] In the right hemisphere, the TPO area is adjacent to the visual-spatial region of the parietal lobe. By use of the splenium, the posterior portion of the corpus callosum, auditory-linguistic information from the left hemisphere can be integrated with the visual-spatial input of the right hemisphere. Musiek[67] provides an excellent review of the auditory aspect of the corpus callosum.

Dyslexia is thought to result from lesions of the TPO region[68,69] and/or the corpus callosum.[70] In particular, the inferior portion of the splenium has been implicated in pure alexia (i.e., without agraphia).[71,72] It is interesting to note that the anterior and middle sections of the corpus callosum are thought to be associated with schizophrenia[73] and depression.[74]

Interpretation from SSW and CES Results

One cannot generalize about the severity of the SSW score in patients with angular gyrus or commissural pathway lesions. Their results vary from the normal-to-severe range, based on the locus of the disorder, the patient's age, and the age at onset.

The Competing Environmental Sound (CES) test is useful in identifying certain lesions of the corpus callosum. The CES is a dichotic procedure in which a sound such as a honking horn is delivered to one ear, and the sound of a person coughing is presented to the other. The patient is asked to identify both sounds from four picture choices.[75] The CES test results are compared with those of the SSW test when there is concern of commissural involvement. The affected ear on the two tests may differ in certain corpus callosum cases because environmental sounds are processed primarily in the right hemisphere.[76] Therefore, the cerebral routing of this information is likely to be the opposite of that for speech information.[77]

Left-ear SSW Peak

The most common characteristic of those with angular gyrus or commissural pathway lesions is a significant left-competing peak of errors on the SSW test. We have consistently seen this left-sided pattern in angular gyrus cases (except in a small percentage of left-handers) and in all of our corpus callosum and anterior commissure cases that have significant SSW scores.

A significant left-ear SSW peak in the absence of AR involvement typically suggests corpus callosum dysfunction.[19,78,79] Katz *et al.*[34] found that lesions of the splenium and body of the corpus callosum were typically associated with moderate C-SSW scores. Similar results were found in cases with lesions of the anterior commissure.[32]

CES Pattern

Anterior corpus callosum patients who have significant CES scores (most often the older subjects) and posterior corpus callosum patients tend to have the majority of CES errors on the right side. This forms a "crossed pattern" when the SSW and CES results are compared (FIG. 6, left panel). In this way, these corpus callosum or anterior commissure cases with moderate or severe C-SSW scores can be differentiated from the right AR cases (FIG. 4, left panel). However, it appears that lesions of the body of the corpus callosum may have left-ear peaks for both the SSW and CES tests.[34]

Interpretations from Response Bias

On the SSW, the Type A pattern is associated with angular gyrus and/or corpus callosum lesions.[32] This response bias has been noted in one-third of corpus callosum cases.[34] A similar percentage has been found in anterior commissure patients. Unfortunately, the Type A pattern is not a strong localizing sign because it may be found in cases with lesions in a variety of cerebral, cerebellar, and brainstem regions. However, if the listener has a severe reading and/or spelling disorder, there is a greater probability that the lesion, if any, involves the angular gyrus and/or the splenium of the corpus callosum.

It is difficult to explain the Type A pattern. However, it is our assumption that Type A patterns relate to defective commissural processes. Because of some type of interference, one auditory channel is slowed. This could produce a temporal condition in which one stimulus is ignored when the task requires rapid switching of attention between the ears. Which competing word is ignored depends on language dominance (i.e., which channel must cross the corpus callosum) and in which ear the materials are presented first. We infer this because column F (left-competing condition when the left ear is leading) is the one affected, except in a small number of cases, usually in left-handers.

Among the 110 cases, 22 had lesions primarily involving the commissural pathways. FIGURE 6 (left panel) shows the results for 18 cases with genu, splenium, and/or anterior commissure damage, and FIGURE 6 (right panel) shows the results for 6 individuals with impairment of the body of the corpus callosum. Of the commissural cases, 27% had Type A patterns.

To summarize, TPO (and/or posterior corpus callosum) lesions produce severe reading and spelling problems. Fewer learning problems but greater numbers of behavioral problems are noted with lesions of the anterior or middle portions of the corpus callosum. For the TPO group, an SSW peak is found in the left ear, as it is in right AR cases. However, unlike the AR group there is a crossed SSW-CES pattern, in which the environmental sound errors are primarily in the right ear. Type A patterns may also be used to differentiate TPO from PT cases. While it is rarely seen in PTs, more than one-quarter of the TPOs had the Type A pattern.

SITE-OF-DYSFUNCTION SIGNS IN CASES WITH AUDITORY-PROCESSING PROBLEMS

Response bias and other SSW indicators, along with CES results, have been used to locate dysfunction in three major cerebral regions. The SSW scores, Order Effects,

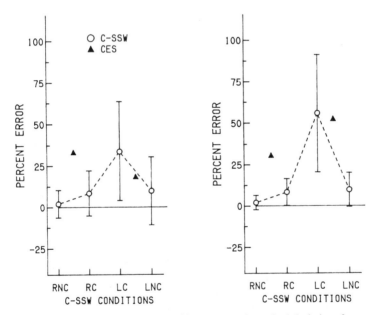

FIGURE 6. Mean corrected (C-SSW) condition scores and standard deviations for corpus callosum and anterior commissure lesion cases. The four conditions are right noncompeting (RNC), right competing (RC), left competing (LC), and left noncompeting (LNC). Separate results are shown for genu and splenium (corpus callosum), and anterior commissure cases (N = 18) (*left panel*), and subjects with lesions of the body of the corpus callosum (N = 6) (*right panel*). Competing environmental sound (CES) test means are displayed for each ear. For left panel the SDs for CES are right ear = 32, left ear = 23; for right panel, right ear = 24, left ear = 28.

and Type A patterns have been discussed as means of identifying problems of the posterior temporal, anterior cerebral, and temporo-parieto-occipital regions. These signs are based on data from adult patients with well-localized, acquired lesions of the brain.

Generally speaking, response bias and the side of the SSW peaks have not been used diagnostically in the evaluation of learning-disabled (LD) cases. Information from brain lesion studies have not been applied to LD and other groups that have auditory-processing (AP) difficulties because they are not thought to have actual CNS damage.[80] Citing brain loci might imply the presence of lesions. Furthermore, SSW signs have not been verified as locus-specific in developmentally disabled (DD) populations. However, there is increasing evidence of anatomical alterations and physiological dysfunction in certain LD groups[81,82] and in the developmentally disabled.[83] These findings have encouraged further consideration of SSW signs to gain insight into locus-specific auditory limitations. Despite our present efforts, we believe that site-of-dysfunction statements from the SSW test in LD and DD cases are premature and of little value in remedial educational planning.

The relationships among auditory tests within our battery have helped in acquiring a better understanding of what the SSW test is able to reveal. By combining the SSW indicators with performance on other tests, we are able to provide evidence of the different types of AP problems. The diagnostic battery will be described briefly.

Audiometric Test Battery

The audiologist is called upon to evaluate the status of the peripheral hearing mechanism as well as to assess central auditory function.[84] The peripheral tests include immittance measurements, puretone thresholds, and word recognition scores in quiet. The central tests that we routinely use are the SSW, phonemic synthesis (PS),[85] and speech-in-noise (S-N).[86]

The SSW is administered and scored in the same manner for AP evaluations of children and adults as it is for site-of-dysfunction testing. The standard that is applied for determining the significance of the scores does differ. The norms for AP evaluations are based on the national sample.[27] The sample is composed of data for 287 normal control subjects that were contributed by over 40 audiologists throughout the United Sates and two provinces of Canada. Means and standard deviations are provided for analyzing the SSW scores by age, for children 5 through 11 yr. Performance for groups aged 12 through 59 yr did not differ statistically, and therefore were combined as the normal adult group. Age-adjusted criteria have also been established for response biases.[87,88]

The PS test has been used as a measure of auditory decoding for many years because it taps phonemic recognition, phonemic memory, and phonemic synthesis skills.[89] S-N tasks have been used as an indication of a general auditory-processing deficit.[90] It has also been considered as a measure of auditory figure-ground difficulty, a common complaint among learning-disabled individuals.[21] The PS and S-N procedures were used to help characterize components of the SSW test.

Three Major Auditory-Processing Categories

The work of Duffy et al.[82] demonstrated significant differences in EEG activity in dyslexics compared to normal controls. Using brain electrical activity mapping (BEAM), a computerized procedure, they found the major differences between the groups to be in the left hemisphere. The specific regions were the occipital lobe, the temporo-occipital region, Wernicke's area (auditory cortex), and Broca's area. In addition, the region of the supplementary motor cortex was implicated, bilaterally.

There are no known SSW signs that identify disorders of the occipital lobe, per se. However, the other regions that were called into question by Duffy *et al.* can be subsumed under the three regions that we have discussed. It is appealing that some of the characteristic behaviors noted with damage to these cerebral zones have also been identified in LD cases with the corresponding SSW signs. This may therefore implicate the specific cerebral regions in certain learning-disabled individuals. While AP problems may help to explain some of the behaviors, we do not mean to imply a cause and effect relationship. For example, the difficulty in inhibiting a response to the introductory phrase, Are you ready?, in frontal lobe cases, may neither cause nor be caused by the auditory figure-ground problems that are seen in the same group. It is more likely that a third factor contributes to both phenomena, or that these may be completely unrelated characteristics. Despite this disclaimer, we do see many instances in which poor auditory skills could underlie the observed behavior. It should be noted that the audiometric signs for the three cerebral regions are not mutually exclusive.

Posterior Temporal Signs—the Auditory-Decoding Group

In children who are referred because of learning disabilities, PT response bias is closely associated with right-competing SSW peaks and delayed responses. They show evidence of faulty phonemic processing on such tests as phonemic synthesis, and not surprisingly, mild-to-moderately depressed performance on speech-in-noise tasks. If one does not have a clear knowledge of the speech sounds that are heard, the confusion will be even greater when background noises mask out critical information and cause an increased challenge to the entire central auditory system.

The poor phonemic discrimination, memory, and synthesis that we see in children who have PT signs, also provide a basis for understanding the observed academic problems. Vague engrams for speech sounds should affect phonic skills (as we typically see in these children), which in turn affects spelling and word accuracy in reading. The difficulty in understanding oral directions stems from confusion rather than from forgetting what is said. As young children, members of this group often have speech-language problems. The speech difficulty is mainly misarticulation, which characteristically affects *r*- and *l*-sounds. Receptive language impairment is commonly found on tests such as the Peabody Picture Vocabulary Test.

Anterior Cerebral Signs—the Auditory Tolerance-Fading Memory Group

Anterior cerebral response bias has been noted in LD cases. On the SSW, these individuals are the ones most likely to have unusually quick responses to items and to get tongue-twisted in giving their answers. Delays in responding often result in errors. Despite instruction and reinstruction, they respond to the introductory phrases on the SSW as though they cannot inhibit the reaction. These individuals tend to be highly distractable and display severe speech-in-noise difficulty in everyday listening situations. Academically, they are not as disabled as the other two groups but often forget the instructions they are given. Their reading problems are more likely to involve comprehension than an inability to sound out words. Language ability is relatively good, although they perform less well in expressive tasks, both written and oral. On occasion, this learning-disabled person is a rapid speaker. The test results for such an individual are very likely to suggest an auditory tolerance-fading memory problem.

Audiometric testing situations produce undue anxiety in these children, and we often note that they are reticent to separate from their parents. These children, especially when young, tend to be outwardly less cooperative and even volatile (e.g., yelling into the talkback microphone). They require a great deal of encouragement and feedback.

Temporo-parieto-occipital Signs—the Auditory Integration Group

Type A patterns, or sharp SSW peaks in the left-competing condition, are commonly associated with poor integration (presumably interhemispheric transfer and combining the information from auditory and visual modalities). In this group, we see especially long delays in responding. Nevertheless, the eventual answer is typically correct and appears effortless despite the extremely long pause.

Test scores alone may not differentiate those with TPO-type integration difficulties from others who appear to have involvement of the middle-anterior portions of the corpus callosum or anterior commissure. Academically, the TPO group has severe reading and spelling problems and are often labeled "dyslexic." They perform poorly in auditory-visual integration tasks such as in phonics.

SUMMARY

We have described three major groupings that encompass most auditory processing difficulties. While the problems may be superimposed upon one another in any individual client, each diagnostic sign is closely associated with particular communication and learning disorders. In addition, these behaviors may be related back to the functional anatomy of the regions that are implicated by the SSW test.

The auditory-decoding group is deficient in rapid analysis of speech. The vagueness of speech sound knowledge is thought to lead to auditory misunderstanding and confusion. In early life, this may be reflected in the child's articulation. Poor phonic skills that result from this deficit are thought to contribute to their limited reading and spelling abilities.

The auditory tolerance-fading memory group is often thought to have severe auditory-processing problems because those in it are highly distracted by background sounds and have poor auditory memories. However, school performance is not far from grade level, and the resulting reading disabilities stem more from limited comprehension than from an inability to sound out the words. Distractibility and poor auditory memory could contribute to the apparent weakness in reading comprehension.[90,91] Many of the characteristics of the auditory tolerance-fading memory group are similar to those of attention deficit disorder cases. Both groups are associated anatomically with the AC region.[83]

The auditory integration cases can be divided into two subgroups. In the first, the subjects exhibit the most severe reading and spelling problems of the three major categories. These individuals closely resemble the classical dyslexics. We presume that this disorder represents a major disruption in auditory-visual integration. The second subgroup has much less severe learning difficulties, which closely follow the pattern of dysfunction of the auditory tolerance-fading memory group.

The excellent physiological procedures to which we have been exposed during this Windows on the Brain conference provide a glimpse of the exciting possibilities for studying brain function. However, in working with individuals who have cognitive impairments, the new technology should be validated by standard behavioral tests. In turn, the new techniques will provide those who use behavioral measures with new parameters and concepts to broaden our understanding.

For the past quarter of a century, the SSW test has been compared with other behavioral, physiological, and anatomical procedures. Based on the information that has been assembled, we have been able to classify auditory processing disorders into three major categories. Each category is based on audiometric findings and appears consistent whether the underlying disorder is a tumor or stroke in the adult, or a developmental disability in a child. Many of the behavioral characteristics are predictable on the basis of pathological findings in humans and extrapolation from animal models.

We must now attempt further validation of these major groups and begin to detail the subcategories. The comparison with physiological procedures, such as those described at this conference, would provide an excellent point of departure for future research.

REFERENCES

1. KATZ, J. 1962. The use of staggered spondaic words for assessing the integrity of the central auditory nervous system. J. Speech Hear. Disord. **33:** 132-146.
2. BOCCA, E., C. CALEARO & V. CASSINARI. 1954. A new method for testing hearing in temporal lobe tumours. Acta Otolarynogol. **44:** 219-221.
3. MATZKER, J. 1959. Two new methods for assessment of central auditory function in cases of brain disease. Ann. Otol. Rhinol. Laryngol. **68:** 1185-1197.
4. FELDMANN, H. 1960. Untersuchungen zur Diskrimination differenter Schallbilder bei simultaner, monauraler und binauraler Darbietung. Arch. Ohren- Nasen- Kehlkupfheilkd. **176:** 600-605.
5. KIMURA, D. 1961. Some effects of temporal lobe damage on auditory perception. Can. J. Psychol. **15:** 157-165.
6. HADAWAY, S. 1969. An investigation of the relationship between measured intelligence and performance on the staggered spondaic word test. Master's thesis, Oklahoma State University. Oklahoma City, OK.
7. WETHERBY, A., R. KOEGEL & M MENDAL. 1981. Central auditory nervous system dysfunciton in echolatic autistic individuals. J. Speech Hear. Disord. **24:** 420-429.
8. YOZAWITZ, A., G. BRUDDER, S. SUTTON, L. SHARPE, B. GURLAND, J. FLEISS & L. COASTA. 1979. Dichotic perception: Evidence for right hemisphere dysfunction in affective psychosis. Br. J. Psychiatry **135:** 224-237.
9. ARNST, D. 1980. Performance of older adults on the SSW test. *In* The SSW Test: Assessment and Clinical Use. D. Arnst & J. Katz, Eds.: 449-456. College Hill Press. San Diego, CA.
10. AMERMAN, J. & M. PARNELL. 1980. The staggered spondaic word test: A normative investigation of older adults. Ear Hear. **1:** 42-45.
11. KEYDAR, B. & J. KATZ. 1976. The Hebrew version of the staggered spondaic word (SSW) test. J. Aud. Res. **16:** 135-142.

12. RUDMIN, F. 1979. Development of a Japanese SSW test. Audiol. Jpn. **22:** 36-40.
13. KATZ, J., R. BASIL & J. SMITH. 1963. A staggered spondaic word test for detecting central auditory lesions. Ann. Otol. Rhinol. Laryngol. **72:** 908-918.
14. KATZ, J. 1968. The SSW test: An interim report. J. Speech Hear. Disord. **33:** 132-146.
15. BERLIN, C., R. CHASE, A. DILL & T. HAGEPANOS. 1965. Auditory findings in patients with temporal lobectomies. ASHA **7:** 386.
16. LYNN, G. & J. GILROY. 1975. Neuro-audiological abnormalities in patients with temporal lobe tumors. J. Neurol. Sci. **17:** 167-184.
17. JERGER, J. & S. JERGER. 1975. Clinical validity of central auditory tests. Scand. Audiol. **4:** 147-163.
18. KATZ, J. & G. PACK. 1975. New developments in differential diagnosis using the SSW test. *In* Central Auditory Processing Disorders. M. Sullivan, Ed.: 84-107. University of Nebraska Press. Omaha, NE.
19. MUSIEK, F. & D. WILSON. 1979. SSW and dichotic digit results pre- and post-commissurotomy: A case report. J. Speech Hear. Disord. **44:** 528-533.
20. GRIMES, A., C. GRADY, N. FOSTER, T. SUDERLAND & N. PETRONAS. 1985. Central auditory function in Alzheimer's disease. Neurology **35:** 352-358.
21. KATZ, J. & R. ILLMER. 1972. Auditory perception in children with learning disabilities. *In* Handbook of Clinical Audiology. J. Katz, Ed.: 540-563. Williams & Wilkins. Baltimore, MD.
22. STUBBLEFIELD, J. & E. YOUNG. 1975. Central auditory dysfunction in learning disabled children. J. Speech Hear. Res. **19:** 561-571.
23. WHITE, E. 1977. Children's performance on the SSW test and Willeford battery: An interim report. *In* Central Auditory Dysfunction. R. Keith, Ed. Grune & Stratton. New York, NY.
24. LUKAS, J. & O. ESCHENHEIMER. 1978. Performance of learning disabled children and language handicapped children on central auditory tests. Paper presented at the American Speech and Hearing Association convention. Nov. 18-21. San Francisco, CA.
25. LUCKER, J. 1980. Diagnostic significance of the Type A pattern of the Staggered Spondaic Word test. Audiol. Hear. Ed. **6:** 21-23.
26. MYRICK, D. 1965. A normative study to assess performance of a group of children age 7-11 on the staggered spondaic word (SSW) test. Master's thesis. Tulane University. New Orleans, LA.
27. KATZ, J. *et al.* 1985. Combined national sample—1985 norms: Ages 5 to 60 years. SSW Rep. **7:** 1-6.
28. ARNST, D. & J. KATZ, EDS. 1982. The SSW Test: Development and Clinical Use. College Hill Press. San Diego, CA.
29. LUKAS, R. & J. GENCHUR LUKAS. 1985. Spondaic word tests. *In* Handbook of Clinical Audiology. J. Katz, Ed. Williams & Wilkins. Baltimore, MD.
30. KATZ, J. 1976. Locating auditory disorders of the brain and brainstem. Presented at the American Speech and Hearing Association meeting. Nov. 20-23. Houston, TX.
31. KATZ, J. 1978. SSW Workshop Manual. Allentown Industries. Buffalo, NY.
32. KATZ, J. 1987. SSW Workshop Manual. (Rev. edit.) JIMM Co. Buffalo, NY.
33. AIR, D. 1980. A study of central auditory functioning in aphasics. Ph.D. diss. University of Cincinnati. Cincinnati, OH.
34. KATZ, J., A. AVELLANOSA & N. AGUILAR-MARKULIS. 1980. Evaluation of corpus callosum tumors using SSW, CES and PICA. Paper presented at American Speech-Language-Hearing Association convention. Nov. 21-24. Detroit, MI.
35. CELESIA, G. 1976. Organization of auditory cortical areas in man. Brain **99:** 403-414.
36. ELLIOTT, H. 1969. Textbook of Neuroanatomy. 2nd edit. J. B. Lippincott. Philadelphia, PA.
37. LURIA, A. 1966. Higher Cortical Functions in Man. Basic Books. New York, NY.
38. MASSARO, D. 1975. Understanding Language. Academic Press. New York, NY.
39. BUTLER, K. 1983. Language processing: Selective attention and mnemonic strategies. *In* Central Auditory Processing Disorders: Problems of Speech, Language and Learning. E. Lasky & J. Katz, Eds.: 297-315. University Park Press. Baltimore, MD.
40. LURIA, A. 1970. Traumatic Aphasia: Its Syndromes. Psychology and Treatment. Mouton. The Hague.

41. BURNS, M. & G. CANTER. 1977. Phonemic behavior of aphasic patients with posterior cerebral lesions. Brain Lang. 4: 492-507.

42. BARU, A. & T. KARASEVA. 1972. The Brain and Hearing: Hearing Disturbances Associated with Local Brain Lesions. New York Consultants Bureau. New York, NY.

43. YOUNG, L. & R. CARHART. 1974. Time-intensity trading functions for pure tones and a high-frequency AM signal. J. Acoust. Soc. Am. 56: 605-609.

44. TALLAL, P. & M. PIERCY. 1973. Developmental aphasia: Impaired rate of nonverbal processing as a function of sensory modality. Neuropsychologica 11: 389-398.

45. TALLAL, P. & M. PIERCY. 1974. Developmental aphasia: Rate of auditory processing and selective impairment of consonant perception. Neuropsychologica 12: 83-93.

46. TALLAL, P. 1976. Rapid auditory processing in normal and disordered language development. J. Speech Hear. Res. 19: 561-571.

47. BLUMSTEIN, S. 1985. The effects of slowed speech on auditory comprehension in aphasia. Brain Lang. 24: 246-265.

48. BALAS, R. 1971. Staggered spondaic word test: Support. Ann. Otol. Rhinol. Laryngol. 80: 134-139.

49. KATZ, J., D. MCCARTHY, L. JACOBS & L. WILSON. 1982. Cross validation of the SSW test using CT scan verification. Unpublished study.

50. OLSEN, W. 1983. Dichotic test results for normal subjects and for temporal lobectomy patients. Ear Hear. 4: 324-330.

51. KAPLAN, H., V. GLADSTONE & J. KATZ. 1984. Site of Lesion Testing: Audiometric Interpretation. Vol. II. 287-307. University Park Press. Baltimore, MD.

52. FUSTER, J. 1980. The Prefrontal Cortex. Raven Press. New York, NY.

53. PENFIELD, W. & L. ROBERTS. 1959. Speech and Brain Mechanisms. Princeton University Press. Princeton, NJ.

54. PENFIELD, W. & B. MILNER. 1958. The memory defect produced by bilateral lesions of the hippocampal zone. Arch. Neurol. Psychiatr. 79: 475-497.

55. MILNER, B. 1959. Memory deficit in bilateral hippocampal lesions. Psychiatr. Res. Rep. 11: 43-58.

56. ISAACSON, R. & K. PRIBRAM. 1986. The Hippocampus. Vol. 4. Plenum Press. New York, NY.

57. JARRELL, T., C. GENTILE, P. MCCABE & N. SCHNEIDERMAN. 1986. Role of the medial geniculate region in differential Pavlovian conditioning of bradycardia in rabbits. Brain Res. 21: 126-136.

58. ELLIS, M. 1985. Amygdala norephrine involved in two separate long-term memory retrieval processes. Brain Res. 2: 254-263.

59. FEDIO, P. & J. VAN BUREN. 1974. Memory deficits during electrical stimulation of the speech cortex in conscious man. Brain Lang. 1: 29-42.

60. STRUSS, D. & F. BENSON. 1984. Neuropsychological studies of the frontal lobes. Psychol. Bull. 95: 3-25.

61. MCALLISTER, T. & T. PRICE. 1987. Aspects of the behavior of psychiatric inpatients with frontal lobe damage: Some implications for diagnosis and treatment. Compreh. Psychiatry 28: 14-21.

62. IVNIK, R., F. SCHARBOUGH & E. LAWS. 1987. Effects of anterior temporal lobectomy on cognitive functions. J. Clin. Psychol. 43: 128-137.

63. EFRON, R., P. CRANDALL, B. KOSS, P. DIVENYL & E. YUND. 1983. Central auditory processing. III. The "cocktail party" effect and anterior temporal lobectomy. Brain Lang. 19: 254-330.

64. EFRON, R. & P. CRANDALL. 1983. Central auditory processing. II. Effects of anterior temporal lobectomy. Brain Lang. 19: 237-253.

65. DEJERINE, J. 1892. Contribution à l'étude d'anatomie-pathologique et clinique verbale. Mem. Soc. Biol. (Paris) 44: 61-90. [Cited by A. Damasio & H. Damasio. 1983. The anatomic basis of pure alexia. Neurology 33: 1573-1583.]

66. GESCHWIND, N. & W. LEVITSKY. 1968. Human brain: Left-right asymmetries in temporal speech region. Science 161: 186-187.

67. MUSIEK, F. 1986. Neuroanatomy, neurophysiology and central auditory assessment. Part III. Corpus callosum and efferent pathways. Ear Hear. 7: 349-358.

68. HENDERSON, Y. 1986. Anatomy of posterior pathways in reading: A reassessment. Brain Lang. **29:** 119-133.
69. DAMASIO, A. & H. DAMASIO. 1983. The anatomic basis of pure alexia. Neurology. **33:** 1573-1583.
70. WEISBERG, L. & M. WALL. 1987. Alexia without agraphia: Clinical-computed tomography correlations. Neuroradiology. **29:** 283-286.
71. GREENBLATT, S. 1973. Alexia without agraphia or hemianopsia: Anatomical analysis of an autopsied case. Brain **96:** 307-316.
72. AJAX, E., T. SCHENKENBERG & M. KOSTELJANETZ. 1977. Alexia without agraphia and the inferior splenium. Neurology **27:** 685-688.
73. GULMANN, N., G. WILDSCHIODTZ & K. ORBEK. 1982. Alteration of interhemispheric conduction through corpus callosum in chronic schizophrenia. Biol. Psychiatry **17:** 585-594.
74. NASRALLAH, H. & M. MCCHESNEY. 1981. Psychopathology of corpus callosum tumors. Biol. Psychiatry **16:** 663-669.
75. KATZ, J., D. KUSHNER & G. PACK. 1975. The use of competing speech (SSW) and environmental sound (CES) test for localizing brain lesions. Paper presented at the American Speech-Language-Hearing Association convention. Nov. 21-24. Washington, DC.
76. KIMURA, D. 1964. Left-right differences in the perception of melodies. Q. J. Exp. Psychol. **16:** 355-358.
77. KIMURA, D. 1961. Speech dominance and the perception of verbal stimuli. Can. J. Psychol. **15:** 166-171.
78. LYNN, G., J. BENITZ, A. EISENBREY, J. GILROY & H. WILNER. 1972. Neuro-audiological correlates in cerebral hemisphere lesions: Temporal and parietal lobe tumors. Audiology **11:** 115-134.
79. LYNN, G. 1975. Dichotic speech discrimination in patients with deep cerebral hemisphere lesions. Paper presented at the Ninth Colorado Medical Audiology Workshop. March. Vail, CO.
80. KINSBOURNE, M. 1983. Pediatric aspects of learning disorders. *In* Central Auditory Processing Disorders: Problems of Speech, Language and Learning. E. Lasky & J. Katz, Eds. Williams & Wilkins Co. Baltimore, MD.
81. HIER, D., M. LEMAY, P. ROSENBERGER & V. PERLO. 1978. Developmental dyslexia: Evidence for a subgroup with reversal of asymmetry. Arch. Neurol. **35:** 90-92.
82. DUFFY, F., M. DENCKLA, P. BARTELS & G. SANDINI. 1980. Dyslexia: Regional differences in brain electrical activity by topographic mapping. Ann. Neurol. **7:** 412-420.
83. LOU, H., L. HENRIKSEN & P. BRUHN. 1984. Local cerebral hyperperfusion in children with dysphasia and/or attention deficit disorder. Arch. Neurol. **41:** 825-829.
84. KATZ, J. & L. WILDE. 1985. Auditory perceptual disorders in children. *In* Handbook of Clinical Audiology. 3rd Edit. J. Katz, Ed. Williams & Wilkins. Baltimore, MD.
85. KATZ, J. & C. HARMON. 1981. Phonemic synthesis: Testing and training. *In* Central Auditory and Language Disorders is Children. R. Keith, Ed. College-Hill Press. Houston, TX.
86. MUELLER, G. 1985. Monosyllabic procedures. *In* Handbook of Clinical Audiology. 3rd edit. J. Katz, Ed. Williams & Wilkins Co. Baltimore, MD.
87. KATZ, J. 1981. The national sample for children: A piece of the pie. SSW Rep. **3:** 4-6.
88. KATZ, J. 1982. The national sample looks at reversals. SSW Rep. **4:** 14.
89. KATZ, J. & C. HARMON. 1982. Phonemic Synthesis: Blending Sounds into Words. Developmental Learning Materials. Allen, TX.
90. LEWIS, N. 1976. Otitis media and linguistic incompetence. Arch. Otolaryngol. **102:** 387-390.
91. JUST, A. & P. CARPENTER. 1980. A theory of reading: From eye fixation to comprehension. Psychol. Rev. **87:** 829.

Index of Contributors